Fundamentals of
applied pathophysiology

For all the students for whom we have had the pleasure of working with, helping them to develop their knowledge and skills.

Fundamentals of applied pathophysiology

An essential guide for nursing students

Edited by

Muralitharan Nair
University of Hertfordshire

and

Ian Peate
University of Hertfordshire

WILEY-BLACKWELL

A John Wiley & Sons, Ltd., Publication

Library of Congress Cataloging-in-Publication Data

Fundamentals of applied pathophysiology/editors, Muralitharan Nair and Ian Peate.
    p. ; cm.
  Includes bibliographical references and index.
  ISBN 978-0-470-51795-6 (pbk.)
  1. Physiology, Pathological. 2. Nursing. I. Nair, Muralitharan. II. Peate, Ian.
  [DNLM: 1. Pathology–methods. 2. Nursing Care–methods. 3. Physiological Processes. QZ 4 F981 2008]
  RB113.F86 2009
  616.07–dc22

      2008033266

A catalogue record for this book is available from the British Library.

Set in 10/13 pt Times by Aptara® Inc., New Delhi, India
Printed in Singapore by Fabulous Printers Pte Ltd

2 2010

Contents

For the Instructor Resources and the Student Companion Website for this book, please visit **www.wileyeurope.com/college/nair**

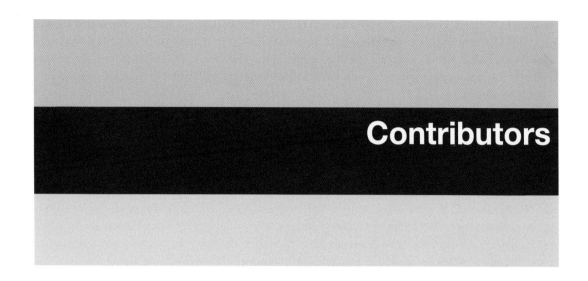

Contributors

Carl Clare RN DipN BSc (Hons) MSc (Lond) PGDE (Lond)

Senior Lecturer, School of Nursing and Midwifery, Faculty of Health and Human Sciences, University of Hertfordshire, Hatfield, Hertfordshire, AL10 9AB

Carl began his nursing career as a Nursing Auxiliary in 1990. He later undertook a 3-year student nurse training at Selly Oak Hospital (Birmingham). He moved to the Royal Devon and Exeter Hospitals, then to the Northwick Park Hospital and finally to the Royal Brompton and Harefield NHS Trust as a Resuscitation Officer and Honorary Teaching Fellow of Imperial College (London). He has worked in nurse education since 2001. His key areas of interest are physiology, sociology, cardiac care and resuscitation. Carl has previously published work in the field of cardiac care and resuscitation.

Janet G. Migliozzi RGN, BSc (Hons), MSc (London), PGD Ed., FHEA

Senior Lecturer, School of Nursing and Midwifery, Faculty of Health and Human Sciences, University of Hertfordshire, Hatfield, Hertfordshire, AL10 9AB

Janet commenced her nursing career in London, becoming a Staff Nurse in 1988. She has worked at a variety of hospitals across London, predominately in vascular, orthopaedic and high dependency surgery before specialising in infection prevention and control. She has worked in nurse education since 1999. Her key interests include microbiology, particularly in relation to health care-associated infection, vascular/surgical nursing, health informatics and nurse education. Janet has previously published work in and the field of minimising risk in relation to health care-associated infection and is a member of the Infection Prevention Society.

Muralitharan Nair SRN, RMN, DipN (Lond) RNT, Cert Ed., Cert., in Counselling, BSc (Hons) MSc (Surrey), FHEA

Senior Lecturer, School of Nursing and Midwifery, Faculty of Health and Human Sciences, University of Hertfordshire, Hatfield, Hertfordshire, AL10 9AB

Muralitharan commenced his nursing career in 1971 at Edgware General Hospital, becoming a Staff Nurse. In 1975, he commenced his mental health nurse training at Springfield Hospital and worked as a

Staff Nurse for approximately 1 year. He has worked at St Mary's Hospital, Paddington, and Northwick Park Hospital returning to Edgware General Hospital to take up the post of Senior Staff Nurse and then Charge Nurse. He has worked in nurse education since 1989. His key interests include physiology, diabetes, surgical nursing and nurse education. Muralitharan has published in journals and written a chapter on elimination.

Ian Peate EN(G) RGN DipN (Lond) RNT BEd (Hons) MA(Lond) LLM

Associate Head of School, School of Nursing and Midwifery, Faculty of Health and Human Sciences, University of Hertfordshire, Hatfield, Hertfordshire, AL10 9AB

Ian began his nursing career in 1981 at the Central Middlesex Hospital, becoming an Enrolled Nurse working in an intensive care unit. He later undertook a 3-year student nurse training at Central Middlesex and Northwick Park Hospitals, becoming a Staff Nurse and then a Charge Nurse. He has worked in nurse education since 1989. His key areas of interest are nursing practice and theory, sexual health and HIV/AIDS. He is currently an Associate Head of School. His portfolio centres on recruitment and marketing and professional academic development within the School of Nursing and Midwifery.

Peter S. Vickers Cert Ed., Dip CD, SRN, RSCN, BA, PhD, FHEA

Senior Lecturer Child Nursing, School of Nursing and Midwifery, Faculty of Health and Human Sciences, University of Hertfordshire, Hatfield, Hertfordshire, AL10 9AB

Peter began teaching in both primary and secondary education in 1961 and was a student at St Luke's Teacher Training College, Exeter. Initially, specialising in the education of children with special needs, and becoming the Deputy Head of a school for children with severe behavioural problems, he then specialised in the teaching of arts and crafts. Following 4 years with the army, he commenced nurse training at the York School of Nursing, followed later by undertaking further studies at the Charles West School of Nursing, Great Ormond Street, London, where he specialised in immunology and infectious diseases. Following his work as a Clinical Nurse Specialist, Peter became the Clinical Nurse Manager for Paediatrics at Newcastle General Hospital, where he commenced his PhD studies, before entering nurse education in 1992. After leaving nurse education in 1996, he again worked in the clinical area, working in the Paediatric Unit at the Luton & Dunstable Hospital, before commencing his present position at the University of Hertfordshire. Peter was awarded his doctorate in 1999 for his research into children who had survived bone marrow transplants for immune deficiency disorders, and their families, in the UK and Germany. Now he teaches biosciences – particularly immunology, children's health and research, as well as undertaking his own research studies.

Anthony Wheeldon RN, Dip HE, BSc (Hons), MSc (Lond), PGDE

School of Nursing and Midwifery Faculty of Health and Human Sciences, University of Hertfordshire, Hatfield, Hertfordshire, AL10 9AB

After qualification in 1995, Anthony worked as a Staff Nurse and a Senior Staff Nurse in the Respiratory Directorate at the Royal Brompton and Harefield NHS Trust. He began teaching on postregistration courses in 2000 before moving into full-time nurse education at Thames Valley University in 2002. Anthony has a wide range of nursing interests including cardiorespiratory nursing, anatomy and physiology, respiratory assessment and nurse education. He is currently a Senior Lecturer at the University of Hertfordshire.

Acknowledgements

We would like to thank all of our colleagues for their help, support, comments and suggestions.

Muralitharan would like to thank his wife, Evangeline, and his daughters, Samantha and Jennifer, for their continued support and patience.

Ian would like to thank his partner Jussi Lahtinen for all of his continued support and encouragement.

Introduction

Ian Peate and Muralitharan Nair

Pathophysiology

Pathophysiology is concerned with the disturbance of normal mechanical, physical and biochemical functions. The disturbance is either caused by disease, an abnormal syndrome or a condition. Porth (2005) looks at the word *pathophysiology* (a combined word) from the Greek *pathos* meaning disease and physiology being related to the various normal functions of the human body. Pathophysiology addresses both the cellular and the organ changes that occur with disease as well as the effects these changes have on body function. When something impacts upon the normal physiological functioning of the body (i.e. disease), this then becomes a pathophysiological issue. It must, however, be remembered that normal health is not and cannot be exactly the same in any two individuals; therefore, the term *normal* must be treated with caution.

This text has been written with the intention of making the sometimes complex subject of pathophysiology accessible and exciting. The human body has an extraordinary ability to respond to disease in a number of physiological and psychological ways; it is able to compensate for the changes that occur as result of the disease process. This text considers those changes (the pathophysiological processes) and the effect they can have on a person.

Health care provision

The provision of health care is in a constant state of flux, and it should aim to respond to the global shift in the burden of disease; this change is seeing a larger number of people affected by long-term conditions. Those who are affected by long-term conditions (patients and families) can often experience physical and mental health problems both at the same time either as a consequence of their illness or independent of it (DH, 2006). There are a number of factors that impinge on the provision of health, the maintenance of health and the prevention of disease, for example:

- health inequalities
- technological advances
- public expectation
- the role and function of the nurse
- the role and function of other health care providers
- personal, social and cultural factors

According to the Nursing and Midwifery Council (NMC, 2007), to be able to care for people, safely and effectively, the nurse must have the knowledge and skills to meet needs:

- in a complex and diverse society where social inequality exists
- inside and outside hospital and across health and social care
- across public, private and voluntary health provider organisations
- of an increasing older population
- of those with long-term conditions
- across the patient care pathway
- in supporting lifestyle changes
- using disease prevention and health promotional interventions
- by treating patients as partners in health care and maximising choice
- through the use of technological advances
- in new and emerging roles which cross professional boundaries
- as leaders and members of multidisciplinary and interdisciplinary teams
- as lifelong learners in an ever-evolving health care environment

In order for the student of nursing to aspire to and provide care that takes the above points into account, there must be a sound understanding of pathophysiological principles.

Fundamentals of applied pathophysiology

This is a foundation text that will enable the reader to grow personally and professionally in relation to the provision of health care. This textbook is primarily intended for nursing students who will come into contact with patients who may have a variety of physically related health care problems such as pneumonia, diabetes mellitus, Alzheimer's disease and many more diseases, in both the hospital and community settings. The focus of the text is on the adult person. Illness and disease are discussed explicitly, emphasising the fact that individuals do become ill and experience disease.

It is the intention of this text to develop knowledge and skills both in theory and practice and to apply this knowledge in order to provide safe and effective high-quality care. The overriding aim is to relate normal body function to pathological changes that may lead to disease processes, preventing the individual leading a 'normal' life.

The level at which the text has been written will provide readers with a straightforward understanding of applied pathophysiology, providing nursing students (and others) with an essential/fundamental understanding of applied pathophysiology in order to deliver high-quality care in any setting.

Fundamentals of Applied Pathophysiology is not only intended as a valuable textbook for students during their lectures but also as a reference resource to be taken with them and used in the practice setting (wherever this may be). It is not our intention that this text be read from cover to cover, the reader is encouraged to delve in and out of it; we aim to entice and encourage the reader to read further and in so doing instill a sense of curiosity. Although the book is written with nursing students in mind, it may also be appropriate for registered health care professionals who may wish to approach pathophysiological issues in a more user-friendly manner. Illustrations are used in abundance to assist the reader in understanding and appreciating complex disease patterns that are being discussed.

Using a fundamental approach will provide readers with an essential understanding of applied pathophysiology. A result of working in a variety of health care settings means that students may find themselves assisting and working with other health care professionals in the care and management of the patient, for example, assisting in radiology departments in the safe preparation of patients for special investigations, such as barium meal or reinforcing the dietary advice given to patients by the dietician. An understanding of pathophysiology 'normal' and 'abnormal' can help the student and the patient.

A note about the terms used

There are a plethora of terms used to describe people who are the recipients of health care and choosing the correct term, one that will be appreciated by all readers, is challenging.

The term 'patient' can refer to all groups and individuals who have direct or indirect contact with all health and social care workers. Patient is the expression that is commonly used within the National Health Service (NHS) and it is a term that has been used throughout this text. It is recognised and respected that not everyone supports the use of the passive concept that can be associated with this term, but it is used here in the knowledge that it is widely understood; it may apply to those who are recipients of health and social care in hospitals, in the person's own home, in the primary care setting and in the independent and voluntary sector. We could have used other expressions, for example service user, client or consumer; however, for the sake of brevity the phrase patient has been used.

The chapters

The format of this text allows the reader to access information regarding pathophysiology as a quick reference guide or in a more in-depth manner; this is an easy-to-use textbook providing the funda-mental concepts associated with pathophysiological processes. The processes of specific diseases are introduced; treatments and nursing care are provided in a clear and concise manner.

The text uses a sound evidence base throughout, drawing on contemporary literature to support discussion. The use of standards/frameworks produced by voluntary and statutory organisations is also included, for example patient safety and risk assessment. Government policy, in the guise of the National Service Frameworks, will be referred to and readers are encouraged to probe deeper to inform their practice with the overriding aim of the provision of safe and effective nursing care. Policy and procedure that is used locally will be referred to encouraging the reader to make reference to local guidance when necessary.

Each chapter begins with key words, by beginning to, introduce the reader at an early stage to terms that will be discussed within the chapter. To assess current knowledge, the reader is invited to test this at the start of each chapter. The intended learning outcomes provide a sample of what the chapters will cover. Illustrations have been included in order to ease and facilitate learning.

At the end of each chapter, multiple choice questions have been formulated for you to answer. There are also another set of questions provided for you to test your knowledge; this can help you determine how far you have progressed after reading and assimilating the contents of the chapter. A glossary of terms is available, providing you with the opportunity to develop your vocabulary further in relation to the terminology being used. This interactive approach is provided in an attempt to prompt thinking and to encourage you to investigate and explore further a field in relation to the pathophysiological issues discussed or even those that have not been discussed.

Our overriding objective is to encourage you and to motivate you as well as instill in you the confidence and competence to become a proficient provider of care. Proving care with a sound knowledge base and the desire to care with compassion and understanding is a hallmark of a professional health care worker.

We believe that understanding and applying this understanding is the key to the provision of high-quality care, safe and effective care as well developing critical thinking, innovation and creativity. The contributors have enjoyed the challenges that the writing of this book has provided them with, and we hope that you find the chapters as stimulating and thought provoking as did when we wrote them; most of all, we hope that those you care for benefit as a result of your learning.

References

Department of Health (2006). *Modernising Nursing Careers*. London: DH.

Nursing and Midwifery Council (2007). *A Review of Pre Registration Nursing Education: A Consultation*. London: NMC.

Porth, C.M. (2005). *Pathophysiology Concepts of Altered States*, 7th edn. Philadelphia: Lippincott.

Copyright information

The following illustrations are reproduced with permission from Tortora and Derrickson (2007) *Principles of Anatomy and Physiology*, 11th edition, John Wiley & Sons, Hoboken, NJ:

1.1, 1.3, 1.6, 1.7, 1.8, 1.9, 1.10, 1.11, 1.12, 1.13, 1.14, 1.15, 3.5, 3.6, 5.1, 5.2, 5.3, 5.5, 5.6, 5.7, 6.1, 6.2, 6.3, 6.4, 6.5, 6.11, 6.12, 7.1, 7.2, 7.3, 7.4, 7.5, 7.6, 7.7, 8.2, 8.6, 8.8, 8.9, 9.7, 9.8, 11.1, 11.5, 11.10, 11.11, 11.14, 13.1, 13.3, 15.6, 15.7, 15.11, 17.2, 17.3

The following illustrations are adapted with permission from Graham-Brown and Burns (2002) *Lecture Notes on Dermatology*, 8th edition, Blackwell Publishing, Oxford:

18.1, 18.2, 18.6

The following illustrations are adapted with permission from Bulstrode and Swales (2007) *The Musculoskeletal System at a Glance*, Blackwell Publishing, Oxford:

16.3, 16.5

Chapter 1

Cell and body tissue physiology

Peter S. Vickers

KEY WORDS

- Plasma membrane
- Organelles
- Connective tissue
- Passive transport

- Nucleus
- Cell cycle
- Muscle tissue
- Active transport

- Cytoplasm
- Epithelial tissue
- Nervous tissue
- Bulk transport

Test your prior knowledge

- What are the three main parts of a human cell?
- Describe the structure and function of a human cell.
- Describe the phases of a cell cycle.

> **Learning outcomes**
>
> On completion of this section the reader will be able to:
> - Outline the structure and function of a human cell.
> - List and describe the functions of the organelles.
> - Explain the phases of a cell cycle.
> - Explain the cellular transport system.
> - Describe the structure and function of epithelial tissue, connective tissue, muscle tissue and nervous tissue.
> - Explain the process of tissue repair (inflammation).

Introduction

To understand the human body and how it works (and also how it fails to work properly), it is important to understand the anatomy and physiology of the cell. There is a very wide diversity amongst living organisms as regards their size, shape, colour, behaviour and habitat. In spite of this, however, there are also similarities, and this fundamental similarity is known as the 'cell theory'. This cell theory states that all living organisms are composed of one or more cells and the products of cells. Despite the fact that the cells belong to different organisms, and even cells within the same organism may have different functions, there are many similarities between them. For example, there are similarities in their chemical composition, their chemical and biochemical behaviour and in their detailed structure.

All cells have many characteristics, but these characteristics can differ from cell to cell, such as:

- Cells are able to carry out certain specific functions. In other words, they are active.
- Cells need to consume food to live and to carry out their functions, but they do not have mouths; however, they are still able to catch and digest their food and use it for growth and reproduction. The correct term for this is **endocytosis** – they surround and engulf organisms such as bacteria and digest them.
- Cells can grow and repair.
- Similarly, cells can reproduce themselves. They do this by a process known as **simple fission**. This means that they reproduce themselves by dividing into two, and then each new cell grows to full size before they themselves divide by simple fission and so on. In other words, they replicate themselves.
- Like humans, cells can get irritable if something upsets or stimulates them.
- The nutrition that the cells have taken in is also used for the storage and release of energy (just like humans), thus enabling them to grow and repair themselves.
- Similarly, just as humans do not utilise all the food they eat – some of it cannot be used and so is excreted – similarly, the cells excrete what they do not need or cannot use.
- Lastly, just as all humans will eventually die, so will cells. Some have a short life, whilst others survive many years – but eventually they will die.

So, cells are not all that different from humans in many respects. They do what humans do – albeit in different ways.

Anatomy of the cell

Each cell has a structure that is almost as complex as the human body (Figure 1.1). For example, each cell contains as many molecules as the body has cells. There is no such thing as a typical cell. However, each cell is surrounded by a **membrane** and contains **protoplasm**. This protoplasm consists of a **nucleus** which is kept separate from the rest of the cell by a **nuclear membrane** (although the nuclear membrane disappears during the process of cell division). As well as the nucleus, the protoplasm consists of a colourless, opaque substance called **cytoplasm** (Watson, 2005). The cells themselves consist of water, proteins, lipids, carbohydrates and the various ions such as potassium (K^+) and magnesium (Mg^{2+}). Within the cytoplasm there are also many complex protein structures called **organelles**.

Cells vary in size from 2 to 20 Micrometer (μm). For example, a lymphocyte (a type of blood cell) is about 8–10 μm in diameter. All the cells in the body, apart from those on the surface of the body, are surrounded by a fluid that is known as **extracellular fluid** (i.e. fluid outside of the cell).

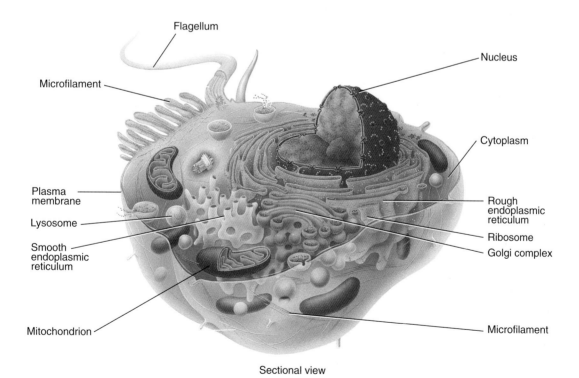

Sectional view

Figure 1.1 Simplified structure of a cell.

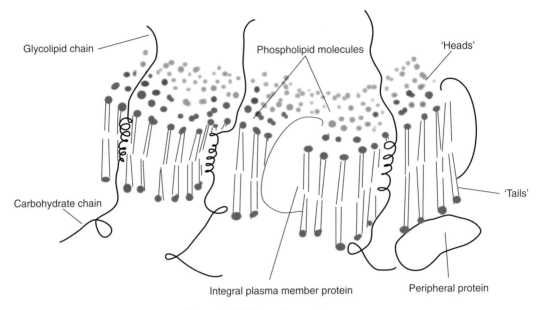

Figure 1.2 The cell membrane.

The cell membrane

The cell membrane is made up of a double layer (bilayer) of phospholipid (fatty) molecules with protein molecules interspersed between them (Figure 1.2). The cell membrane can vary from 7.5 to 10 nanometer (nm) in thickness.

The cell membrane acts just like a 'skin' that protects the cell from the outside environment. In addition, it regulates the movement of water, nutrients and waste products into and out of the cell. A phospholipid molecule consists of a polar 'head' which is hydrophilic (water loving) and 'tails' which are hydrophobic (water hating). The hydrophilic 'heads' are attracted to water and are found on the inner and outer surfaces of the cell (water is the main component of both extracellular and intracellular environments), whilst the hydrophobic 'tails' are found in the middle of the cell membrane where they can avoid water. These phospholipid molecules are arranged as a bilayer with the heads facing outwards. This means that the bilayer is self-sealing. It is the central part of the plasma membrane, consisting of hydrophobic 'tails' that makes the cell membrane impermeable to water-soluble molecules, and so prevents the passage of these molecules into and out of the cell (Marieb, 2006). If the membrane just consisted of these phospholipid molecules, then cells would not be able to function. However, within the cell membrane there are also plasma member proteins (PMPs) which can be either integral or peripheral.

Some of the integral PMPs are embedded amongst the tails of the phospholipid molecules, whilst others penetrate the membrane completely (see Figure 1.2). Subunits of some of these integral proteins can form channels which allow for the transportation of materials into and out of the cell. Other subunits are able to bind to carbohydrates to form receptor sites. These **receptor sites** are important, as will be discussed in the chapter 3 – inflammation, immune response and healing.

Peripheral PMPs bind loosely to the surface of the cell membrane and so can easily be separated from it. Some of them function as enzymes to catalyse cellular reactions, whilst others are receptors for hormones and other chemical membranes, or function as binding sites for attachment to other structures (Marieb, 2006).

Functions of the cell membrane

- **Endocytosis** and **exocytosis** – concerned with the transport of fluids and other matter into and out of the cell.
- **Endocytosis** is the intake of extracellular fluid and particulate material (small particles) ranging in size from macromolecules to whole cells (e.g. the bacteria engulfed and destroyed by macrophage cells).
- **Exocytosis** is the bulk transport of material out of the cells.

There are three types of endocytosis:

- **Phagocytosis** – involves the ingestion of large particles, even whole microbial cells.
- **Pinocytosis** – involves the ingestion of small particles and fluids.
- **Receptor-mediated endocytosis** – involves large particles, notably proteins, but also has the important feature of being highly selective.

Endocytosis involves part of the cell membrane being drawn into the cell along with the particles or fluid to be ingested (see Figure 1.3). This membrane is then pinched off to form a membrane-bound **vesicle** within the cell, while at the same time the cell membrane as a whole reseals itself. Inside the cell, the fate of this vesicle depends upon the type of endocytosis involved as well as the material it contains. In some cases, the endocytic vesicle ultimately fuses with an organelle called a **lysosome**, after which processing of the ingested material can occur. Endocytosis is also the means by which many simple organisms obtain their nutrients.

The cell membrane and transport

One of the key properties of the cell membrane in regards to transport is its **selective permeability**. This refers to its ability to let certain materials pass through, whilst preventing others from doing so. This selective permeability is based on the hydrophobicity (water hatred) of its component molecules. Because the phospholipid tails in the centre of the bilayer are composed entirely of hydrophobic fatty acid chains (lipids are fats), it is very difficult for water-soluble (hydrophilic) molecules to penetrate to the membrane interior. The result is a very effective permeability barrier.

However, this barrier can be penetrated, but only by way of specific transport systems. These control what goes into and out of the cell, or what crosses from one subcellular compartment to another. Cell membranes control **metabolism** by restricting the flow of glucose and other water-soluble **metabolites** in and out of cells and between subcellular compartments. This is known as compartmentation. The cells store energy in the form of **transmembrane ion gradients** by allowing high concentrations of particular **ions** to accumulate on one side of the membrane.

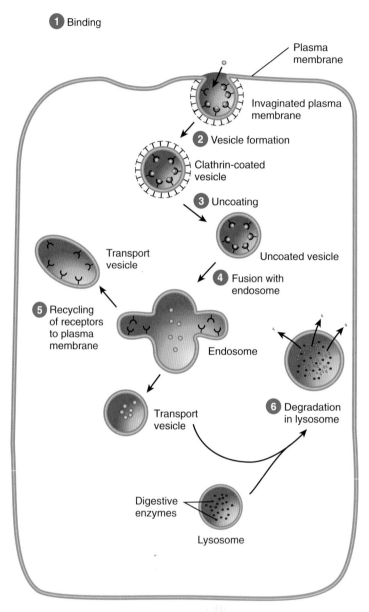

Figure 1.3 Endocytosis.

Ions pass from inside to outside of the cell (or the other way round) so that there are more supplies of these ions just outside the cell or inside it and the membrane controls the speed/rate at which these ions pass through the membrane. The controlled release of such ion gradients can be used to:

- extract nutrients from surrounding fluids
- pass electrical messages (known as nerve excitability)
- control cell volume and stop cells bursting with excess fluid

To return to the cell membrane itself, there are four factors that decide the degree of permeability of a membrane:

■ Size of molecules – large molecules cannot pass through the integral membrane proteins, but small ones such as water and **amino acids** can.
■ Solubility in lipids (fats) – substances that easily dissolve in lipids can pass through the membrane more easily than non-lipid soluble substances. Lipid-soluble substances include oxygen, carbon dioxide and steroid hormones.
■ If an ion has an electrical charge opposite to that of the membrane, then it is attracted to the membrane and can more easily pass through it.
■ Carrier integral proteins can carry substances across the membrane, regardless of size, ability to dissolve in lipids or membrane electrical charge.

There are two ways in which substances can move across the membrane: **passive** or **active**.

   Passive processes are:

■ diffusion
■ facilitated diffusion
■ osmosis
■ filtration

   Active processes are:

■ active transport pumps
■ endocytosis
■ exocytosis

   A **passive process** is one in which the substances move on their own down a concentration gradient from an area of higher to one of lower concentration. The cell does not expend any energy on the process. Think of it as rolling down a hill from an area of high altitude to one of lower altitude. Little energy is expended just rolling down a hill.

   Diffusion is the most common form of passive transport in which a substance of higher concentration moves to an area where there is a lower concentration of that substance (Colbert *et al.*, 2007). This difference between the area of high concentration and low concentration is known as a **concentration gradient**. This process of diffusion is essential for respiration. It is through diffusion that oxygen is transported from the lungs to the blood and carbon dioxide makes the opposite journey from blood to the lungs (Colbert *et al.*, 2007).

   Facilitated diffusion is similar to diffusion, but with one exception. For this process to take place, there needs to be a substance that helps – a facilitator. **Glucose** is moved using this process. Although glucose can move part of the way through the membrane on its own, it needs something else (a **carrier/transport protein**) to give it that extra push to get it completely through the membrane (Colbert *et al.*, 2007; McCance and Huether, 2006; Rangarajan and Shaw, 2004).

   Osmosis is the process in which water travels through a selectively permeable membrane so that concentrations of a substance that is soluble in water (known as a **solute**) are the same on both sides of that membrane. This is known as **osmotic pressure** (see Figures 1.4 and 1.5). The higher the concentration of the solute on one side of the membrane, the higher the osmotic pressure available for the movement of the water (Colbert *et al.*, 2007).

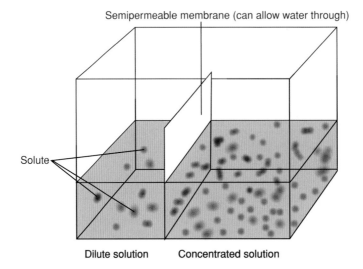

Figure 1.4 Osmosis.

Filtration is similar to osmosis, except that pressure is applied in order to 'push' water and solutes across that membrane. The heart is a major supplier of the force that can lead to one type of filtration (renal filtration) as it pushes blood into the kidneys where filtration of the blood can take place (Colbert *et al.*, 2007).

An **active process** is one in which substances move against a concentration gradient from an area of lower to higher concentration. The cell must expend energy that is released by splitting **adenosine**

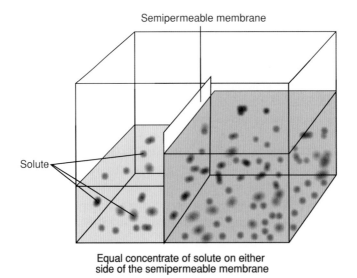

Figure 1.5 Osmosis and movement of solute.

triphosphate (ATP) into **adenosine diphosphate** (ADP) and phosphate. Think again of a hill. When walking up a hill, a lot of energy is expended. The steeper the hill, the more the energy used. ATP is a compound of a base, a sugar and three phosphate groups (triphosphate). These phosphate groups are held together by high-energy bonds, which when broken release a high level of energy. Once, one of these phosphate bonds has been broken and a phosphate group has been released, that compound now has only two phosphate groups (diphosphate) and there is now also a spare phosphate group which in turn will join up with another ADP group, so forming another molecule of ATP (with energy stored in the phosphate bonds), and the whole process continues recurring.

Active transport pumps can only work if they have a source of energy. This energy occurs as a result of a reaction involving ATP. The energy is required because the cell is attempting to move a substance to an area that already has a high concentration of that substance – similar to requiring energy to climb a hill rather than roll down it. Obviously, the higher the concentration already present, the more energy required to move further molecules of the particular substance into that area. For example, cells contain a lot of potassium (K^+); therefore, to get more potassium into the cell requires energy to transport it through the membrane.

Now, to turn to what is inside the cell membrane, starting with cytoplasm.

Cytoplasm

Cytoplasm is a ground substance (also known as a matrix) in which various cellular components are found. '**Cyto**' means cell, so any word that has 'cyto' in it is to do with cells.

Cytoplasm, itself, is a thick, semitransparent, elastic fluid containing suspended particles and the cytoskeleton. The cytoskeleton provides support and shape to the cell. In addition, it is involved in the movement of structures in the cytoplasm because some cells can change shape, for example phagocytic cells (see Figure 1.3).

What is the role of the cytoplasm?
- Chemically, cytoplasm is 75–90% water plus solid compounds – mainly **carbohydrates**, **lipids** and **inorganic substances**, and it is the substance in which **chemical reactions** occur.
- The cytoplasm receives raw materials from the external environment (such as from digested food) and converts them into usable energy by decomposition reactions.
- As well as the breakdown of raw materials to make energy, the cytoplasm is also the site where new substances are synthesised (produced) for the use of the cell.
- It is the place where various chemicals are packaged for transport to other parts of the cell, or to other cells in the body.
- Finally, it is in the cytoplasm that various chemicals facilitate the excretion of waste materials.

Nucleus

What is a nucleus?
The simple analogy is to think of it as the brain of the cell.

Do all cells have a nucleus?

Prokaryotic cells do not have a nucleus, but eukaryotic cells do. **Eukaryotic cells** are found in animals and plants, whilst prokaryotic cells are very typical of bacteria. In many ways, prokaryotic cells are less complex and often smaller than are eukaryotes.

However, not all human cells possess a nucleus. An example of a cell without a nucleus is the red blood cell. The chapter on blood demonstrates that mature red blood cells are concave in shape. That is because they have lost their nucleus and so the cell has 'collapsed in' on itself. Also, just to make it more confusing, some cells can have more than one nucleus, for example some muscle fibre cells (see Figure 1.12).

Some facts about the **nucleus** are:

- The nucleus is the largest structure in the cell.
- It is surrounded by a nuclear membrane. This nuclear membrane has two layers and, like the cell membrane, is selectively permeable.
- The protoplasm within the nucleus is not called cytoplasm, but is called **nucleoplasm**.
- The nucleus assumes a great responsibility for both **mitosis** and **meiosis**.
- Inside the nucleus is found the **genetic material**, consisting principally of **DNA** (deoxyribonucleic acid). When a cell is not reproducing, the genetic material is a threadlike mass called **chromatin**.
- Before cell division, the chromatin shortens, and coils into rod-shaped bodies called **chromosomes**.
- The basic structural unit of a chromosome is a **nucleosome** – composed of the DNA and protein.
- DNA has two main functions:
  - □ It provides the genetic blueprint which ensures that the next generation of cells is similar to existing ones.
  - □ It provides the plans for the synthesis of protein in the cell itself.
- All this information is stored in **genes**.
- Also, inside the nucleus are little spherical bodies called **nucleoli** and these are responsible for the production of **ribosomes** from ribosomal RNA depicted as **rRNA** (RNA = ribonucleic acid).
- In humans, there are 23 pairs of chromosomes in each cell with a nucleus, with the exception of the spermatozoa and ova (sperm and eggs).
- Sperm and ova only have 23 single chromosomes (i.e. one of each).
- The chromosomes are the same for males and females except for one pair – the X and Y chromosomes. It is these chromosomes that determine whether a baby is going to be male or female.

Mitosis and meiosis

These are the processes by which the cell reproduces itself. Most human cells reproduce asexually by mitosis, but the spermatozoa and ova reproduce by meiosis. Whereas the cells reproducing by mitosis finish up as exact copies of the parent cells with a pair of each of the 23 chromosomes, the cells reproducing by meiosis just finish up with one each of the 23 chromosomes.

In order for the body to grow, and also for the replacement of body cells that die, our cells must be able to reproduce themselves, but in order for genetic information not to be lost, they must be able to reproduce themselves accurately. They do this by cloning themselves. In some organisms, this can occur by **simple fission**, where the nucleus in a single cell becomes elongated and then divides to form two nuclei in the same cell, each new nucleus carrying identical genetic information. The cytoplasm then divides in the middle between the two nuclei, and so two identical daughter cells result, each with its own nucleus and other essential **organelles**.

In humans, cell reproduction is a complex process called **mitosis**, in which the number of chromosomes in the daughter cells has to be the same as in the original parent cell.

Mitosis can be divided into four stages:

- prophase
- metaphase
- anaphase
- telophase

- Before and after it has divided, the cell enters a stage known as **interphase** – this was thought to be a resting period for the cell, but the cell is actually very busy during this period because it has to get ready for replication.
- Extra **organelles** are manufactured by the replication of existing **organelles**.
- Also, the cell builds up a store of energy which is required for the process of division.

Prophase

The first stage after interphase is **prophase**:

- During prophase (Figure 1.6), the **chromosomes** become shorter, fatter and more easily visible, and each chromosome now consists of two **chromatids**, each containing the same genetic information (in other words, the DNA has replicated itself during interphase).
- The nucleolus and nuclear membrane disappear, leaving the chromosomes in the cytoplasm.

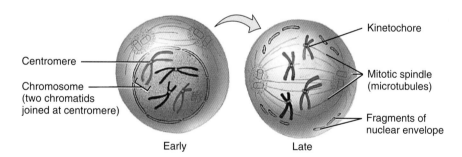

Figure 1.6 Prophase.

Metaphase

- During metaphase (Figure 1.7), the 46 chromosomes (2 of each of the 23 chromosomes) each consisting of two chromatids become attached to the spindle fibres.

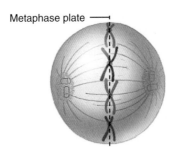

Figure 1.7 Metaphase.

Anaphase

■ During anaphase (Figure 1.8), the chromatids in each chromosome are separated.

■ One chromatid from each chromosome then moves towards each pole of the spindle.

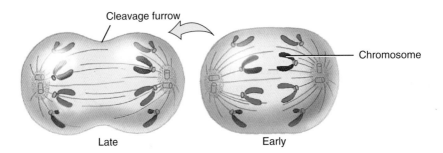

Figure 1.8 Anaphase.

Telophase

■ There are now 46 chromatids at each pole, and these will form the chromosomes of the daughter cells.

■ The cell membrane constricts in the centre of the cell dividing it into two cells.

■ The nuclear spindle disappears, and a **nuclear membrane** forms around the chromosomes in each of the daughter cells (Figure 1.9).

■ The chromosomes become long and threadlike again, and are very difficult to see.

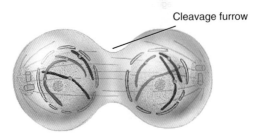

Figure 1.9 Telophase.

Cell division

Cell division is now complete, and the daughter cells themselves enter the **interphase** stage in order to prepare for their replication and division.

Cell cycle

Looking now at the cell cycle (Figure 1.10) and supposing that one full cycle represents 24 hours, then the actual process of replication (mitosis) would only last for about 1 hour out of those 24 hours. The rest of the time, the cell is undertaking the replication of its DNA. It also has to produce two of everything that is in the cell. In addition, it has to go through the process of obtaining and digesting nutrients so that it has the raw materials for this duplication, as well as for the energy required in order to carry out various functions of the cell.

Reproduction

During the reproduction of humans, the egg is penetrated by a sperm, which then releases its DNA to combine with the DNA of the egg, so that the resulting embryo will have two copies of each of the 23 chromosomes in nucleated cells. If the sperm and eggs had two copies of each chromosome (like other cells), the resulting fusion and developing embryo would have four copies of each chromosome. This means that the next generation would have four copies of each chromosome. The generation after that would have eight copies, and so on. This is obviously not practical, so the sperm and eggs undergo

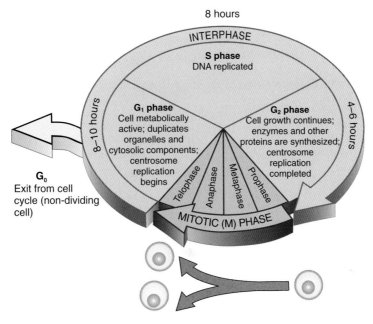

Figure 1.10 Cell cycle.

a process known as **meiosis** to ensure that the resulting embryo will only carry two copies of each chromosome in each cell with a nucleus.

Meiosis

For descriptive purposes, meiosis can be divided into eight stages (not the four of mitosis). However, they have the same names, but are known as either I or II.

First meiotic stage	Second meiotic stage
■ Prophase I	Prophase II
■ Metaphase I	Metaphase II
■ Anaphase I	Anaphase II
■ Telophase I	Telophase II

As with **mitosis**, these phases are continuous with one another. However, there are differences as well as similarities between mitosis and meiosis.

First meiotic stage
Prophase I
- This is similar to prophase in mitosis.
- However, instead of being scattered randomly, the chromosomes are arranged in 23 pairs. For example, the two chromosome number ones will pair up, as will the two chromosome number twos.
- Within each pair of chromosomes, genetic material may be exchanged between the two chromosomes.
- It is these exchanges that are partly responsible for the differences between children of the same parents.
- This process is called 'gene crossover'.

Metaphase I
As in mitosis, the chromosomes become arranged on the spindles at the equator. However, they remain in pairs.

Anaphase I
One chromosome from each pair moves to each pole, so that there are now 23 chromosomes at each end of the spindle.

Telophase I
The cell membrane now divides the cell into two halves, as in mitosis. Each daughter cell now has half the number of chromosomes that each parent cell had.

Second meiotic stage
- The cells produced by the first meiotic division now divide again.
- Prophase II, metaphase II, anaphase II and telophase II are all similar to their equivalent stage in mitosis, with the exception that the DNA has not been replicated before prophase II, so there are only 23 single chromosomes in each of the granddaughter cells.

Fusion of the gametes

- When the gametes, each with 23 chromosomes, fuse together, a cell known as a **zygote** with 23 paired chromosomes (i.e. 46 in all) is formed.
- One chromosome in each pair comes from the mother and one from the father.
- The zygotic cell then divides (by mitosis) many times to form the embryo.

The organelles

All cells contain many **organelles** (little organs).

Endoplasmic reticulum

This is the first of the organelles to be discussed (see Figure 1.11). The endoplasmic reticulum (ER) consists of membranes that form a series of channels (called **cisternae**) dividing the cytoplasm into compartments.

There are two types of cisternae:

1. Granular (rough) ER – associated with **ribosomes**
2. Agranular (smooth) ER – free of ribosomes

Ribosomes include tiny particles of RNA on which the synthesis of proteins needed by the cell takes place, and they are formed in the nucleoli:

- It is believed that ER is formed from the nuclear membrane.
- The membranes of the ER also contain many **enzymes** that speed up chemical reactions within the cells.

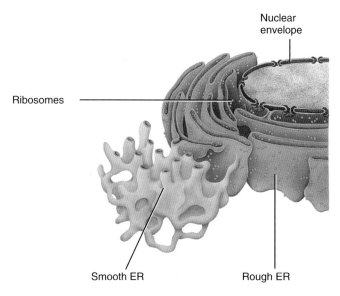

Figure 1.11 Endoplasmic reticulum.

- ER is a series of channels (cisternae) concerned with the transport of materials, primarily proteins; however, it also contains a number of enzymes of importance in cell metabolism, such as digestive enzymes as well as enzymes involved in the synthesis of steroids and some enzymes that are responsible for a variety of reactions leading to the removal of toxic substances from the cell (McCance and Huether, 2006).
- The alteration or addition of proteins for export from the cell can occur within the cisternae.
- Granular ER is particularly well developed in cells that actively synthesise (produce) and export proteins.
- Agranular ER is found in steroid hormone secreting cells, such as the cells of the adrenal cortex or the testes.
- ER is also present in liver cells, and here it has a role in drug detoxification.

Golgi apparatus

The Golgi apparatus is a collection of membranous tubes and elongated sacs – actually flattened cisternae stacked together. It plays a part in concentrating and packaging some of the substances that are made in the cell, for example lysosomal enzymes. The complex also plays a part in the assembly of substances for secretion outside of the cell. Secretory cells (such as those found in the mucus membrane) have many Golgi stacks, whereas non-secretory cells have few Golgi stacks per cell.

Proteins for export from the cell are synthesised on the ribosomes, and then travel through the ER to the Golgi vesicles (a vesicle is a fluid-filled sac). Vesicles leaving the Golgi fuse with the cell membrane by the process of **exocytosis**. The contents of the vesicles are then exported out of the cell. In addition, the Golgi is itself involved in the formation of **glycoproteins**.

Lysosomes

Lysosomes are organelles bound to the membrane that contain a variety of enzymes. Lysosomes have a number of functions:

- They are responsible for the digestion of material taken up by endocytosis, e.g. pathogenic organisms.
- They also break down cell components, for example during embryological development, the fingers and toes are webbed – the cells between the toes and fingers are removed by the lysosomal enzymes.
- After the baby's birth, the uterus, which weighs around 2 kg at full term, is invaded by **phagocytic cells** that are rich in lysosomes – these reduce the uterus to its non-pregnant weight of about 50 g within about 9 days.
- In normal cells, some of the synthesised proteins may be faulty – **lysosymes** are responsible for their removal.

It is important that lysosomes do not rupture and release their contents inside living cells; otherwise the lysosomal enzymes would start to digest the cell. In certain degenerative diseases, such as rheumatoid arthritis, enzymes released by the breakdown of lysosomes from macrophages may be a significant factor in attacking living cells and tissues.

Lysosomes also contribute to hormone production, e.g. thyroxine – a hormone affecting a wide range of physiological activities including metabolic rate.

Peroxisomes

These are organelles similar in structure to lysosomes, but much smaller. They are particularly abundant in liver cells. They contain several enzymes that are toxic to body cells. The role of peroxisomes in cells appears to be one of detoxification of harmful substances, such as alcohol and formaldehyde. More importantly, they neutralise dangerous free radicals. Free radicals are highly reactive chemicals that contain electrons that have not been paired off, and so are 'free' to disrupt the structure of molecules (Marieb, 2004).

Mitochondria (single = mitochondrion)

Mitochondria (often known as the power houses of the cell) consist of three membranes, the inner one of which has many folds that increase the surface area available for chemical reactions to occur. This process is collectively known as **internal respiration**. The mitochondrial matrix (the space surrounded by the inner membrane) contains enzymes of the **tricarboxylic acid** (TCA) cycle, as well as those enzymes involved in fatty acid oxidation. The inner membrane is of the same thickness as the outer membrane and is responsible for **oxidative phosphorylation**. The mitochondria themselves are often found concentrated in regions of the cell associated with intense metabolic activity.

By using ATP, the mitochondria are able to generate the energy needed by the cell for it to be able to function by converting the chemical energy contained in molecules of food. The production of ATP requires the breakdown of food molecules, and it occurs in several stages, each requiring the appropriate enzyme. An enzyme is a protein that can initiate and speed up a chemical reaction (it acts as a **catalyst**). The enzymes in the mitochondria are stored in the membranes in the required order so that the reactions occur in the correct sequence. This is very important, as it would be disastrous if the chemical reactions occurred out of sequence.

Mitochondria are self-replicating – just like the cells. DNA that is incorporated into the mitochondrial structure controls the replication process.

The cytoskeleton

The cytoskeleton is a lattice-like collection of fibres and fine tubes that occur in the cytoplasm, and it is involved in the cell's ability to maintain and alter its shape as required.

There are three components of the cytoskeleton:

- microfilaments
- microtubules
- intermediate filaments

Microfilaments

These are rod-like structures, 6 nm in diameter, consisting of a protein called actin. In muscle, both actin (thick) and myosin – another protein (thin) are involved in the contraction of muscle fibres. In non-muscle cells, microfilaments help to provide support and shape to the cell, and also assist in the movement of cells as well as movement within the cells.

Microtubules

- These are relatively straight, slender, cylindrical structures that range in diameter from 18 to 30 nm. They consist of a protein called tubulin.

- Microtubules and microfilaments help to provide shape and support for cells.
- They also provide conducting channels through which various substances can move through the cytoplasm.
- They also assist in the movement of pseudopodia.

Intermediate filaments

- These range in size from 8 to 12 nm in diameter and help to determine the shape of the cell.
- Examples of intermediate filaments are neurofilaments found in the nerve.

Centrioles, cilia and flagella

Centrioles

- They are found in most animal cells and are cylindrical in structures. They are composed of nine sets of microtubules arranged in a circular pattern.
- They are involved in cell reproduction.

Cilia and flagella

- These structures extend from the surface of some cells and can bend, thus causing movement.
- In humans, cilia generally have the function of moving fluid or particulates over the surface of the cells.
- Ciliated cells of the respiratory tract move mucous that has trapped foreign particles over the surface of respiratory tissues.
- A flagellum is usually a much larger structure than a cilium and is often used like a tail to propel the cell forward.
- The only example of a cell in the human body with a flagellum is the sperm, where the flagellum acts as a tail and propels the sperm towards the ova.

Types of cells

Figure 1.12 demonstrates some of the cells that make up certain tissues.

Tissues

A human begins as a single cell – the fertilised egg. As soon as fertilisation takes place, the egg divides continuously. However, these cells do not divide endlessly and haphazardly. They divide and grow together in such a way that they become specialised, for example muscle cells, skin cells, cells of the lens of the eye and blood cells (Marieb, 2006). These group together to become tissues. Tissues are basically groups of cells that are similar in structure and generally perform the same functions (McCance and Huether, 2006). There are four primary types of tissues:

- epithelial
- connective
- muscle
- nervous

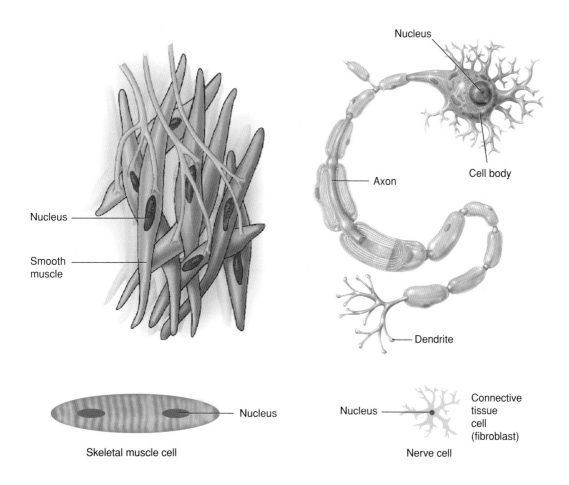

Figure 1.12 Types of cells.

These four primary tissue types 'interweave to form the fabric of the body' (Marieb, 2006, p. 85). In simple terms:

- Epithelial tissue is concerned with 'covering'.
- Connective tissue is concerned with 'support'.
- Muscle tissue is concerned with 'movement'.
- Nervous tissue is concerned with 'control' (Marieb, 2006).

Specialised cells form themselves into tissue in one of the two ways.

The first way is by means of mitosis. Cells formed as a result of mitosis are clones of the original cell. Therefore, if one cell with a specialised function undergoes mitosis, and subsequent generations of daughter cells continue to undergo mitosis, then the resulting hundreds of cells will all be the same type and have the same function – they will become tissue. For example, epithelial cell sheets (such as skin) are formed as a result of mitosis (McCance and Huether, 2006).

The second way in which specialised cells can form tissues involves their migration to the site of tissue formation and then assembling there. This is particularly seen during the development of the

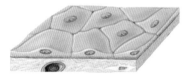

Figure 1.13 Simple epithelium.

embryo when, for example, cells migrate to sites in the embryo where they differentiate and assemble into a variety of tissues (McCance and Huether, 2006). This movement of cells is known as chemotaxis. Chemotaxis is discussed in detail in Chapter 3, but put simply, it is 'movement along a chemical gradient caused by chemical attraction' (McCance and Huether, 2006, p. 33).

Types of tissues

Epithelial tissue

Epithelial tissue lines and covers areas of the body, as well as forming the glandular tissue of the body. So, the exterior of the body (skin) is covered by one type of epithelial tissue, whilst another type of epithelial tissue lines some digestive system organs such as the stomach, the small intestines and the kidneys (Marieb, 2006). In effect, epithelial tissue covers most of the internal and external surfaces of the body.

Epithelial tissue is classified into two ways:

1. The number of cell layers:
    - ■ Simple – where the epithelial is formed by a single layer of cells (Figure 1.13).
    - ■ Stratified – where the epithelium has two or more layers of cells (Figure 1.14).
2. Shape:
    - ■ squamous
    - ■ cuboidal
    - ■ columnar

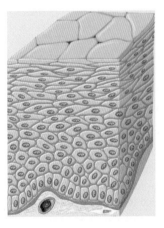

Figure 1.14 Stratified epithelium.

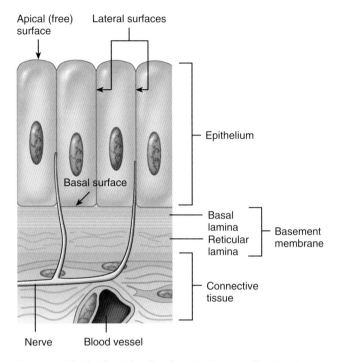

Figure 1.15 Epithelial cells classified according to shape.

Simple epithelial tissue is most concerned with absorption, secretion and filtration, but because they are usually so thin, they are not involved in protection.

Simple squamous epithelium rests on a basement membrane (basal layer) – the basement membrane is 'a structureless material secreted by the cells' (Marieb, 2006, p. 86). The basement membranes provide a layer of cells that supports and separates epithelial tissue from underlying connective tissue. Squamous epithelial cells fit very closely together to give a thin sheet forming the tissue. It is this type of epithelial tissue that is found in the alveoli of the lungs and the walls of capillaries. Rapid diffusion of filtration can take place through this very thin tissue. Oxygen and carbon dioxide exchange takes place through the epithelial tissue lining the alveoli of the lungs, whilst nutrients and gases can pass through the epithelial tissue from the cells into and out of the capillaries. In addition, simple squamous epithelial cells form serous membranes that line certain body cavities and organs.

Simple cuboidal epithelial tissue consists of one layer of cells resting on a basement membrane. However, because cuboidal epithelial cells are thicker than squamous epithelial cells, they are found in different places of the body and perform different functions. This epithelial tissue is found in glands, such as the salivary glands and the pancreas, as well as forming the walls of kidney tubules and covering the surface of the ovaries (Marieb, 2006, p. 87).

The third type of simple epithelial tissue – **simple columnar epithelium** (Figure 1.15), whilst being composed of single layer of cells, is made up of a single layer of quite tall cells that, like the other two types, fit closely together. This epithelial tissue lines the entire length of the digestive tract from the stomach to the anus and contains **goblet cells**. Goblet cells produce **mucus**, and those simple columnar epithelial tissues that line all the body cavities that are open to the body exterior are known as **mucous membranes** (Marieb, 2006).

Stratified epithelial tissue, unlike the simple epithelial tissue, consists of two or more cell layers. Because these stratified epithelial tissues have more than one layer of cells, they are stronger and hardier than the simple epithelia. This means that a primary **function of stratified epithelia is protection**.

Stratified squamous epithelial tissue (Figure 1.14) is the most common stratified epithelium that is found within the human body, and it consists of several layers of cells (Marieb, 2006). Although this epithelial tissue is called squamous epithelium, in actual fact, it is not made up entirely of squamous cells. It is the cells at the free edge of the epithelial tissue that is composed of squamous cells, whilst those cells that are close to the basement membrane are composed of either cuboidal or columnar cells. It is found in places that are most at risk of everyday damage, including the oesophagus, the mouth and the outer layer of the skin (Marieb, 2006).

Stratified cuboidal epithelial tissue only has two cell layers and is fairly rare in the human body, only being found in the ducts of large glands. The same can be said of the stratified columnar epithelial tissue.

There is a fourth type of epithelial tissue, known as **transitional epithelium**. This is a highly modified stratified squamous epithelium and it forms the lining of just a few organs/structures – all of which form part of the urinary system – the urinary bladder, the ureters and part of the urethra. This type of tissue has been modified in such a way that it can cope with the considerable stretching that takes place with these organs. So, when one of these organs or structures is not stretched, the tissue has many layers with the superficial (those in the top layer) cells being rounded and looking like domes. However, when one of these organs or structures is distended with urine, then the epithelium becomes thinner, the surface cells flatten and they become just like squamous cells. These transitional cells are able to slide past one another and change their shape, allowing the wall of the ureter to stretch as a greater volume of urine flows through. Similarly, it allows for more urine to be stored in the bladder (Marieb, 2006).

Glandular epithelium

Glandular epithelial tissue is found within glands. According to Marieb (2006), a gland consists of several cells that make and secrete a particular product.

There are two major types of glands developed from epithelial sheets:

- exocrine glands
- endocrine glands

Exocrine glands have ducts leading from them, and their secretions empty through these ducts to the surface of the epithelium. Examples of exocrine glands include the sweat glands, the liver and the pancreas.

Endocrine glands, on the other hand, do not possess ducts. Instead, their secretions diffuse directly into the blood vessels that are found within the glands. All endocrine glands secrete hormones. These glands include the thyroid, the adrenal glands and the pituitary gland.

Connective tissue

Connective tissue is found everywhere in the body and it connects body parts to one another. It is the most abundant and widely distributed of all four primary tissue types, and although connective tissues perform many functions and vary considerably in their structure, they do have four main functions, which can be summarised quite simply as:

- protection
- support
- binding together other tissues (Marieb, 2006)
- acting as storage sites for excess nutrients (McCance and Huether, 2006)

However, the most common structure and function of connective tissue is to act as the framework on which the epithelial cells gather in order to form the organs of the body (McCance and Huether, 2006).

There are several common characteristics of connective tissue, and one is that there are few cells in the tissue, but surrounding these few cells there is a great deal of what is known as **extracellular matrix**. This extracellular matrix is composed of **ground substance** and **fibres** and it varies in consistency from fluid to a semisolid gel, whilst the fibres that are made up of **fibroblasts** – one of the connective tissue cells – are of three types:

- collagenous (white) fibres
- elastic (yellow) fibres
- reticular fibres

The ground substance is composed largely of water plus some adhesion proteins and large polysaccharide molecules, and it is these adhesion proteins that serve as a glue that allows connective tissue cells to attach themselves to the fibres. The change of consistency within the ground substance from fluid to a semisolid gel depends upon the number of polysaccharide molecules that are present. An increase in polysaccharide molecules causes the matrix to move from being a fluid to being a semisolid gel. The ground substance can store large amounts of water, so it serves as a water reservoir for the body (Marieb, 2004).

Collagen fibres have great strength, whilst elastic fibres are able to be stretched and then to recoil. Finally, the reticular fibres form the internal 'skeleton' of soft organs such as the spleen.

Connective tissue forms a 'packing' tissue around organs of the body (very much like the packing that can surround a delicate object in a parcel in transit) and so protects them. It is able to bear weight, and to withstand stretching and various traumas, such as abrasions. There is a wide variation in types of connective tissue, for example fat tissue is composed mainly of cells and a soft matrix. Bone and cartilage have very few cells but do contain large amounts of hard matrix and that is what makes them so strong (Marieb, 2006).

There are also variations in the blood supply to the tissue. Although most connective tissues have a good blood supply, there are some types, for example tendons and ligaments that have a poor blood supply, whilst cartilages have no blood supply. That is the reason why these structures heal very slowly when they are injured – often a broken bone will heal much quicker than a damaged tendon or ligament (Marieb, 2006).

Types of connective tissue
Bone
Bone is the most rigid of the connective tissues and it is composed of bone cells surrounded by very hard matrix containing calcium and large numbers of collagen fibres. Because of their hardness, bones provide protection, support and muscle attachment (Marieb, 2006).

Cartilage
Cartilage, which is not as hard, but is more flexible than bone, is found in only a few places in the body, for example hyaline cartilage, which is found supporting the structures of the larynx. It attaches the ribs to the sternum and covers the ends of the bones where they form joints (Marieb, 2004). Other types of cartilage include fibrocartilage which, because it can be compressed, forms the discs between the vertebrae of the spinal column, and elastic cartilage where some degree of elasticity is required, for example in the external ear.

Dense connective tissue
Dense connective tissue forms strong, stringy structures such as tendons (which attach skeletal muscles to bones) and the more elastic ligaments (that connect bones to other bones at joints). Dense connective tissue also makes up the lower layers of the skin (known as the dermis). These tissues have collagen fibres as the main matrix element, with many fibroblasts found between the collagen fibres (Marieb, 2006). These fibroblasts are cells that are involved in the manufacture of the fibres.

Loose connective tissue
Loose connective tissues are softer and contain more cells, but fewer fibres, than other types of connective tissue (with the exception of blood). There are four types of loose connective tissues, namely:

- areolar tissue
- adipose tissue
- reticular tissue
- blood

Areolar tissue
Areolar tissue is the most widely distributed connective tissue type in the body. It is a soft tissue that cushions and protects the body organs that it surrounds. It helps to hold the internal organs together. It has a fluid matrix that contains all types of fibres which form a loose network, so giving it its softness and pliability. It provides a reservoir of water and salts for the surrounding tissues. All body cells obtain their nutrients from this tissue fluid and also release their waste into it. It is also in this area that, following injury, swelling can occur (known as oedema) because the areolar tissue soaks up the excess fluid just like a sponge does causing it to become puffy (Marieb, 2004).

Adipose tissue
This tissue is commonly known as 'fat' and is actually areolar tissue in which there is a preponderance of fat cells. It forms the subcutaneous tissue which lies beneath the skin where it insulates the body and can protect it from the extremes of both heat and cold (Marieb, 2004). In addition, adipose tissue protects some organs, such as kidneys and eyeballs.

Reticular connective tissue

Reticular connective tissue consists of a delicate network of reticular fibres that are associated with reticular cells (similar to fibroblasts). It forms an internal framework to support many free blood cells – mainly the lymphocytes – in the lymphoid organs such as the lymph nodes, the spleen and bone marrow (Marieb, 2004).

Blood

'Blood, or vascular tissue, is considered a connective tissue because it consists of blood cells, surrounded by a nonliving, fluid matrix call blood plasma' (Marieb, 2004). Blood is concerned with the transport of nutrients, waste material, respiratory gases (such as oxygen and carbon dioxide), as well as many other substances throughout the body.

Muscle tissue

There are three types of muscle tissue and these are responsible for helping the body to move, or to move substances within the body. The three types of muscle tissue are:

- skeletal muscle
- cardiac muscle
- smooth muscle

Skeletal muscle

This muscle is attached to bones and is involved in the movement of the skeleton. These muscles can be controlled voluntarily and form the 'bulk' of the body (the flesh). The cells of skeletal muscle are long, cylindrical and have several nuclei. In addition, they appear striated (have stripes). They work by contracting and relaxing, with pairs working antagonistically against each other – i.e. one muscle contracts and the opposite muscle relaxes. So, for example, if the muscles in the front of the arm contract and the ones at the back of the arm relax, then the arm bends.

Cardiac muscle

Cardiac muscle is only found in the heart and it acts as a pump to pump blood around the body. It does this by contracting and relaxing, just like skeletal muscles, and it appears striated. However, unlike skeletal muscles, it works in an involuntary way – the activity cannot be consciously controlled. The cells of cardiac muscle do not have a nucleus.

Smooth muscle

Also known as visceral muscle, smooth muscle (see Figure 1.12) is found in the walls of hollow organs, for example the stomach, bladder, uterus and blood vessels (hence 'visceral' because these organs are also known as 'viscera'). Smooth muscle has no striations, and like cardiac muscle it works in an involuntary way. Smooth muscle causes movement in the hollow organs, for example as smooth muscle contracts the cavity of an organ becomes smaller (constricted) and when smooth muscle relaxes the organ becomes larger (dilated). This allows substances to be propelled through the organ in the right direction, for example faeces in the intestines. Because smooth muscle contracts and relaxes slowly, it forms a wavelike motion (known as peristalsis) to push, in the case of the intestines, the faeces through the intestines (Figure 1.16).

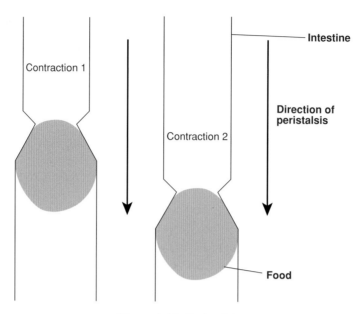

Figure 1.16 Peristalsis.

Nervous tissue

Nervous tissue is concerned with control and communication within the body by means of electrical signals. The main type of cell that is found in nervous tissue is the **neuron** (see Figure 1.12). All neurons receive and conduct electrochemical impulses around the body. The structure of neurons is very different from other cells. The cytoplasm is found within long processes or extensions – some in the leg being more than a metre long. These neurons receive and transmit electrical impulses very rapidly from one to the other across **synapses** (junctions). It is at the synapses that the electrical impulse can pass from neuron to neuron, or from a neuron to a muscle cell. The total number of neurons is fixed at birth, and cannot be replaced if they are damaged (McCance and Huether, 2006).

In addition to the neurons, nervous tissue includes some cells that are known as **neuroglia-supporting cells**. These supporting cells insulate, support and protect the delicate neurons. The neurons and supporting cells make up the structures of the nervous system, namely:

- the brain
- the spinal cord
- the nerves

Tissue repair

The many tissues of the body are always at risk of injury or disease. Inflammation is the body's immediate reaction to tissue injury or damage, because when tissue injury or damage does occur, this stimulates the body's inflammatory and immune responses to spring into action so that the healing process can begin almost immediately.

There are four major signs and symptoms of an inflammatory response (Nairn and Helbert, 2002), namely:

- pain
- swelling
- heat
- redness

There may also be nausea, sweating, a raised pulse, a lowered blood pressure and even a loss of consciousness. These symptoms are the body's response to the pain and to shock.

Inflammation is usually initiated by damage to a cell. Following this damage, three simultaneous processes occur:

- **Mast cell degranulation**. Mast cells are tissue cells which contain granules in their cytoplasm. These granules are similar to, but smaller than, the granules found in basophils in the blood. These granules contain, amongst other substances, histamine which, during the process of degranulation, is released into the tissues. It causes some inflammatory symptoms, and works with the two other processes (below) to provide full inflammatory symptoms.
- **The activation of four plasma protein systems**. These systems are the complement, clotting and kinin systems, and immunoglobulins (antibodies). The complement system activates and assists inflammatory and immune processes. It also plays a major role in the destruction of bacteria. The clotting system traps bacteria that have entered the wound and also interacts with platelets to stop any bleeding. The kinin system helps to control vascular permeability, whilst immunoglobulins help in the destruction of bacteria.
- **The phagocytic cells** move to the area of damage in order to **phagocytose** bacteria or any other non-self debris in the wound.

A typical inflammatory response to tissue in injury is:

- Arterioles near the injury site constrict briefly, followed by vasodilation which increases blood flow to the site of the injury (**redness** and **heat**).
- Dilation of the arterioles at the site increases the pressure in the circulation, which increases the movement of plasma proteins and blood cells into the tissues in the area, so causing oedema (**swelling**).
- The nerve endings in the area are stimulated, partly by pressure (**pain**).
- The clotting and kinin systems, along with platelets, move into the area and block any tissue tears by commencing the clotting process.
- Phagocytes and lymphocytes move into the area and start to destroy any infectious organisms found there and remove pus.
- These blood cells remain in the area until tissue regeneration (repair) takes place – known as resolution.

Thus, inflammation can be summed up as the presence of:

- vasodilation – redness/heat
- vascular permeability – oedema
- cellular infiltration – pus
- thrombosis – clots
- stimulation of nerve endings – pain

Conclusion

This chapter has looked at the building blocks of the human body, namely the cells. Cells are extremely complicated parts of the body, but an understanding of them and their functions is important in order to understand how the human body itself functions. Cells form tissues, which then form all the structures, systems and organs of the body. Therefore, it is necessary to also have an understanding of tissues. The remainder of this book will look at the various systems, structures and organs of the body – how they function as well as what can go wrong with them.

Multiple choice questions

1. The three types of endocytosis are:
(a) phagocytosis, pinocytosis, exocytosis
(b) phagocytosis, exocytosis, cytolysis
(c) cytolysis, receptor-mediated endocytosis, pinocytosis
(d) pinocytosis, receptor-mediated endocytosis, phagocytosis

2. The commonest form of passive transport of substances into and out of the cell is:
(a) filtration
(b) diffusion
(c) facilitated diffusion
(d) osmosis

3. The splitting of which molecule causes the release of energy in the cell?
(a) ADP
(b) ADH
(c) ATP
(d) AMP

4. Which cells reproduce by meiosis?
(a) white and red blood cells
(b) spermatozoa and ova
(c) cardiac and muscle cells
(d) squamous and cuboidal

5. The process of mitosis includes which phases?
(a) telophase II, anaphase I, prophase, metaphase
(b) prophase, metaphase, telophase, anaphase
(c) innerphase, prophase, anaphase, metaphase
(d) metaphase II, prophase II, anaphase II, telophase II

6. Granular endoplasmic reticulum is associated with:
(a) lysosomes
(b) peroxisomes
(c) chromosomes
(d) ribosomes

7. Put simply, connective tissue is concerned with:
(a) covering
(b) support

(c) movement

(d) control

8. Simple epithelial tissue is mainly concerned with:

(a) absorption, protection, filtration

(b) protection, absorption, secretion

(c) secretion, filtration, absorption

(d) secretion, filtration, protection

9. Why do bones heal faster than tendons following injury? Is it because:

(a) they are harder

(b) they are more rigid

(c) they have many free blood cells

(d) they have a better blood supply

10. The four major signs and symptoms of an inflammatory response following damage to tissue are:

(a) pain, swelling, redness, heat

(b) swelling, pain, depression, redness

(c) pain, pus, heat, blood clots

(d) blood clots, depression, pus, itching

Answers: 1.d, 2.b, 3.c, 4.b, 5.b, 6.d, 7.b, 8.c, 9.d, 10.a.

Test your knowledge

❷ How does the cell membrane control metabolism?

❷ Explain briefly the differences between phagocytosis, receptor-mediated endocytosis and pinocytosis.

❷ How does the process of cellular reproduction ensure that there are only 46 (23 pairs) chromosomes in a fetus?

❷ Describe the function of connective tissue.

❷ Briefly explain the roles of the four plasma protein systems in the process of tissue repair.

Glossary of terms

Active transport: The process in which substances move against a concentration gradient from an area of low concentration to one of higher concentration. It requires the release and use of energy.

Active transport pumps: Also known as sodium pumps, these are the mechanisms situated in plasma membranes that use the energy produced by the ATP reaction to pump sodium ions (Na^+) out of the cell and potassium ions (K^+) into it.

Adenosine diphosphate (ADP): Found inside cells, it helps to produce ATP during reactions which produce cellular energy and is itself formed from ATP at a later stage. It is this continual synthesis and breaking down of ADP and ATP that produces the energy.

Adenosine triphosphate (ATP): The compound that is essential for the production of cellular energy.

Amino acid: The building block of proteins. The type of protein that is produced depends upon the number and types of amino acids that are used to construct it.

Carbohydrates: An organic compound that is composed of carbon, hydrogen and oxygen. Sugars (including glucose) are carbohydrates. They are very important as an energy store.

Carrier/transport protein: Small molecules that help in the movement of ions across a cell membrane.

Catalyst: A catalyst is a substance that speeds up a reversible chemical reaction. Enzymes are catalysts.

Chemical reactions: Reactions that involve molecules, in which the molecules are formed, changed, or broken down.

Chromatid: One of the two strands of chromatin. Two identical chromatids form a chromosome after nuclear reproduction.

Chromatin: The material which makes chromosomes. It consists of DNA and proteins.

Chromosomes: Tightly coiled chromatin. This is the form in which the genetic material of all cells is organised.

Concentration gradient: The gradient that demonstrates the difference between an area of high concentration and low concentration of substances.

Cytoplasm: Collective name for all the contents of the cell, including the plasma membrane, but not including the nucleus.

Deoxyribonucleic acid (DNA): Found in the nucleus, it contains all the genetic information of an organism.

Diffusion: The most common form of passive transport of materials, it is the ability of gases, liquids and solutes to disperse randomly and to occupy any space available, so that there is an equal distribution.

Endocytosis: The general name for the various processes by which cells ingest foodstuffs and infectious microorganisms.

Enzymes: Molecules that speed up chemical reactions.

Eukaryotic cells: These are cells that normally include, or have included, chromosomal material within one or more nuclei.

Exocytosis: The system of transporting material out of cells.

Extracellular fluid: Fluid outside of the cell, but surrounding it.

Extracellular matrix: Found in connective tissue, this is non-living material that is made up of ground substance and fibres. It separates the living cells found in this tissue.

Facilitated diffusion: Similar to diffusion, this requires the help of another substance – a carrier protein – for the process to take place, i.e. a facilitator.

Fibres: These are any long, thin structures. The body contains many of them, including nerve fibres and muscle fibres.

Fibroblasts: These are the typical cell type of connective tissue. They are responsible for the production and secretion of extracellular matrix materials.

Genes: The smallest physical and biological units of heredity that encode for a molecular cell product.

Genetic material: Mainly DNA (deoxyribonucleic acid) that contains genetic information.

Glucose: Also known as dextrose, it is the principal sugar found in the blood. It is essential for life. An absence can lead to diabetes, coma and even death.

Glycoproteins: Proteins linked to carbohydrates.

Goblet cells: Individual cells found in mucosal membranes that produce mucus.

Ground substance: The name given to that part of the extracellular matrix (found in connective tissue) that is composed mainly of water, with some adhesion proteins and large polysaccharide molecules.

Hormones: Chemical messengers that are linked to the endocrine system.

Inorganic substances: Compounds that do not contain carbon. Water is an inorganic compound.

Internal respiration: The use of oxygen by cells in the enzymatic release of energy from organic compounds. This is known as aerobic respiration. Anaerobic respiration does not require oxygen, but does require a substance such as nitrate or iron to do the same job as oxygen (accept electrons during the chemical reaction). Only human cells with mitochondria can undertake aerobic respiration.

Ion: An atom that contains either a positive or a negative electrical charge.

Lipids: Organic compounds that are soluble in organic substances such as alcohol and benzene. They include fats, waxes, oils, steroids and phospholipids.

Lysosome: Organelles within the cell that are an important part of the cell's digestive system because they secrete lysosyme and other similar enzymes – very important in the phagocytosis of microorganisms.

Lysosyme: A bacteria-destroying enzyme found in lysosomes, sweat, tears, saliva and other bodily secretions.

Meiosis: The process by which the gametes (spermatozoa and ova) are reproduced.

Membrane: The outer covering of a cell and of a nucleus within a cell.

Metabolism: The collective name for all the physical and chemical processes occurring within a cell/living organism, but often referring only to reactions involving enzymes.

Metabolites: A substance involved in the process of metabolism – either to cause it, assist it, or occurring as a result of the process.

Mitosis: The process by which cells (other than the gametes) are reproduced by simple division of the nucleus and the cell itself.

Neuroglia-supporting cells: These cells are found in nervous tissue and their role is to support the delicate neurons by insulating, supporting and protecting them.

Nuclear membrane: The outer shell of the nucleus within the cell.

Nucleoli: Small spherical bodies found in the cell nucleus that are involved in the production of ribosomes.

Nucleoplasm: The name given to the protoplasm that is found within the nucleus.

Nucleosome: The basic structural unit of a chromosome.

Organelles: Structural and functional parts of a cell that act like human organs to fulfil all the needs of the cell so that it can grow, reproduce and carry out its functions.

Osmosis: The process by which water travels through a selectively permeable membrane so that concentrations of substances in water are the same on either side of the membrane.

Osmotic pressure: The pressure that must be exerted on a solution to prevent the passage of water into it across a semipermeable membrane from a region of higher concentration of solute to a region of lower concentration of solute.

Oxidative phosphorylation: This is the process by which energy released during aerobic respiration and is linked to the production of adenotriphosphate (ATP).

Passive transport: The process by which substances move on their own down a concentration gradient from an area of high concentration to one of lower concentration. No cellular energy is required for this process.

Phagocytosis: The method by which cells ingest large particles, including whole microorganisms.

Pinocytosis: The method by which the cell ingests small particles and fluids.

Prokaryotic cells: The opposite of eukaryotes, their DNA/RNA is not contained within a discrete nucleus. They are generally very small and include bacteria.

Protoplasm: The collective name for everything within the cell, including cytoplasm, nucleus and the organelles, as well as the plasma membrane.

Receptor-mediated endocytosis: A highly selective method by which the cell is able to ingest large particles (particularly proteins).

Receptor sites: Also known as membrane receptor molecules. These are proteins on the membrane of cells that are able to receive certain other proteins that match them, for example hormones and antibodies.

Ribosomal ribonucleic acid (rRNA): Involved in the translation of the genetic material encoded in DNA into proteins. They work in conjunction with ribosomes and messenger RNA (mRNA) and transfer RNA (tRNA).

Ribosomes: Organelles found in cytoplasm that play a major role in the synthesis of proteins from RNA.

Selective permeability: The ability of the cell membrane to allow only certain substances to pass through into or out of the cell.

Simple fission: The asexual reproduction of cells by means of division of the nucleus and the cell body.

Solute: A substance that is dissolved in a solution.

Transmembrane ion gradient: The gradient involving the concentration of ions on either side of a plasma membrane. It is involved in the production of cellular energy.

Tricarboxylic acid (TCA) cycle: The TCA cycle is also known as Krebs cycle. This is an aerobic pathway that occurs in the mitochondria and is necessary for the production of energy there.

Vesicle: A spherical space within the cell cytoplasm that is involved in storage and transfer of substances for the cell.

References

Colbert, B.J., Ankney, J. and Lee, K.T. (2007). *Anatomy and Physiology for Health Professionals: An Interactive Journey*. New Jersey: Pearson Prentice Hall.

Marieb, E.N. (2004). *Human Anatomy and Physiology*, 6th edn. San Francisco: Pearson Benjamin Cummings.

Marieb, E.N. (2006). *Essentials of Human Anatomy and Physiology*, 8th edn. San Francisco: Pearson Benjamin Cummings.

McCance, K.L. and Huether, S.E. (2006). *Pathophysiology: The Biologic Basis for Disease in Adults and Children*, 8th edn. St. Louis: Mosby.

Nairn, R. and Helbert, M. (2002). *Immunology for Medical Students*. St. Louis: Mosby.

Rangarajan, D. and Shaw, D. (2004). *One Stop Doc: Cell and Molecular Biology*. London: Arnold.

Watson, R. (2005). Cell structure and function, growth and development. In: Montague, S.E., Watson, R. and Herbert, R.A. (eds) *Physiology for Nursing Practice*, 3rd edn. Edinburgh: Elsevier, pp. 49–69.

Chapter 2

Cancer

Peter S. Vickers

KEY WORDS

- Cancer
- Tumour
- Oncogene
- Chemotherapy

- Carcinogen
- Malignant
- Radiotherapy
- Immunotherapy

- Carcinoma
- Neoplasm
- Cytotoxic

Test your prior knowledge

- What is the difference between a malignant tumour and a benign tumour?
- Name three methods of treating cancer.
- What can cause lung cancer?

Introduction

According to McLannahan (2001), approximately one in five people living in industrial countries will die of cancer, most of whom will be over 65 years of age.

Cancer is a disease of abnormal cell growth, **cell division** and **cell differentiation**. The disease 'cancer' actually consists of a group of diseases, all of which are underpinned by (and caused by) uncontrolled abnormal cell growth. Cancers are always life-threatening but not always fatal. There are many causes of cancers, just as there are many types of cancers.

According to McCance and Roberts (2006), cells of multicellular organisms are not concerned just with the individual cell, but rather with the survival of the entire multicellular organism. These cells can be thought of as specialised members of a society – a cellular society. This means that all cells work for the good of the organism. Because of this, the processes of cell division, proliferation and differentiation are normally regulated so that they are in balance – particularly a balance between the rate of cell birth and the rate of cell death (see Chapter 1).

However, as in any society, there are always some abnormal cells that disobey all social control mechanisms, in this case, the social control mechanisms of cell division, proliferation and differentiation. These are the cells that will proliferate to form tumours in the body, and indeed, as McCance and Roberts (2006) point out, virtually every cell in the body has the potential to become a tumour if it mutates.

Carcinogenesis is a multi-step mechanism and is caused by an accumulation of cellular and chemical errors, particularly concerning the deoxyribonucleic acid (**DNA**) of a cell. Altered DNA bases – known as **mutations** – are the cause of any changes that lead to cells becoming cancers, and it requires several mutations within the DNA to occur in order for carcinogenesis to happen (King, 2000). Carcinogenesis always begins with a single cell whose DNA has been damaged for some reason. This cell starts to grow in an abnormal and uncontrolled way. Following the process of division and reproduction, as discussed in Chapter 1, each new **daughter cell**, because it has inherited its parent's DNA, also grows in an uncontrolled way. Normally, a cell is programmed to stop growing when it reaches its correct size, but because of the DNA abnormality (**mutation**), it continues past this point and grows ever larger.

The body does have mechanisms to deal with cells that are abnormal, which means that these cells that carry a genetic mutation causing uncontrolled growth should either commit suicide (**apoptosis**) or should be killed by the body's own defences (see Chapter 3). In order to become a cancer, these abnormal cells have to be multiplied literally billions of times (King, 2000). For a single cell to develop billions of daughter cells takes a long time, and this is why cancers are generally considered to be diseases of old age. Unfortunately, there are exceptions to this, and some cancers develop in children (some even in babies). Examples of these are some cancers of the eye – retinoblastoma, and of the blood – certain leukaemias (King, 2000). However, the idea that cancer is generally a disease linked with old age still holds true, and there is a high incidence of cancer occurring after the age of 40 years.

Cancer can occur in almost any cell, but the most common cancers are to be found in the:

- skin
- lung
- colon
- breast
- prostate gland

Over the past few years, there have been some changes in the incidence rates of the various cancers. For example, the incidence of stomach and colon cancer has reduced, whilst the incidence of skin and lymphoid cancers have increased (Marieb, 2004). Marieb (2004) also points out that despite all the advances in diagnosis, care and treatment of cancer, the overall rate of cancer deaths has increased. This may be accounted for by the fact that life expectancy has also increased (at least in the developed world), and, as was mentioned above, cancers are more prevalent in older people.

Biology of cancer

For whatever reason, the DNA of a cell becomes altered, causing the cell to grow uncontrollably. This is known as the initiation period. What happens after the cell starts to grow uncontrollably determines whether or not cancer will occur.

Apoptosis (or cell suicide) is a process that is continually occurring within the body. This is because altered and damaged cells are constantly being produced in the body. To understand why this should be so, one only needs to look at the process in which DNA and cells are replicated (see Chapter 1). This process is an extremely rapid one (as it needs to be to keep pace with the needs of the body in terms of replacing altered and damaged cells). For example, skin cells are constantly being replaced because of damage caused by being worn away and dislodged every time the skin comes into contact with any surface. Because of the speed at which this very complicated process of DNA replication occurs, it can be no surprise when mistakes occur.

The second mechanism that the body possesses in order to try and prevent the development of damaged cells is the destruction of these cells by the body's own immune system. One of the many functions of the immune system is called immune surveillance, and this does just what it says. Certain white blood cells of the immune system (known as **T-cytotoxic lymphocytes**) move through the body looking for any abnormal or 'alien' (e.g. bacteria and viruses) cells. Each cell carries receptors on the outer membrane of cells, and some of these receptors are specific identification (ID) receptors that identify them as belonging to that particular body. If these T-cytotoxic cells come across a cell in the body that does not carry these particular ID receptors for that body, then they will kill it. Now, although cancerous cells will belong to the same body as the T-cytotoxic lymphocytes, because of the alteration in the cancerous cells, due to the altered DNA, the ID receptors on these cancerous cells may have slight alterations to their formation. Luckily, even though there is only a slight alteration to the ID receptors carried by cancerous cells, they are still different enough for the T-cytotoxic cells to recognise them as not being 'correct' cells, and destroy them. However, unfortunately, some of the cells (known as **precancerous** cells) are able to develop strategies to hide their differences from the immune system, and so escape being destroyed by the T-cytotoxic cells. Once the precancerous cells have achieved this evasion of the body's immune system, they can then proceed to divide and replicate in order to cause cancers, because all their daughter cells will also have this ability to evade the T-cytotoxic lymphocytes (Gorczynski and Stanley, 2006; Janeway *et al.*, 2005; King, 2000; Lydyard *et al.*, 2004; Nairn and Helbert, 2002; Vickers, 2005).

Once the precancerous cell has developed a strategy for avoiding both apoptosis and the T-cytotoxic lymphocytes, it can then proceed to **clone** itself, and the cancer starts to develop. To transform a single precancerous cell into a cancer requires more than just a straightforward cloning of this cell, because, in addition to the cell cloning itself, there needs to be the formation of new blood vessels (known as **angiogenesis**). The reason for the necessity of these new blood vessels developing is that all cells require a good blood supply so that oxygen and nutrients can reach them and keep them alive (as well as allowing for the removal of carbon dioxide and other toxins). In order for these new blood vessels to develop, the cancerous cell needs to produce **angiogenic growth factors** (i.e. substances produced in the cell to allow for the development of new blood vessels). The other thing to consider is that the cancerous cells need extra blood flow (more than a normal cell) because they are growing so rapidly and to such a great size that they require extra oxygen and nutrients for the growth to continue and for the extra **metabolism** that is required by the cancerous cell to take place.

There are several models that demonstrate the development of cancers, and the two that are of most relevance at the moment are described below.

■ **Molecular biology model**: Figure 2.1 describes the process of the development of cancer from the cellular perspective. A normal cell can become precancerous as a result of DNA changes (1) during reproduction/cloning. The precancerous cell can then become a cancer as a result of further alteration in its DNA (2) during cloning, and the final DNA change (3) can cause the cancerous cell to become metastatic and to spread throughout the body. Thus, it can be seen that the DNA needs to continue to mutate for a normal cell to reach the metastatic stage – it is not just a single mutation.

■ **Clinical model**: In this model (Figure 2.2), that looks at the actual clinical disease as opposed to the biochemical underpinning, the cancer commences with a normal cell, that starts to overproliferate (i.e. reproduce/clone excessively) so that although these cells are 'normal', they are dividing rapidly. The next stage occurs when there are sufficient cancerous cells to be able to say that a cancer is present, although it is still only situated in one place within the body. The third stage is when the cancerous cells start to invade the surrounding tissue (aggressive behaviour), and finally the cancer spreads to other, often remote, parts of the body – metastasis.

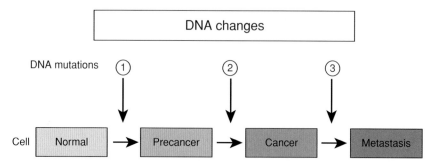

Figure 2.1 Molecular biology model (after King, 2000).

Often once a cancer can be detected it is already at an advanced stage and thus the prognosis is poorer than if it had been diagnosed at an earlier stage.

Causes of cancer

The main causes of cancer appear to be linked to interactions between genes and the environment.

Genes

The role of genes in the development of cancer is very important, and there are three types of genes that are involved:

- proto-oncogenes
- oncogenes
- tumour suppressor genes

Proto-oncogenes possess the genetic codes for the proteins that are needed for normal cell division and growth, whilst **oncogenes** are proto-oncogenes that have mutated and so have become

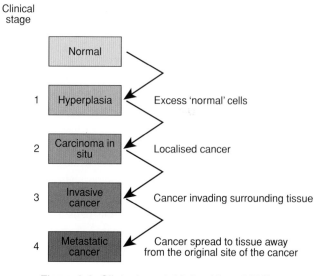

Figure 2.2 Clinical model (after King, 2000).

cancer-causing genes that increase the rate at which cells divide and proliferate. One of the problems with proto-oncogenes is that many of them have fragile sites that can easily break once they are exposed to **carcinogens**. Once this occurs, then the proto-oncogenes are converted into oncogenes. Unfortunately, since oncogenes have been discovered in only 15–20% of cancers found in humans, there has to be something else which causes cancerous cells to develop, and **tumour suppressor genes**, for example *p*53, provide the answer. Tumour suppressor genes work to suppress or even prevent cancer by repairing any damaged cell DNA, as well as slowing down or even stopping cell division. These tumour suppressor genes also help to inactivate **carcinogens** as well as improving the ability of the immune system to destroy cancer cells (Marieb, 2006). These tumour suppressor genes are also capable of improving the ability of the immune system to destroy cancer cells (Marieb 2006)

When these mutated cancer-causing cells occur in **germline cells** (i.e. sperm and ova), then these cancer-causing genes can be inherited from one generation to the next, and so produce families in which there is a predisposition for certain cancers, such as breast cancer (Jorde *et al.*, 2006). Therefore, it is now known that certain forms of cancer oncogenes can be inherited within some families. However, if the oncogene is only to be found in **somatic cells**, then they would not be inherited by future generations. Examples of inherited cancers, for which a specific oncogene has been isolated, include:

- retinoblastoma (cancer of the eye – found in children)
- Wilm's tumour (cancer of the kidney – also found in children)
- familial breast cancer

Environmental factors

Turning now to the link between cancer genes and environmental factors, the frequency of the cancer-causing mutations, and the seriousness of their effects, can be altered by a large number of environmental factors (Jorde *et al.*, 2006). Chemicals that cause mutations in cells can cause cancers, and so it is appropriate to describe these particular chemicals as carcinogens. In addition, there are other environmental agents that may enhance the development of genetically altered cells but do not cause new mutations. So, Jorde *et al.* (2006, p. 229) conclude that 'it is often the interaction of genes with the environment that determines carcinogenesis; both play key roles in this process'.

- Environmental agents, such as chemicals, radiation and viruses, can cause cancer by increasing the frequency with which cells mutate. Environmental agents that cause cancer are known as **carcinogens**, and most carcinogens are **mutagens** (they increase the frequency of mutations). What is apparent is that most of the agents that are known to cause cancer (carcinogenesis) also cause genetic changes (mutagenesis), whilst agents that cause genetic change also cause cancer (McCance and Roberts, 2006).

Many environmental agents are known to be carcinogenic, and include things such as:

- radiation
- alcohol
- chemicals
- some foods
- air pollution
- smoking
- viruses

At the same time, however, most human cancers appear to arise spontaneously, and develop without any known prior exposure to a carcinogenic agent, but this may be because the carcinogenic agents have not yet been identified.

Radiation

- Ultraviolet radiation: Ultraviolet (UV) sunlight (or solar radiation) causes **basal cell carcinoma** and **squamous cell carcinoma**. These are two common cancers that are found in people who have pale skins with light complexions. This type of radiation causes mutations in two tumour suppressor genes. In addition, the very **malignant** pigmented moles known as **melanomas** are linked to the amount of exposure to UV light.
- Ionising radiation: The list of carcinomas caused by ionising radiation is extremely long and extensive, and includes:

- acute leukaemias in adults and children
- thyroid cancer
- breast cancer
- lung cancer
- stomach cancer
- cancer of the colon
- oesophageal cancer
- urinary tract cancers
- multiple **myelomas**

Ionising radiation is thought to inhibit cell division. This is of particular importance where the cells only live for a short time, which leads to rapid cell division, for example:

- lymphocytes
- cells of lymphoid tissue
- bone marrow cells
- intestinal epithelial cells

The developing fetus is especially at risk, even at such low doses that may not cause any problems to adults. This is because during pregnancy, fetal organ development occurs very early and at an extremely rapid rate therefore; even small doses of radiation can completely alter the integrity of the cells and hence normal development (McCance and Roberts, 2006). This is why pregnant women – especially in the early stage of pregnancy – should not have X-rays taken (unless there is no alternative and their condition is life-threatening).

Smoking

It has been known for a long time that cigarette smoking is carcinogenic, and that it remains one of the most important causes of cancer. A hundred years ago, lung cancer was a rare disease, but as the incidence of cigarette smoking increased, so the incidence of lung cancer rose to epidemic proportions. Smoking not only leads to lung cancer, it also increases the incidence of cancer of the bladder, pancreas, kidney, larynx, oral cavity and oesophagus (McCance and Roberts, 2006). The reason for this is that there are 20 carcinogens in tobacco smoke that can cause tumours.

Diet

Many **toxic**, **mutagenic** and **carcinogenic** chemicals can be found in the human diet. Sources of toxic carcinogenic substances within our diet include various compounds that are produced during the cooking of fat, meat or protein. In addition, there are naturally occurring carcinogens that are associated with plant food substances, for example **alkaloids** and by-products of moulds/fungi.

Alcohol

Alcohol is linked with increased rates of incidence of oral cancer and cancer of the pharynx, larynx, oesophagus and liver – particularly if taken with large quantities of tobacco in the form of cigarettes, cigars and in pipes. Alcohol interacts with smoke, and this increases the risk of malignant tumours. Although the rationale for this is not proven, it is thought that it acts possibly as a **solvent** for the carcinogenic smoke products. Alcohol consumption has also been linked to breast cancer and **colorectal** cancer.

Sexual and reproductive behaviour

The possible mechanism for the carcinogenesis of cervical and other cancers of the sexual organs is a viral infection transmitted between sexual partners. According to Murphy and Mathew (2000), the age of first sexual intercourse allied to the number of sexual partners (or the number of sexual partners of a partner) are the major factors leading to the risk of the development of cervical cancer.

Certain types of the human papillomavirus (HPV) are known to be a cause of cervical cancer (Hausen, 2000). Another virus that has been identified with cancers of this area is the Herpes simplex virus (HSV) – many types of which are associated with cancers of the cervix, vulva, penis and anus (Hausen, 1991).

Environmental pollution

Because of the huge quantities of air that humans inhale every day (about 20 000 litres), even small amounts of carcinogens and other pollutants in the atmosphere can cause problems. There is particular concern with the industrial emissions of pollutants, such as arsenics, benzene, chloroform and vinyl chloride, but there are many others (Blair and Kazerowni, 1998; Katsouyanni and Pershagon, 1997). Consequently, it is known that living close to certain industries is a recognised risk factor for developing certain cancers, although, again, other factors have to be taken into account – particularly lifestyle factors (such as drinking and smoking as discussed above). According to McCance and Roberts (2006), indoor pollution is generally considered to be a greater risk than outdoor pollution, partly because of second-hand or environmental tobacco smoke.

Along with smoke, another indoor air pollutant of significance is radon gas – this is a natural radioactive gas that is present in certain soils (e.g. granite). It can get trapped in houses and produce carcinogenic radioactive decay products (Krewski et al., 1999; Neuberger and Allen, 1997; Polpong and Borornkitti, 1998).

Occupation

Exposures to carcinogenic substances as a result of one's occupation have been recognised for a long time as being a cause of cancer. In Victorian times, for example, there was a high incidence of testicular cancer amongst boy chimney sweeps.

Asbestos accounts for the largest number of occupational cancers in recent years, although that is improving as the risks of asbestos have become common knowledge. What is particularly of concern is that a combination of asbestos exposure and cigarette smoking can actually lead to a staggering 53-fold increase in the risk of lung cancer (Humphrey *et al.*, 1995). In actual fact, a large percentage of cancers of the upper respiratory tract, lung, bladder and peritoneum can be linked causally to various occupational factors (McCance and Roberts, 2006).

Hormones

The relationship between hormones and human cancer has been widely studied since 1919. Hormones, such as steroids, can be immunosuppressive. However, much of the current research on hormones and cancer focuses on the sex steroids, which include:

- oestrogen
- progesterone
- testosterone

According to McCance and Roberts (2006), most evidence to date supports the role of hormones as promoters of carcinogenesis in target tissues rather then as primary carcinogens. However, oestrogen is now being seen as a cause of cancer, but its exact mechanism is unknown.

Oral contraceptives

Some studies have found that oral contraceptives have no effect on the risk of breast cancer in most women (Paul *et al.*, 1995), whilst other studies (Hulka, 1997; Kelsy and Gammon, 1991) have identified subgroups of women using oral contraceptives who have an increased risk of breast cancer. These subgroups include:

- women who have used oral contraceptives for many years prior to the age of 25 years
- those who used them before 1971
- extended use before the first full-term pregnancy
- use of oral contraceptives at the age of 45 years, or older
- history of biopsy-confirmed benign breast disorders
- **nulliparous**, **premenopausal** women, with an early **menarche**
- women with only one child
- family history of breast cancer
        (McCance and Roberts, 2006).

By in contrast, complete/incomplete pregnancies and the use of oral contraceptives reduce the risk of ovarian cancer. This is because ovarian cancer appears to develop from the epithelial cells on the ovarian surface, and the main stimulus for division of these cells is **ovulation** itself. What happens is that after each ovulation, epithelial cells then replicate in order to ensure that the exposed surface of the ovary (following ovulation and release of the egg) is covered. So, those factors that help to prevent ovulation also help to protect against ovarian cancers (Hulka, 1997; McCance and Roberts, 2006). The risk of endometrial cancer is reduced by 55% in women who have taken oral contraceptives for 5 years, as opposed to those who have not used oral contraceptives (McCance and Roberts, 2006). In addition, it is also thought that oral contraceptive usage may reduce colorectal cancers (Franceschi and LaVecchia, 1998).

Male hormones

According to McCance and Roberts (2006), the male sex hormones (i.e. testosterone) actually stimulate the growth of target tissues for cancers, such as the prostate – hence the risk of **benign** or **malignant** prostate tumours.

Viruses

There are a group of viruses, known as **oncogenic viruses**, that can cause cancers, for example:

- papovaviruses
- adenoviruses
- herpesviruses
- hepadenoviruses

Burkitt lymphoma and nasopharyngeal carcinoma are caused by the Epstein-Barr virus (EBV), whilst HPV is found in cervical cancer (Nairn and Helbert, 2002).

Staging of cancers

Following the diagnosis of a cancer, the patient will be told the stage that the cancer has reached. The stage a cancer has reached at the time of diagnosis can give an indication of the likely prognosis for the patient. The staging system is linked to the spread of the cancer (metastasis).

There are four general cancer stages – although most types of cancer also have specific staging criteria (Colbert *et al.*, 2007):

- **Stage 1**: no spread of the cancer from the original site of the cancer.
- **Stage 2**: the cancer has spread to neighbouring tissues.
- **Stage 3**: the cancer has spread to nearby **lymph nodes**.
- **Stage 4**: the cancer has spread to tissues and organs in other parts of the body.

Cancers that have started to spread have a much poorer prognosis than do cancers that are still confined to their original site. Stage 1 cancers have a much better chance of responding to treatment, whilst Stage 4 cancers are very often **terminal**. Consequently, the earlier a patient is diagnosed, the better the chances of overcoming cancer.

Signs and symptoms of cancer

Cancers can present in many ways depending upon the type of cancer and where it is situated, e.g. brain, kidney, blood, breast, but there are some common factors to most of them. These are:

- General run-down condition (**general malaise**, **anorexia**/loss of appetite, loss of weight.
- Marked change in bowel or bladder habits.
- Nausea or vomiting for no apparent reason.
- Bloody discharge of any kind; failure to stop bleeding in the usual time.
- Presence of swelling, lump or mass anywhere in the body.

- Any change in the size or appearance of moles or birthmarks.
- Unexplained stumbling.
- Unexplained pain (or persistent crying of an infant or child).

The problem that the doctor has in diagnosing cancer is that these signs and symptoms can be related to many other medical conditions. This is why there is sometimes a delay in diagnosing cancer until the cancer has developed and may have started to metastasise.

Treatment of cancer

Whilst there are different treatments for different cancers, there are certain principles and types of treatment that are generally accepted as standard. There are six types of treatment that are used at the moment – depending upon the individual cancer and patient. These are:

1. drug therapy
2. radiation therapy
3. immunotherapy
4. surgical removal
5. hormone therapy
6. photodynamic therapy

The first, very important, point to make is that the earlier the cancer is diagnosed and treatment begins, the better will be the prognosis. If the cancer is still localised (i.e. it has not spread to other parts of the body) at the time of diagnosis, then the plan would be the removal of the primary cancer by surgery, accompanied by drug therapy and/or radiation therapy (King, 2000). Unfortunately, not all cancers are amenable to surgery, for example the blood cancers such as leukaemias and lymphomas.

If the cancer is detected late, or if surgery does not remove all of the **primary cancer** and metastasis occurs, then other forms of treatment are necessary – mainly drug therapy and radiotherapy. In this scenario, then it is often not possible to cure the cancer and the treatment is based on preventing the growth of the cancer, or at least slowing it down (King, 2000).

Drug therapy

The other name for drug therapy is chemotherapy, and there are two different types of chemotherapy that are used in the treatment of cancer, namely:

- cytotoxic chemotherapy
- cytostatic chemotherapy

The difference between the two types of chemotherapy is that cytotoxic chemotherapy has the potential to cure a patient whereas cytostatic drugs are not able to get rid of the cancer but can prevent it growing too large.

Side effects of chemotherapy

Unfortunately, because all these drugs affect normal cells as well as cancerous cells, treatment using these drugs can cause many severe side effects (Robinson, 1993). These side effects can include:

- Secondary cancers, including leukaemia – this can occur because the normal blood cells, including the white blood cells which form a major part of the immune system (see Chapter 3), are particularly sensitive to many of these drugs, and a reduction in white blood cells can lead to further tumours arising because of a lack of immune surveillance.
- Infections – a reduction in white blood cells can leave the body open to serious infections including septicaemia because the immune system has been compromised.
- Sterility – the germ cells in the ovary and testes are also very sensitive to these chemotherapeutic drugs and young people in particular can become sterile as a result of the treatment.
- Hair loss – this occurs because the cells of the hair follicles are rapidly dividing (as can be seen from the speed at which hair grows), and as some chemotherapeutic drugs target rapidly dividing cells because cancerous cells are themselves rapidly dividing cells, normal rapidly dividing cells are also destroyed.
- Nausea and vomiting – these are frequent side effects of chemotherapy because the drugs can activate the centres in the brainstem that can cause vomiting.
- Skin damage – these occur in the same way that hair loss occurs because skin cells have to rapidly replicate to replace the skin cells that are damaged with normal wear and tear (King, 2000).

Radiation therapy

Ionising radiation damages cell DNA. Once the DNA of a cell is damaged, one of three results could occur, namely:

- the death of the cancerous cell
- the cell becomes so severely damaged that any changes in its environment will cause it to die
- the cell becomes damaged but can eventually repair itself

Radiation therapy attempts to kill the cancer cell, but as with chemotherapy, normal cells can also be killed by the radiation.

Immunotherapy

According to Nairn and Helbert (2002), all attempts at using immunotherapy to cure tumours are based on the idea that the immune system already can eradicate existing tumours by means of immune surveillance, but they agree with Male *et al.* (2006) that most of these attempts have failed.

Surgical removal

Surgical therapy is used when the cancer has not yet spread. In addition, it is generally agreed that if there is any chance that local lymph nodes may be involved and at the same time there is no evidence that the disease has spread, then the lymph nodes should also be removed.

As with chemotherapy, there are two types of surgery. There is surgery to cure the disease and there is **palliative** surgery. Palliative surgery which means alleviating the symptoms without curing the cancer has two purposes (McCance and Roberts, 2006):

- to prevent symptoms that would have occurred without the surgery
- to relieve symptoms that are already present

Hormonal therapy

Hormonal therapy has been used for some years now and although the way in which this works is not really known, but it is thought that it works by blocking receptors on the cancerous cells, it prevents a cell from receiving normal growth stimulation signals (McCance and Roberts, 2006).

Examples of hormones being used in cancer therapy include:

- corticosteroids – used with leukaemias, malignant lymphomas, Hodgkin disease and breast cancer
- androgens – used with breast cancer
- oestrogens – used with breast cancer and prostate cancer

Photodynamic therapy

Light on its own does not damage the cells, whether they are malignant cells or normal cells. However, when light combines with oxygen, it can have a serious effect on photosensitive chemicals such as **porphyrins** (an example of porphyrin is **haemoglobin** which binds and transports oxygen in the body). It is now possible to produce a drug consisting of a modified porphyrin which is given systemically and then the target cancer can be eliminated by using a special light that is focused on the cancer and not the surrounding tissues. This can cause the death of the malignant cells of the cancer (King, 2000). Photodynamic therapy has now been successfully used to treat:

- cancers of the bladder
- head and neck cancers
- cancer of the oesophagus

Gene therapy

This is still experimental, but there is work ongoing that is looking at using the fact that genetics plays an important part in the causes of cancer. The eventual hope is that it would be possible to replace the affected genes with normal ones.

Prevention of cancer

Although the treatment of cancers has improved dramatically over the last 20 years or so, it is still better to try and prevent cancers occurring in the first place. As was discussed earlier, there are many environmental factors that play a part in causing the development of cancers. These include factors such as smoking, diet, alcohol, occupation, sexual behaviour and UV radiation. By reducing or even removing these environmental factors it is possible, to a large extent, to prevent many cancers occurring, although, because of the genetic factors previously mentioned, cancers will never go away.

Increasing fruit and vegetable intake has the potential to reduce the risk of getting several cancers, including bowel cancer, breast cancer, cancer of the mouth, larynx, and nasopharynx cancer, and even lung cancer (King, 2000). In addition, bowel cancer and breast cancer, amongst others, can be prevented by reducing smoking as well as the intake of alcohol. A reduction in meat and alcohol intake, along with an increase in eating more fruits and vegetables can reduce bowel cancer by as much as 70% (King, 2000). A diet which includes increased amounts of fruits and vegetables and reduced amounts of fat and alcohol can reduce breast cancer by as much as 40% if started before puberty (15% if started after puberty), whilst a diet high in fruits and vegetables can prevent an estimated 25% of lung cancers – in both smokers and non-smokers (King, 2000). So, it can be seen that diet is one environmental factor that can be used to reduce the incidence of many cancers.

For many years now, the link between smoking and lung cancer has been well known and well documented, although there are still many arguments about the role of passive smoking as a cause of lung cancer.

Taking sensible precautions in strong sunshine can prevent a lot of skin cancers, particularly the very malignant melanomas.

In addition to looking at environmental factors as a means of preventing cancer, there are also certain drugs that can help to reduce cancers. For example, the drug tamoxifen has been found to achieve the prevention of breast cancers particularly in women from families who carry a genetic defect that causes breast cancer. The major risk factor for breast cancer is excessive oestrogen production and tamoxifen is an anti-oestrogen drug, which is why it helps to prevent breast cancer (King, 2000). However, in a major trial in the United States, it was found that women who took tamoxifen had twice as many endometrial cancers than did the control group, in addition to a higher-than-expected incidence of problems such as pulmonary embolus and deep vein thrombosis. However, because the risk probability of developing breast cancer for some women in families who carry the breast cancer gene defects is as high as 80%, many of them believe that the risk of developing these other problems is outweighed by the risk of developing breast cancer if tamoxifen is not taken (King, 2000).

The fifth most common cause of cancer deaths in women is ovarian cancer and oral contraceptive pills have been found to be effective against endometrial and ovarian cancer (King, 2000). In fact, it is so effective against ovarian cancer that oral contraceptive pills have now halved the risk of developing it.

Another drug that appears to prevent a particular type of cancer, in this case colon cancer, is aspirin. Colon cancer is the third most important cause of cancer-related deaths in both men and women (King, 2000). It is not only aspirin that is effective, but also non-steroidal anti-inflammatory drugs that are taken for arthritis and similar diseases.

Finally, in this section, it is necessary to look at the potential role of **vaccines** in preventing various cancers. There have been many approaches that have been used to develop vaccines for use in the treatment of cancer. At present, **prophylactic** approaches to cancer focus on the use of vaccines that will induce immunity to viruses that are known to be associated with the development of a tumour, in the same way that any vaccination induces immunity to the causative organism, e.g. measles, mumps or rubella. An example of a vaccine in use to give immunity to a cancer is the HPV vaccine. HPV vaccines prevent the development of cervical carcinoma because HPV is a known cause of cervical cancer (Leggatt and Frazer, 2007).

Another possible vaccine against a virus that causes cancer would be a vaccine against hepatitis B, and such a vaccine would reduce the incidence of liver cancer.

As we are able to identify other cancers that are caused by viruses, this prophylactic measure of vaccination against those particular viruses could help to prevent these cancers and save so many lives.

In contrast to the use of vaccines against viruses that cause cancer, most other tumour vaccine approaches are designed to enhance or to initiate effective tumour immunity in patients who already have cancer.

Examples of cancers

Acute lymphoblastic leukaemia

Acute lymphoblastic leukaemia (ALL) is a primary disorder of the bone marrow in which the normal marrow cells are replaced by immature or **undifferentiated blast** cells (King, 2000). When the quantity of normal marrow is depleted to below the level necessary to maintain peripheral blood cells within normal ranges then the following occur:

- anaemia
- neutropaenia
- thrombocytopaenia

The exact cause of ALL is unknown, but the following are suspected of being involved in the development of this disease:

- environmental causes
- infectious agents (especially viruses)
- genetic factors
- chromosomal abnormalities

Acute leukaemia is the most common malignancy in children, with over 400 new cases in children under the of 15 years being diagnosed each year in UK, with the incidence of ALL being more common amongst Caucasian children. ALL is classified according to the cell type involved.

ALL results from the growth of an abnormal type of leucocyte in the bone marrow, the **spleen** and the **lymph nodes**. These abnormal cells have little **cytoplasm** and a round nucleus – it resembles a **lymphoblast**. With ALL, the normal bone marrow cells may be displaced or replaced. The changes that occur in blood and bone marrow result from an accumulation of leukaemic cells and a deficiency of normal cells:

- Red cell **precursors** and **megakaryocytes** from which platelets are formed are decreased, leading to anaemia, bleeding and bruising.
- Normal white cells are decreased, which makes the patient liable to pick up infections.
- The leukaemic cells may infiltrate into the lymph nodes, spleen and liver, so causing a diffuse **adenopathy** and **hepatosplenomegaly**.
- The increase in the size and amount of marrow and/or this infiltration of leukaemic cells causes bone and joint pain.
- Invasion of the central nervous system (CNS) by leukaemic cells can lead to headaches, vomiting, cranial nerve palsies, convulsions and coma.
- Weight loss, muscle-wasting and fatigue occur when the body cells are deprived of nutrients because of the immense metabolic needs of the proliferating leukaemia cells.

Therefore the signs and symptoms of ALL are:

- an increase in lethargy and general malaise
- persistent fever of unknown cause
- recurrent infection
- prolonged bleeding (e.g. after dentistry)

- bruising easily
- pallor
- enlarged lymph nodes
- pain, particularly abdominal, bone and joint
- CNS involvement leading to headache and vomiting

(Manson and McCance, 2006).

Treatment and prognosis of ALL

The treatment for ALL includes:

- supportive therapy, including:
  - ☐ control of infections, anaemia, bleeding, etc.
- specific therapy, including:
  - ☐ cytotoxic chemotherapy – e.g. dexamethasone, vincristine, imatinib, asparaginase, methotrexate (Pui and Evans, 2006)
  - ☐ radiation therapy
  - ☐ bone marrow transplantation (BMT) to replace the damaged marrow with non-cancerous marrow

The prognosis of ALL is good these days:

- almost 80% of children and 40% of adults survive more than 5 years (Pui *et al.*, 2004)

However, later relapses can still occur after long remissions.

Lung cancer

- Lung cancer affects the lung tissue.
- It is the most common cause of death from cancer in men and the second most common cause of death from cancer in women (WHO, 2004), and in 2006, it was calculated that it is responsible for 1.3 million deaths each year throughout the world (WHO, 2006).

The causes of lung cancer:

- The greatest cause of lung cancer is long-term exposure to inhaled carcinogens, particularly tobacco smoke (Samet *et al.*, 1988).
- People who do not smoke tobacco may still get lung cancer, due to a combination of genetic factors (Gorlova *et al.*, 2007) and exposure to passive smoking (Hackshaw *et al.*, 1997; Sasco *et al.*, 2004).
- Radon gas (Catelinois *et al.*, 2006) may also play a part in the development of lung cancer, as may air pollution (Kabir *et al.*, 2007; King, 2000).

Signs and symptoms of lung cancer are:

- dyspnoea (difficulty in breathing)
- haemoptysis (coughing up blood)
- chronic cough and wheezing
- chest or abdominal pain
- cachexia, fatigue and loss of appetite

- dysphonia (hoarse voice)
- difficulty in swallowing

(Harrison *et al.*, 2005).

Unfortunately, for many patients, by the time that they have sought medical attention because the symptoms have become so apparent, the cancer has already metastasised.

Treatment of lung cancer depends upon the particular type of lung cancer and how far it has metastasised, but common treatments include:

- surgery (El-Sherif *et al.*, 2006)
- chemotherapy – e.g. cisplatin and vinorelbine (Tsuboi *et al.*, 2007)
- radiation therapy (Wagner, 1998)

The 5-year survival rate for all types of lung cancer is very low (14%) (Minna, 2005), although again the earlier it is diagnosed and treated the better the long-term prognosis. Consequently, this makes the prevention of this particular cancer a real priority (Vineis *et al.*, 2007).

Breast cancer

Throughout the world, breast cancer is the fifth most common cause of death from cancer (after lung cancer, stomach cancer, liver cancer and colon cancer), whilst among women throughout the world, breast cancer is the most common cancer (WHO, 2006). The incidence of breast cancer has increased significantly since the 1970s, and this is partly explained by the modern lifestyles in the Western world. Breast cancer is not purely a cancer of women, because males can also have breast cancer, although this is less common than it is in females (National Cancer Institute, 2006). The reason for this phenomenon is that the breast is composed of exactly the same tissues in both males and females. The lifetime risk for getting breast cancer is 1 in 11 for women and 1 in 1000 for men (King, 2000). The 5-year survival rates for breast cancer are 80% without metastasis, but only 40% once the cancer has metastasised (King, 2000).

There are different sorts of breast cancer (although these can overlap), including (Figure 2.3):

- ductal carcinoma (where the milk ducts become cancerous)
- lobular carcinoma (cancer of the lobules attached to the ducts)
- inflammatory breast carcinoma (diffuse cancer of the breast)

The causes of breast cancer have already been mentioned earlier in this chapter, particularly with regard to hereditary breast cancer. In addition to those, however, the younger a woman is when her first child is born, the lower the risk of her developing breast cancer (American Cancer Society, 1995).

Signs and symptoms of breast cancer can include (Robinson and Huether, 2006):

- painless/painful lump in the breast
- a lump under the arm or above the collar bone
- nipple discharge/bleeding from the nipple
- **oedema** of the arms
- nipple retraction

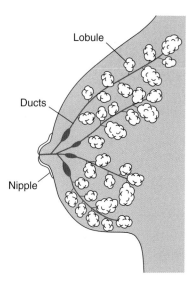

Figure 2.3 Diagram of breast showing lobules and ducts.

■ pitting of the skin of the breast (known as 'peau d'orange' because it resembles the skin of an orange).

The ideal treatment for breast cancer is surgery – the main treatment when the tumour is localised and has not metastasised, followed by:

■ chemotherapy – before, after, or instead of surgery where patients are unsuitable for surgery
■ hormonal therapy (e.g. tamoxifen) – once chemotherapy has been completed
■ immunotherapy – e.g. Herceptin (a monoclonal antibody that slows the growth of breast cancer cells)
■ radiation therapy – to eliminate any microscopic cancer cells that may remain near the site of the primary tumour following surgery

Surgery can range from a simple lumpectomy (just involving the cancerous lump itself) to a radical mastectomy – removal of the whole breast tissue and neighbouring lymph nodes (Marieb, 2004).

Conclusion

Cancer is always an emotional subject because of the historically very high mortality rate associated with it. Over the past few years, great strides have been made in the prevention and treatment of many cancers, but it still remains a tremendous challenge to researchers and clinical staff. Greater knowledge of the biochemical, economic, social and psychological aspects of these diseases has lead to a greater understanding of them and, in some parts of the world, an ability to defeat, or at least ameliorate many of them. However, it is certainly true that the incidences of many of them are increasing (even though they can be better treated). This is related to the fact that many of them are diseases linked with old age because they take so long to develop, and because people in many countries, because of better environmental and health reasons, are living much longer. In the past, they would have died from other causes before the cancers caused problems. So, there have been, and are, many triumphs in the treatment and prevention of cancers, but there is no room for complacency.

Multiple choice questions

1. Cancer is a disease of:
(a) cell growth, cell differentiation, cell division
(b) cell differentiation, cell death, cell dispersal
(c) cell metabolism, cell dispersal, cell activity
(d) cell death, cell differentiation, cell division

2. Apoptosis is:
(a) cell differentiation
(b) cell metabolism
(c) cell suicide
(d) cell evasion of the immune system

3. The biochemical processes leading up to the development of a cancer are known as:
(a) carcinomas
(b) carcinogens
(c) carcinogenesis
(d) cancer mutations

4. What does the cell need to develop new blood vessels?
(a) tumour necrosis factor
(b) dedifferentiation
(c) autonomous growth
(d) angiogenic growth factors

5. According to the molecular biology model of cancer development, the two stages that a cell has to pass through from being a normal cell to metastasis are:
(a) hyperplasia, reproduction
(b) precancer, cancer
(c) precancer, cancer mutation
(d) hyperplasia, cancer

6. Which of the following may cause cancer?
(a) genes, carcinogens, mutagens, lymphocytes
(b) genes, viruses, tobacco smoke, antigens
(c) genes, UV radiation, hormones, tobacco smoke
(d) genes, antigens, tobacco smoke, lymphocytes

7. The cancer-causing genes are known as:
(a) translocation genes
(b) germline genes
(c) oncogenes
(d) tumour suppressor genes

8. Several subgroups of women who use oral contraceptives have been identified as having an increased risk of breast cancer. Which of the ones below are included in those subgroups?
(a) women who used oral contraceptives before 1971
(b) nulliparous, premenopausal women who had an early menarche
(c) women with a family history of lung cancer
(d) women with more than one child

9. Chemotherapy stands for:
(a) immunotherapy
(b) radiation therapy
(c) photodynamic therapy
(d) drug therapy

10. Which of the following are side effects of chemotherapy?
(a) sterility
(b) hair loss
(c) nausea and vomiting
(d) secondary cancers

11. Which of the following are suspected of being a cause of acute lymphoblastic leukaemia?
(a) viruses
(b) smoking
(c) alcohol
(d) chromosomal abnormalities

12. Which cancers are the five most common causes of death from cancer throughout the world?
(a) lung cancer, stomach cancer, breast cancer, prostate cancer, liver cancer
(b) breast cancer, prostate cancer, lung cancer, pancreatic cancer, colon cancer
(c) prostate cancer, lung cancer, breast cancer, stomach cancer, colon cancer
(d) lung cancer, stomach cancer, liver cancer, colon cancer, breast cancer

Answers: 1.a, 2.c, 3.c, 4.d, 5.b, 6.c, 7.c, 8.a,b, 9.d, 10.a,b,c,d, 11.a,d, 12.d.

Test your knowledge

- ❓ How would the body normally prevent abnormal cells from growing and developing into cancer cells?
- ❓ What are the key steps in carcinogenesis (from a molecular biology standpoint as well as clinically)?
- ❓ Describe the contrasting roles of oncogenes and tumour suppressor genes in the development of cancers.
- ❓ Briefly discuss how ionising radiation can cause cancers, particularly with regard to the fetus.
- ❓ Explain how cancer drug therapy is related to the cell cycle.
- ❓ Discuss the many ways of prevention of cancer.

Glossary of terms

Adenopathy: Enlargement of lymph nodes.

Alkaloid: A substance that is basic (i.e. not acidic).

Allele: A gene on one of a paired chromosome that codes for the same physical or other feature as its corresponding one on the other chromosome.

Anaemia: Blood is lacking in iron – often used to mean a deficiency in red blood cells.

Angiogenesis: The growth of new blood vessels.

Angiogenic growth factors: Substances within the body that are involved in the development of new blood vessels.

Anorexia: Loss of appetite/loss of weight.

Antibiotic: A drug used to kill bacteria.

Antibody: An antibody is a protein that binds specifically to a particular substance (its antigen) – it is a major part of the immune system.

Antigens: Substances that can be recognised by the immune system and generate an antibody response.

Apoptosis: Apoptosis, or programmed cell death, is a form of cell death in which the cell activates an internal death programme – it is a form of cell suicide.

Basal cell carcinoma: A cancer involving the surface epithelium of the skin.

Benign: Causes no problem. In cancer, it means a growth that is not malignant.

Blast cell: Immature cell.

Cachexia: This is a syndrome that includes anorexia, weight loss, anaemia, marked weakness, altered protein, lipid and carbohydrate metabolism. This most severe form of malnutrition is often associated with the later stages of cancer.

Cancer: Unregulated growth of cells and tissue that are invasive and able to metastasise. Cancer is 'a set of diseases characterised by unregulated cell growth leading to invasion of surrounding tissues and spread (metastasis) to other parts of the body' (King, 2000, p. 1).

Carcinogen: Something capable of causing cancer.

Carcinogenesis: The biochemical processes involved in producing cancers, including their initiation and generation.

Cell differentiation: The process by which cells take on different roles.

Cell division: The reproduction of cells to cause the production of two identical daughter cells. Also known as binary fission.

Colorectal cancer: A cancer that involves the colon and the rectum.

Cytoplasm: Collective name for all the contents of the cell, including the plasma membrane, but not including the nucleus.

Cytotoxicity: Lethal to cells.

Daughter cell: The resultant cells following cell division.

Dysphonia: Hoarse voice.

Dyspnoea: Difficulty in breathing.

General malaise: Generally lethargic, with loss of appetite and loss of weight. Just generally unwell.

Germline cell: A sperm or egg that possess genes that can be passed on to offspring.

Gray: This is the unit that defines the amount of energy released from radiation. It is usually abbreviated to Gy, and it replaces the older unit of radiation energy, the 'rad' which was equivalent to 0.01 Gy.

Haemoglobin: Occurs, linked to red blood cells and binds oxygen to the cell so that it can carry it around the body to where it is required.

Haemoptysis: Coughing up of blood.

Hepatosplenomegaly: Enlarged liver and spleen.

Lymph node: Part of the lymphatic system, they contain lots of white cells to destroy bacteria that are trapped within the lymph node.

Lymphoblast: An immature lymphocyte (a white blood cell).

Malignant: The collective name for all the physical and chemical processes occurring within a cell/living organism, but often referring only to reactions involving enzymes.

Megakaryocyte: A large bone marrow cell that will give rise to platelets.

Melanoma: Cancerous outgrowth of melanocytes (pigmented cells of the skin).

Menarche: The time when the first menstruation occurs.

Metastasise: The spread of cancerous cells to other parts of the body – often distant to the site of the original cancer.

Mutagen: Something that can affect genes and cause changes (mutations).

Mutagenic: Something capable of causing mutations.

Mutation: A change in one or several bases in DNA.

Neoplasm: A new growth of tissue. It may or may not be malignant.

Nucleotide sequence: Sequences of the bases of DNA that make up genes.

Nulliparous: Never been pregnant.

Oncogene: A gene that contains proteins that contribute to carcinogenesis.

Oncogenic viruses: Viruses that cause cancers.

Ovulation: The release of eggs from the ovary.

Palliative: Easing the situation – making it better, but not a cure.

Porphyrins: An important group of several protein pigments involved in various processes – bound to the iron in haemoglobin.

Precancerous cell: A cell that is at the stage before it becomes cancerous.

Precursor: Something that will eventually turn into something else. For example, a red cell precursor will eventually become a red cell.

Premenopausal: The period before the end of menstruation (i.e. the menopausal period).

Primary cancer: The tumour that first appears – the site of this first cancer.

Prognosis: The likely outcome of a disease or treatment.

Prophylactic: Preventative.

Proto-oncogene: A gene that, due to mutation, can become an oncogene.

Radiation therapy: The use of ultraviolet or ionising radiation to treat cancer.

Solute: Substances that can be dissolved in liquid (solvent).

Solvent: The liquid in which solutes are dissolved.

Somatic cell: A cell that possesses genes that are not passed on to offspring; in other words, cells of the body other than sperm and ova.

Spleen: An organ in the abdomen that removes and destroys old, damaged, or fragile red blood cells. Also, it has an important role to play in immunity.

Squamous cell carcinoma: A cancer involving squamous cells, usually of epithelial tissue.

T-cytotoxic lymphocyte: A specialised white blood cell that is capable of destroying other cells of the body that are damaged or have become infected.

Terminal cancer: Cancer that cannot be cured and leads to death.

Thrombocytopaenia: A deficiency in thrombocytes (platelets).

Toxic: A substance that is poisonous or damaging to something else.

Tumour: Lumps in and on the body caused by the abnormal growth of cells. They can be either malignant or benign.

Tumour suppressor gene: A gene whose function is to suppress the growth and development of tumours.

Vaccine: Substances that can be given to a host in order to provoke an immune response and therefore confer immunity on the host without making the host severely ill, e.g. polio vaccine.

Vector: A means of carrying a substance so that it can be transferred to somewhere else. Viruses are often used as vectors to transfer genes to where they are required in gene therapy.

References

American Cancer Society (1995). Facts on breast cancer. In: *Cancer Response System Document* # 407002–407038. New York: American Cancer Society.

Blair, A. and Kazerowni, N. (1998). Reactive chemicals and cancer. *Cancer Causes and Control*, 8, 437.

Catelinois, O., Rogel, A., Laurier, D. *et al.* (2006). Lung cancer attributable to indoor radon exposure in France: Impact of the risk models and uncertainty analysis. *Environmental Health Perspectives*, *114*(9), 1361–1366.

Colbert, B.J., Ankney, J. and Lee, K.T. (2007). *Anatomy and Physiology for Health Professions: An Interactive Journey*. New Jersey: Pearson/Prentice Hall.

El-Sherif, A., Gooding, W.E., Santos, R. *et al.* (2006). Outcomes of sublobar resection versus lobectomy for stage I non-small cell lung cancer: A 13 year analysis. *Annals of Thoracic Surgery*, *82*(2), 408–415.

Franceschi, S. and LaVecchia, C. (1998). Oral contraception and colorectal tumors. A review of epidemiological studies. *Contraception*, *58*(6), 335.

Gorczynski, R.M. and Stanley, J. (2006). *Problem-Based Immunology*. Philadelphia: Saunders Elsevier.

Gorlova, O.Y., Weng, S.F., Zhang, Y. *et al.* (2007). Aggregation of cancer among relatives of never-smoking lung cancer patients. *International Journal of Cancer*, *121*(1), 2865–2872.

Hackshaw, A.K., Law, M.R. and Wald, N.J. (1997). The accumulated evidence on lung cancer and environmental tobacco smoke. *BMJ*, *18*(315), 980–988.

Harrison, T.R., Kasper, D., Braunwald, E. *et al.* (2005). *Harrison's Principles of Internal Medicine*, 16th edn. New York: McGraw-Hill.

Hausen, H.Z. (1991). Viruses in human cancer. *Science*, *254*, 1167.

Hausen, H.Z. (2000). Papillomavirus causing cancer: Evasion from host-cell control in early events in carcinogenesis. *Journal of the National Cancer Institute*, *92*(9), 690.

Hulka, B.S. (1997). Epidemiologic analysis of breast and gynaecologic cancers. *Progressive Clinical Biological Research*, *396*, 17.

Humphrey, E.W., Ward, H.B. and Perri, T. (1995). Lung cancer. In: Murphy, G.P., Lawrence, W. and Lenhard, R.E. (eds) *Clinical Oncology*, 2nd edn. New York: American Cancer Society.

Janeway, C.A., Travers, P., Walport, M. and Shlomchik, M.J. (2005). *Immunobiology: The Immune System in Health and Disease*, 6th edn. New York: Garland Science.

Jorde, L.B., Carey, J.C., Bamshad, M.J. and White, R.L. (2006). *Medical Genetics*, 3rd edn. St. Louis: Mosby Elsevier.

Kabir, Z., Bennett, K. and Clancy, L. (2007). Lung cancer and urban air-pollution in Dublin: A temporal association. *Irish Medical Journal*, *100*(2), 367–369.

Katsouyanni, K. and Pershagon, G. (1997). Ambient air pollution exposure and cancer. *Cancer Causes and Control*, *8*(3), 284.

Kelsy, J. and Gammon, M.D. (1991). The epidemiology of breast cancer. *CA Cancer Journal Clinics*, *41*, 146.

King, R.J.B. (2000). *Cancer Biology*, 2nd edn. Harlow: Pearson/Prentice Hall.

Krewski, D., Rai, S.N., Zielinski, J.M. and Hopke, P.K. (1999). Characterization of uncertainty and variability in residential radon cancer risks. *Annals of the New York Academy of Science*, *895*, 245.

Lydyard, P.M., Whelan, A. and Fanger, M.S. (2004). *Instant Notes in Immunology*, 2nd edn. Oxford: Garland Science/Bios Scientific Publishers.

Leggatt, G.R. and Frazer, I.H. (2007). HPV vaccines: The beginning of the end for cervical cancer. *Current Opinion in Immunology*, *19*, 232–238.

Male, D., Brostoff, J., Roth, D.B. and Roitt, I. (2006). *Immunology*, 7th edn. St. Louis: Mosby Elsevier.

Manson, T.J. and McCance, K.L. (2006). Alterations of leukocyte, lymphoid and hemostatic function. In: McCance, K.L. and Huether, S.E. (eds) *Pathophysiology: The Biologic Basis for Disease in Adults and Children*. St. Louis: Mosby.

Marieb, E.N. (2004). *Human Anatomy and Physiology*, 6th edn. San Francisco: Pearson/Benjamin Cummings.

Marieb, E.N. (2006). *Essentials of Human Anatomy and Physiology*, 8th edn. San Francisco: Pearson/Benjamin Cummings.

McCance, K.L. and Roberts, L.K. (2006). Biology of cancer. In: McCance, K.L. and Huether, S.E. (eds) *Pathophysiology: The Biologic Basis for Disease in Adults and Children*. St. Louis: Mosby.

McLannahan, H. (2001). On living longer. In: Davey, B., Halliday, T. and Hirst, M. (eds) *Human Biology and Health: An Evolutionary Approach*, 3rd edn. Buckingham: Open University Press.

Minna, J.D. (2005). Neoplasms of the lung. In: Kasper, D.L., Braunward, E., Fauci, A.S. *et al.* (eds) *Harrison's Principles of Internal Medicine*, Vol. 1, 16th edn. New York: McGraw Hill, p. 506.

Murphy, N.S. and Mathew, A. (2000). Risk factors for pre-cancerous lesions of the cervix. *European Journal of Cancer Prevention*, *9*(1), 5.

Nairn, R. and Helbert, M. (2002). *Immunology for Medical Students*. St. Louis: Mosby.

National Cancer Institute (2006). *Male Breast Cancer Treatment*. National Cancer Institute. Available at http://www.cancer.gov/cancertopics/pdq/treatment/malebreast. Accessed 6 September 2008.

Neuberger, T. and Allen, A. (1997). Lung cancer risk from residential radon: Meta-analysis of eight epidemiologic studies. *Journal of the National Cancer Institute*, *89*, 663.

Paul, C., Skegg, D.C.G. and Spears, G.F.S. (1995). Oral contraceptive use and risk of breast cancer in older women. *Cancer Causes and Control*, *6*, 485.

Polpong, E. and Borornkitti, S. (1998). Indoor radon. *Journal of the Medical Association of Thailand*, *81*, 47.

Pui, C.-H. and Evans, E.E. (2006). Treatment of acute lymphoblastic leukemia. *New England Journal of Medicine*, *354*(2), 166–178.

Pui, C.-H., Relling, M.V. and Downing, J.R. (2004). Acute lymphoblastic leukemia. *New England Journal of Medicine*, *350*(15), 1535–1548.

Robinson, S. (1993). Principles of chemotherapy. *European Journal of Cancer*, *2*, 55–65.

Robinson, K.M. and Huether, S.E. (2006). Structure and function of the reproductive system. In: McCance, K.L. and Huether, S.E. (eds) *Pathophysiology: The Biologic Basis for Disease in Adults and Children*. St. Louis: Mosby.

Samet, J.M., Wiggins, C.L., Humble, C.G. and Pathak, D.R. (1988). Cigarette smoking and lung cancer in New Mexico. *American Review of Respiratory Disease*, *137*(5), 1110–1113.

Sasco, A.J., Secretan, M.B. and Straif, K. (2004). Tobacco smoking and cancer: A brief review of recent epidemiological evidence. *Lung Cancer*, *45*(Suppl 2), S3–S9.

Tsuboi, M., Ohira, T., Saji, H. *et al.* (2007). The present state of postoperative adjuvant chemotherapy for completely resected non-small cell lung cancer. *Annals of Thoracic Cardiovascular Surgery*, *13*(2), 73–77.

Vickers, P.S. (2005). Acquired defences. In: Montague, S.E., Watson, R. and Herbert, R.A. (eds) *Physiology for Nursing Practice*, 3rd edn. Edinburgh: Elsevier.

Vineis, P., Hoek, G., Kryzyzanowski, M. *et al.* (2007). Lung cancers attributable to environmental tobacco smoke and air pollution in non-smokers in different European countries: A prospective study. *Environmental Health*, *6*, 7. http://wwwehjournal.net.

Wagner, H. (1998). Radiation therapy in the management of limited small cell lung cancer: When, where, and how much? *Chest*, *113*(Suppl 1), 92S–100S.

WHO (2004). *Deaths by Cause, Sex and Mortality Stratum*. Geneva: World Health Organization.

WHO (2006). *Fact Sheet No. 297: Cancer*. Geneva: World Health Organization.

Winter, P.C., Hickey, G.I. and Fletcher, H.L. (2002). *Instant Notes: Genetics*, 2nd edn. Abingdon: Garland Science/BIOS Scientific Publishers.

Chapter 3

Inflammation, immune response and healing

Peter S. Vickers

Test your prior knowledge

- ❖ How does a virus cause disease?
- ❖ Describe the roles of tears within the immune system.
- ❖ What are the physical signs of inflammation?

> ## Learning outcomes
>
> On completion of this section, the reader will be able to:
>
> ■ List and describe the various types of infectious microorganisms that affect humans.
> ■ Discuss how infectious diseases are transmitted to humans.
> ■ Outline the components of the immune system and their functions.
> ■ Explain the process of inflammation and its role in tissue repair.

Introduction

From the moment that someone is born, and for the rest of their life, they are constantly in danger. Some of the dangers come from inside the body and are known as genetic defects, whilst others come from external sources. Two of the dangers that beset everyone throughout life are infectious diseases and injuries. Fortunately, the human body has inbuilt mechanisms to protect it from these dangers, namely the immune system and wound healing.

Infectious diseases occur as a result of invasion of the body by **microorganisms** which cause damage to the tissues of the body. Every infectious disease is characterised by an interaction between the responses of both the infected human host and the infecting organism. Microorganisms are everywhere – they colonise humans, animals, food, water and soil, and infectious diseases are acquired by humans following contact with an **exogenous pathogen** present within a **reservoir of infection**.

The immune system, which is actually an intricate system of cells, **enzymes** and proteins, is the system that has evolved within humans (and other animals) to protect against these infectious **pathogenic micro-organisms**. In particular, the white blood cells are essential to the functioning of the immune system and this chapter will explain about these, and the other elements of the body that constitute the immune system.

This chapter commences by looking at the microorganisms that can cause disease and then looks at how the immune system fights these microorganisms and how it helps to heal injuries.

Infectious microorganisms

Microorganisms are microscopic cells that either live in the environment, on the skin, or inside bodies. They can cause infectious diseases, and this they do as long as two conditions are met:

■ they are allowed to grow and reproduce in the right conditions for that microorganism
■ they are in the right location for their growth and reproduction

These conditions are important because different microorganisms have differing and sometimes exacting needs for their growth and reproduction. If environmental conditions are not right they will not flourish. However, once the conditions are right for them, microorganisms multiply at an astonishing rate within the host tissues, causing destruction or degeneration so that the host becomes unwell and cannot function properly.

It is not actually the presence of microorganisms that is the problem, rather it is the fact that during their growth and reproduction (as well as part of the protection against the immune system) they produce waste products known as toxins, and it is these that cause the problems. However, not all of microorganisms pose problems for humans. In actual fact, humans need bacteria to help to break down food and digest it. These bacteria are known as **commensal** bacteria.

Unfortunately, even **commensal** microorganisms can become pathogenic if they find themselves in the wrong place. For example, microorganisms that live in the colon and are beneficial may invade the urinary bladder where they become pathogenic microorganisms because they are in the wrong place. A good example of one of these is *Escherischia coli* which normally lives in the gut. If, however, it migrates to the bladder then it causes **cystitis**. When infections are caused in this way, they are known as **endogenous infections** ('endogenous' means 'from within' – in this case the body). All other infections are known as **exogenous infections** – they come from outside of the body.

Spread of infection

The causative organisms of infectious disease in humans can be transmitted from the **reservoir of infection** by one of ten ways:

- droplet spread
- air currents (airborne transmission)
- aerosol
- water
- direct contact
- soil
- inoculation
- faecal–oral route
- vector
- **contaminated intermediates**

Droplet spread

Microbial organisms are spread in mucous droplet nuclei that travel only short distances – less than 1 m from the reservoir to the host. This spread can come from coughing and sneezing (as discussed below), but also by talking or laughing. In one sneeze, 20 000 droplets may be produced and expelled from the person who is the reservoir. Droplet transmission should not be confused with airborne transmission – although there are many similarities. Disease-causing organisms that do not spread more than 1 m from the host reservoir are not regarded as airborne, because they are not carried on currents of air, but just rely upon the force of the expulsion to travel the short distance to a new host. Examples of disease spread by droplet transmission include:

- influenza
- pneumonia
- pertussis (whooping cough)

Air currents (airborne transmission)

Airborne transmission refers to the spread of agents of infection by droplet nuclei in dust. These droplets may spread more than 1 m from the reservoir to the host.

A good example of airborne transmission occurs, as it does for droplet transmission, during the act of coughing and sneezing. Coughing and sneezing expels fine spray into the air which contain mucous and infectious organisms. Consequently, anyone coming into contact is likely to breathe in the mucus/bacteria/virus droplets, and so become infected in turn. Infectious microorganisms that can be spread in this way include:

- measles
- tuberculosis (TB)
- staphylococcal and streptococcal infections
- certain fungal diseases – spread by the spores – such as **histoplasmosis**

Aerosol transmission

Both domestic and industrial water supplies are sources of aerosol transmission. It has a similar action to that which occurs with droplet transmission, except the reservoir is water rather than another human. For example, when someone with asthma requires **salbutamol** via an aerosol, it that works quickly because the drug carried in the tiny droplets of water is able to work on the lining of the respiratory tract very quickly. The same principle happens with aerosol transmission of infectious organisms.

Examples of diseases that are spread by this method include:

- **Legionnaire's disease**
- Tuberculosis (TB)

Water transmission

In waterborne transmission, **pathogens** are usually spread by water that has been contaminated with untreated, or poorly treated, sewage. The pathogenic organisms enter the host either by contact with the mucosa, or by contact with broken skin. Examples of infections spread through water include:

- **Leptospirosis** – often picked up from rat urine whilst swimming in a river.
- **Schistosomiasis** (commonly known as bilharzia) – caused by a **fluke** (similar to a worm) which is a parasite found in fresh water snails that inhabit the edges of major waterways, such as the River Nile (Davey *et al.*, 2001; Re, 2004).

Direct contact

Contact transmission is the spread of an infectious organism by direct, or indirect, contact. Direct contact transmission is also known as 'person-to-person transmission'. This is the direct transmission of an infectious organism by physical contact between its present host and a susceptible recipient host. The most common forms of direct contact transmission are:

- touching
- kissing
- sexual intercourse

There are many diseases that can be transmitted by direct contact and these include:

■ viral respiratory tract diseases (e.g. the common cold, influenza)
■ staphylococcal infections (e.g. septicaemia)
■ hepatitis A
■ measles
■ scarlet fever
■ sexually transmitted diseases (e.g. syphilis, gonorrhoea, genital herpes)
■ infectious mononucleosis (glandular fever)
■ HIV (human immunodeficiency virus) which causes AIDS (acquired immunodeficiency syndrome)

Potential pathogens can also be transmitted by direct contact from animals (or animal products) to humans, e.g. rabies and anthrax.

Indirect contact transmission occurs when the infectious microorganism is transmitted from its present reservoir to a potential susceptible host by means of a non-living object.

Soil

Soil has already been mentioned in the introduction as a potential reservoir for infectious microorganisms. The route of entry from the soil into the body is usually by a skin lesion. Infection can occur:

■ when playing sport on a contaminated playing field
■ whilst gardening on soil that has been contaminated by the use of animal manure
■ whilst farming on land that has been fertilised with animal manure
■ any fall on contaminated ground in which the skin becomes broken

Examples of infectious diseases that can occur from soil include:

■ tetanus
■ gas gangrene

Inoculation

Inoculation can also be accidental, for example by being bitten or scratched. Examples of infections caused this way include:

■ cat scratch disease
■ rabies

Inoculation can occur following an injection as can occur with health care professionals not taking proper precautions, or by someone injecting themselves with drugs. Examples of infections caused this way include:

1. HIV
2. Hepatitis B

Faecal–oral route

This transmission route of infectious microorganisms can occur in several ways, including:

■ hand-to-mouth – this is seen particularly in young children who may be exploring the anal area, and then put their hands in their mouths
■ sewage-contaminated food or water – this can occur, particularly if fresh vegetables, salads and fruit are not properly washed before being eaten. It is a problem in certain countries, where human sewage is used to fertilise fields in which salads are grown
■ certain sexual practices, in which there is oral-anal stimulation ('rimming')

Examples of infectious diseases transmitted via this route, include:

■ gastro-enteritis
■ enteric fevers

Vector transmission

This is commonly held to be inoculation by the bite of a sucking arthropod (such as a 'tick') which is also a host, but there are other types of vector transmission. Vectors are animals that carry pathogens from one host to another. Arthropods are the most important group of disease vectors. Examples include malaria and lyme disease.

Contaminated intermediates

This is caused by indirect contact transmission, and it occurs when the infectious microorganism is transmitted from its initial reservoir to a potential susceptible host by means of a non-living object. These non-living objects, or inanimate intermediates, are called **fomites**. Examples of fomites include:

■ clothes, bedding and towels
■ tissues and handkerchiefs
■ drinking cups and eating utensils
■ toys

Other fomites can transmit infections such as:

■ chicken pox
■ staphylococci and streptococci infections
■ tetanus

(Tortora *et al.*, 2004).

Types of infectious microorganisms

There are many different types of microorganism that can infect humans (Box 3.1), and each of them require different environmental conditions in which to survive and to grow and reproduce, as well as different modes of transfer to humans. Some of them are more well known to humans than are some of the others, and perhaps the three most well-known microorganisms are:

■ bacteria
■ viruses
■ fungi

Box 3.1 Other types of infectious microorganisms

Protozoa
Rickettsiae
Chlamydiae
Helminths

Bacteria

Bacteria come in a great many sizes and shapes, and their diameter ranges from 0.2 to 2.0 micrometer (μm), whilst their length ranges from 2 to 8 μm.

There are three basic shapes of bacteria (Figure 3.1), namely:

- spherical (known as a coccus), e.g. streptococcus, staphylococcus
- rod-shaped (known as a bacillus), e.g. diplobacillus, streptobacillus
- spiral (known as a spiral), e.g. vibrio, spirochetes

Cocci

Cocci are usually round, but they can also be oval, elongated, or even flattened on one side. When cocci divide to reproduce, the cells can remain attached to one another. Cocci that remain in pairs after dividing are called diplococci. Cocci that divide and remain attached in chain-type patterns are called streptococci. Cocci that divide and form grape-like clusters are known as staphylococci (see Figure 3.1).

Bacilli

Most bacilli appear as single rods. However, some that appear in pairs after they have divided are called diplobacilli. Those that occur in chains are known as streptobacilli, whilst those bacilli that have a more oval shape are called coccobacilli (see Figure 3.1).

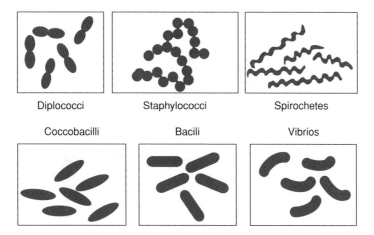

| Diplococci | Staphylococci | Spirochetes |
| Coccobacilli | Bacili | Vibrios |

Figure 3.1 Shapes of bacteria.

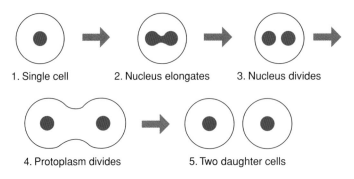

1. Single cell   2. Nucleus elongates   3. Nucleus divides

4. Protoplasm divides   5. Two daughter cells

Figure 3.2 Bacterial reproduction – simple fission.

Spiral

Spiral bacteria have one or more twists – they are never straight. Bacteria that look like curved rods are called vibrios. Spirella have a helical shape. Spirals that are helical and flexible are known as spirochetes (see Figure 3.1).

Bacterial reproduction

Bacteria reproduce quite simply by means of simple fission, also known as binary fission (Figure 3.2). Initially in reproduction DNA divides into two and then a transverse wall or septum divides the cytoplasm of the cell which eventually divides into two, so that there are two daughter cells from each cell, which are clones of the parent cell (see Chapter 1).

Viruses

Viruses are **obligate intracellular parasites**, and they vary from 20 to 200 nanometer (nm) in size, for example the polio virus is 30 nm in size, whilst vaccinia virus (the cause of chicken pox) is 400 nm in size – as big as a small bacterium.

Viruses have varied shapes and chemical composition, but unlike bacteria (or human body cells), they do not contain both RNA and DNA – but only contain either RNA or DNA.

Infection of host cells

Figure 3.3 illustrates the stages involved in viral replication.

First of all, the virus has to be transmitted, and the commonest ways in which viruses as transmitted are:

- via inhaled droplets (e.g. rhinovirus – causes the common cold)
- in food and/or water (e.g. hepatitis A – causes hepatitis)
- by direct transfer from other infected hosts (e.g. HIV – causes AIDS)
- from the bites of arthropods (such as mosquitoes) that are acting as **vectors** (e.g. yellow fever)

Fungi

Fungi are characteristically multicellular organisms with a thick cell wall. They may grow as threadlike filaments known as **hyphae**, although there are many other forms of growth that occur with fungi.

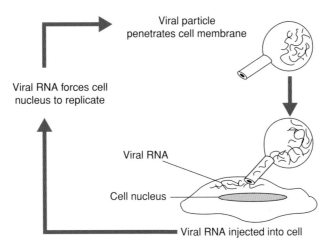

Viral particle
penetrates cell membrane

Viral RNA forces cell
nucleus to replicate

Viral RNA

Cell nucleus

Viral RNA injected into cell

Figure 3.3 Viral replication.

Of these other forms of fungi, the more familiar to us are the single-celled yeasts, and of course the mushrooms.

Fungi are free-living organisms and are common causes of local infections on skin and hair. However, a number of fungi are also associated with significant disease, and many of these are acquired from the external environment. Pathogenic species invade tissues and digest material externally by releasing enzymes. They also take up nutrients directly from host tissues – as do all good parasites. The various forms of fungi can be seen in Figure 3.4.

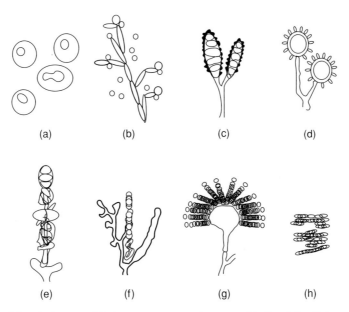

(a)   (b)   (c)   (d)

(e)   (f)   (g)   (h)

Figure 3.4 Typical fungi shapes. (a) *Cryptococcus neoformans*, (b) *Candida albicans*, (c) *Microsporum canis*, (d) *Histoplasma capsulatum*, (e) *Epidermophyton floccosum*, (f) *Trichophyton mentagrophytes*, (g) *Aspergillus fumigatus* and (h) Ringworm infection of the hair.

Protozoa

Protozoa are single-cell microorganisms that range in size from 2 to 100 μm. Many species of protozoa are free-living (i.e. they can exist outside of a cell). Some protozoa are important parasites of humans. Infections are most prevalent in tropical and subtropical regions, but they can also occur in temperate regions.

Although protozoa can cause disease directly (e.g. by the rupture of red cells in malaria), usually the pathology of a protozoal infection is caused by the immunological response of the infected host. Most protozoal infections are actually not life-threatening, unless if the infected host has a compromised immune system. The very obvious exception to the previous statement concerns malaria, which kills more than 1.5 million people every year (most of whom are young children, with an immature immune system).

Rickettsiae, chlamydiae and mycoplasmas
Rickettsiae

Rickettsiae belong to a group of pathogens that, whilst physically/anatomically belonging to bacteria, also have certain similarities with viruses. They are Gram-negative rod-shaped bacteria or coccobacilli. Perhaps the best-known disease that they cause is Typhus. They are maintained in animal reservoirs, and they are transmitted by the bites of ticks, fleas, mites and lice.

Chlamydiae

Chlamydiae are very small bacteria that are also **obligate intracellular parasites**. The majority of chlamydial infections are genital and acquired during sexual intercourse. **Asymptomatic** infection is common, especially in women; however, in men it is usually **symptomatic**. Chlamydiae enter the host through minute abrasions in the mucosal surface, where they bind to specific receptors on the host cells and enter the cells by 'parasite-induced' **endocytosis**.

Mycoplasmas

Mycoplasmas are also tiny bacteria (actually smaller than large viruses), which differ from normal bacteria by the fact that they lack cell walls, and consequently are not rigid structures. They can produce filaments that resemble fungi. Because of their small size and the fact that they lack rigid cell walls and therefore have a degree of plasticity, they were originally considered to be viruses. In fact, according to Tortora *et al.* (2004, p. 324), 'they may represent the smallest cell type and replicating organisms that are capable of a cell-free existence'.

There are several species of Mycoplasma, and in humans, some species may cause atypical pneumonia, **pelvic inflammatory disease**, **pyelonephritis** and **puerperal fever**. *Mycoplasma pneumoniae* is transmitted from person to person by the airborne route, whilst *Mycoplasma hominis* and *Mycoplasma genitaleum* are transmitted by sexual contact (Mims *et al.*, 2004; Tortora *et al.*, 2004).

Helminths

'Helminths' is the correct term for all sorts of parasitic worms that infect the body. As far as human bodies are concerned, there are three main groups of parasitic worms that cause disease:

- tapeworms
- flukes
- roundworms

Tapeworms and flukes are also known as flatworms, because they have flattened bodies. They also have muscular suckers and/or hooks to enable them to attach themselves to the host. Roundworms, on the other hand, have long cylindrical bodies, and they generally lack any specialised attachment organs.

Helminth infestations are commonest in warmer countries, although in terms of intestinal species of helminth, they may also occur in temperate regions.

Transmission

Infestation by helminths can occur after:

- swallowing eggs or larvae via the faecal–oral route
- swallowing larvae in the tissues of another host (e.g. beef, pork, and fish)
- active penetration of the skin by larval stages
- the bite of an infected blood-sucking insect vector

Many helminths live in the intestines, whilst others live in the deep tissues, but almost any part of the body can be infested by these parasitic helminths. Flukes and nematodes (roundworms) actively feed on the host tissues or on the contents of the intestines. Tapeworms, on the other hand, have no digestive system and therefore have to absorb pre-digested nutrients from the host.

The immune system

Immunology is the study of the immune system and its effects on the body and on invading microorganisms. However, the immune system does more than just protect the body from invasion by microorganisms and it is linked to many different organs and cells of the body. The immune system is an intricate system of cells, enzymes and proteins, which together protect the body by making it resistant (i.e. immune to infection by microorganisms (bacteria, viruses, fungi) as well as larger organisms such as worms.

Organs, cells and proteins of the immune system

The lymphatic system:

- the tonsils and adenoids
- the thymus gland
- the lymph nodes
- the spleen
- the appendix
- patches of lymphoid tissue in the intestinal tract

The circulatory system:

- the bone marrow
- lymphocytes (white blood cells)
- phagocytic cells (white blood cells)
- dendritic cells
- thrombocytes (platelets)
- complement proteins

The lymphatic system

The lymphatic system is similar to the blood system and consists of a specialised system of lymph vessels (similar to blood vessels) and specialised lymph nodes and tissue. Unlike the circulatory system, the lymphatic system does not use the heart to pump the lymph around. Instead the lymph (which fills the lymph vessels) is pushed around the body by a combination of contractions of the smooth muscular walls of the lymph vessels, as well as the flexing and relaxing of striated muscle in the body due to the movement of the individual.

The peripheral lymphatic system consists of lymphatic vessels, lymphatic capillaries and encapsulated organs. These organs include the:

- spleen
- tonsils
- lymph nodes

The lymph vessels and capillaries form an extensive network throughout the body and connect the organs of the body to the lymphoid organs, such as the spleen, and the lymph nodes. Lymph originates from plasma that leaks from the blood capillaries, and it drains into the lymphoid organs from nearby organs of the body. The lymph nodes act like fishing nets that trap harmful toxins and infectious organisms from the blood, and allow the very high concentrations of immune cells (in this case lymphocytes) to destroy them.

The lymphatic capillaries join together to form larger lymphatic vessels, and throughout the lymphatic system are to be found in lymph glands – like railway stations on a railway network. All the lymph eventually arrives at two large lymph ducts, called the thoracic duct and the right lymphatic duct. These two lymph ducts then empty into the great veins of the neck, and this restores fluid and proteins to the venous circulation.

Lymphoid tissue

Lymphoid tissue consists of lymph glands (lymph nodes – Figure 3.5) which are the size and shape of a broad bean, and lymphoid tissue which is found in specific organs, such as the spleen, bone marrow, lung and liver.

A lymph node is made up of a meshwork of cells, and the lymph containing any **antigen** from infected tissues and antigen-bearing cells passes through this meshwork. Within the lymph gland, lymphocytes and phagocytes are found in large numbers, so that they can destroy invading microorganisms that have been trapped in the lymph node.

Other lymphoid organs

The spleen collects **antigens** from the blood for presentation to phagocytes and lymphocytes. The spleen also collects, and disposes of, dead red blood cells.

Types of immunity

There are two types of immune defence systems:

- non-specific (or innate) immunity
- specific (or acquired) immunity

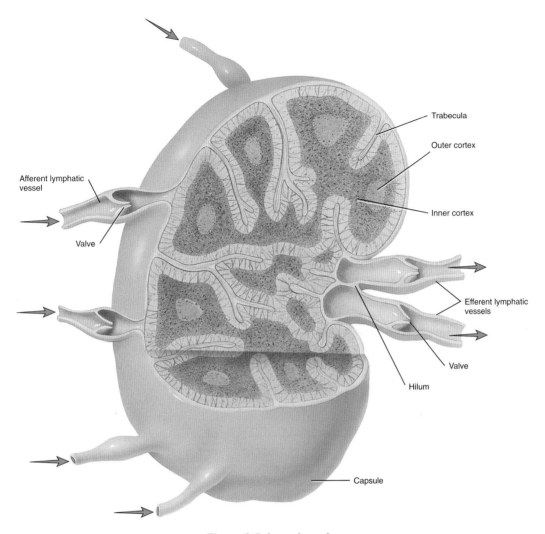

Figure 3.5 **Lymph node.**

Non-specific immunity

Non-specific immunity is the immunity with which we are born; hence its more common name is 'innate immunity'.

The innate immune system can be divided into four different components although there is some overlapping of functions:

- physical barriers
- mechanical barriers
- chemical barriers
- blood cells

Physical barriers

This includes skin and **mucosal membranes**.

The skin acts as a physical barrier to prevent infectious organisms and other materials, such as dirt, from getting to the more delicate and undefended organs within our body. However, skin is not only a physical barrier, but it is also a chemical barrier in that sweat produced from the skin is **bactericidal**. Unfortunately, skin as a physical barrier does have weaknesses, namely the various orifices that connect the internal body to the outside, including the mouth, nose, urethral opening and anus.

Thus, there needs to be some other type of protection for these at risk areas, and the body has that in the form of **mucosal membranes** which coat all the passageways between the internal organs and the outside world. Mucosal membranes contain secretions that are also bactericidal as well as secreting large amounts of **antibodies**.

Mechanical barriers

Actions involving cilia, coughing, sneezing and tears are included in this section as are mechanical barriers.

Cilia are the tiny hairs that are found in the nose. They are constantly moving like coral under the sea and they move mucus-containing dirt and microorganisms away from the inside of the body where they can cause problems to the outside of the body. Alternatively, they can move the mucous inwards to meet the parts of the immuns system that can effectively deal with the microorganisms in particular.

Sneezing and coughing work by pushing any microorganisms or irritants out of the body and into the atmosphere. With each sneeze or cough, millions of viruses are expelled into the atmosphere, and this means that there are fewer viruses in the body to cause even worse problems. This is very effective for the person who is coughing and sneezing, but unfortunately it means that there are all these viruses in tiny droplets suspended in the air, just waiting for someone else to come along and breathe them in, and in turn becoming infected with these viruses.

Tears are a mechanical barrier. They wash any dirt particles or microorganisms away from the eyes. Tears are also a chemical barrier because they contain a bactericidal enzyme known as lysozyme.

Chemical barriers

Some of the components that are involved as chemical barriers have already been mentioned above.

Chemical barriers include:

- tears
- breast milk
- sweat
- saliva
- acidic secretions, including stomach acid
- semen

Most of these secretions contain either bactericidal **enzymes** (such as lysozyme) or antibodies. In addition, bacteria have great difficulty in surviving acidic secretions and are often killed if the environment is too acidic.

Blood cells

As well as the defences mentioned above, the innate system includes certain blood cells, namely leucocytes (white cells) and thrombocytes (platelets).

The actual white cells involved in the innate immune system are known as:

- neutrophils
- monocytes and tissue macrophages
- eosinophils
- basophils
- mast cells

There are several different types of blood cells that are involved with the innate immune system.

Phagocytic cells

Phagocytic cells include:

- mononuclear phagocytes (these are the monocytes and macrophages)
- polymorphonuclear phagocytes (neutrophils)
- eosinophils

A phagocyte is a cell that ingests microorganisms, such as bacteria, as well as other foreign matter, such as dirt in a wound and wood splinters, as well as any of the body's cells that are recognised by the immune system as being 'foreign' or 'non-self' cells through a process called phagocytosis (see Figure 3.6). The neutrophils and eosinophils contain enzymes which are released when the phagocyte ingests a microorganism. These enzymes help to break down the ingested microorganism, so that the cell can utilise what it wants for its own needs, and expel the rest as waste matter.

Mediator cells

A second group of cells of the innate immune system (the basophils and mast cells) are more accurately described as the helper cells of the immune system. They do not actually destroy the invading microorganisms by phagocytosis, but they help the phagocytes to do so. These mediator cells work by releasing various chemicals that have several actions. For example, some of these chemicals improve the inflammatory response to infection and injury, whilst others help the phagocytic cells to reach the microorganisms. Although not usually thought of as being part of the immune system, platelets are included because they help to block off and close any cuts and breaks in the skin, and thus prevent invading microorganisms from getting inside the body.

Specific immunity

It is specific immunity that gives the body immunity to specific **pathogenic microorganisms**, and it consists of lymphocytes (white blood cells) that target specific invading microorganisms. This allows

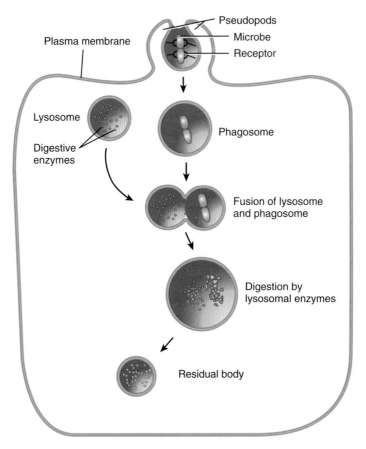

Figure 3.6 Phagocytosis.

for a much more concentrated attack on **pathogenic microorganisms** that have broken through the body's initial defences. It is not the remit of this chapter to discuss specific immunity in detail.

Immune problems

The immune system underpins just about all of health and so if anything goes wrong with it, then there can be serious problems for the body. The things that can go wrong include:

Immunodeficiencies – the immune system not working properly.
Autoimmune diseases – the immune system in a person is working too well and attacking cells of the that person's own body.

There are two types of immune deficiencies: primary and secondary. Primary immunodeficiencies occur as a result of genetic mutations, whilst secondary immunodeficiencies have an external cause, such as infection (HIV) or chemicals. Both types of immunodeficiency can range from very mild to life-threatening, and the treatment consists of supportive care – antibiotics and other similar drugs, as well as improvement of nutrition and general well-being. In addition, some immunodeficiencies may be helped by the injection of **immunoglobulins** (antibodies) to replace the patient's own. With secondary immunodeficiencies, it may be possible to remove the cause of the immunodeficiency. For example, if the immunodeficiency is caused by a drug (such as is given in chemotherapy for cancer – see Chapter 2), once the drug has been discontinued, then the immunodeficiency resolves.

Autoimmunity is often caused by an overreaction of the immune system to an **antigen** which can lead to the immune system attacking the body's own cells. Examples of autoimmune diseases include:

■ Diabetes (the immune system attacks the cells in the pancreas that secrete insulin).
■ Rheumatoid arthritis (the cells of joints, such as fingers and knees, are attacked by the immune system).

There is a third type of disease caused by a malfunctioning immune system, and that is allergy. An allergy is a raised immune response to an allergen (something that causes an allergy, such as peanuts, dust or pollen). As with immunodeficiencies, allergies can range from very mild to life-threatening.

Inflammatory response

Inflammation is the body's immediate reaction to tissue injury or damage. This damage can be caused by:

■ physical trauma
■ intense heat
■ irritating chemicals
■ infection by **viruses, fungi** or **bacteria**.

The inflammatory process (Figure 3.7) involves the movement of white cells, **complement** and other plasma proteins into a site of infection or injury (Roitt and Rabson, 2000).

There are fundamental signs and symptoms of any tissue or bony injury, and these include at the site of the injury to the following four classic signs of inflammation:

■ swelling
■ pain
■ heat
■ redness

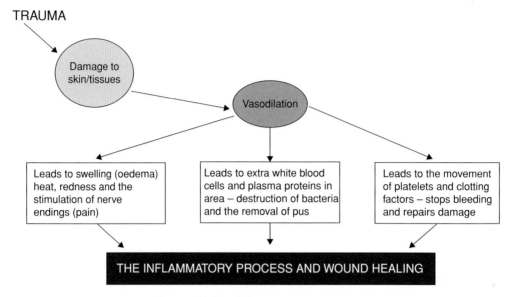

Figure 3.7 The inflammatory process.

There may also be:

■ nausea
■ sweating
■ raised pulse
■ lowered blood pressure

These last few symptoms and signs are the body's response to the pain and to shock, but in terms of immunology, the first four signs and symptoms are important.

Although inflammation does cause pain and other problems, it actually has beneficial properties and effects, namely:

■ the prevention of the spread to nearby tissues of infectious microorganisms and other damaging agents
■ the disposal of killed pathogens and cell débris
■ preparation for repair of the damage
  (Marieb, 2006).

According to Nairn and Helbert (2002), inflammation can be defined clinically as the presence of swelling, redness and pain.

Inflammation is usually initiated by injury to cells and tissues of the body and that following this injury/damage, three processes occur at the same time:

■ Mast cell **degranulation** – the release from the mast cells into the tissues of granules containing **serotonin** and **histamine**. These work with the other two processes below to provide the complete inflammatory signs and symptoms.

■ The activation of four plasma protein systems – complement (helps to orchestrate the inflammatory response), clotting (stops bleeding and repairs damage), **kinin** (involved in **vascular permeability**) and immunoglobulins (destroys bacteria), all of which work together to support the inflammatory process system – activates and assists inflammatory and immune processes, and also plays a major role in the destruction of bacteria.

■ The movement of phagocytic cells to the area in order to phagocytose bacteria or any other non-self débris in the wound.

Summary of inflammation

The timetable of a typical inflammatory response to tissue in injury is:

■ Arterioles near the injury site constrict briefly.
■ This vasoconstriction is followed by vasodilation which increases blood flow to the site of the injury (redness and heat).
■ Dilation of the arterioles at the injury site increases the pressure in the circulation.
■ This increases the exudation of both plasma proteins and blood cells into the tissues in the area.
■ This exudation then causes oedema (swelling).
■ The nerve endings in the area are stimulated, partly by pressure (pain).
■ The clotting and kinin systems, along with platelets move into the area and block any tissue damage by commencing the clotting process.
■ White blood cells – phagocytes and lymphocytes – move into the area and start to destroy any infectious organisms in the vicinity of the trauma.
■ These phagocytes and protein cells, along with the substances they produce, act at the site of the trauma in order to kill any bacteria or other microorganisms in the vicinity, but just as importantly they will remove the debris which results from the coming together of the microorganisms/other non-self matter and the forces of the immune system; this includes exudates and dead cells, also known more commonly as pus.
■ These systems/blood cells/tissue cells will remain in the area until tissue regeneration (repair) takes place. This is known as resolution.

Thus inflammation can be summed up as the presence of:

■ vasodilation – redness/heat
■ vascular permeability – oedema
■ cellular infiltration – pus
■ thrombosis – clots
■ stimulation of nerve endings – pain
  (Traske *et al.*, 2006).

Conclusion

This chapter commenced by looking at infectious diseases. An infection is the result of invasion of the body by microorganisms which cause damage to its tissues. Infectious diseases are characterised by the interaction of the responses of both the infected human host and the infecting organism.

Microorganisms are everywhere – they colonise humans, animals, food, water and soil. Infectious diseases are acquired by humans following contact with an **exogenous pathogen** present within a **reservoir of infection**. Such reservoirs include:

- active human carriers of the disease
- human carriers of the causative organism
- animal cases of disease or carriers of the organism
- the inanimate environment

More than 70 **bacteria**, **viruses**, **fungi** and **parasites** have been identified as pathogenic infecting organisms that are capable of causing serious diseases in humans (Ada and Ramsey, 1997). Vaccines are available against some of these, and work is in progression to find vaccines for almost all the **bacteria** and **viruses**, and about half of the parasites (Ada, 2001).

Vaccines tend to mimic and enhance the body's own defences against invading microorganisms – the immune system. The immune system is an extraordinary system, with the continued cooperation of all its components with each other being necessary for continued good health and for our protection against infecting microorganisms.

Multiple choice questions

1. Which of the following microorganisms force a cell's DNA to replicate its own DNA?
(a) fungi
(b) protozoa
(c) viruses
(d) bacteria

2. Which of the following are reservoirs of infection?
(a) the inanimate environment
(b) active human carriers of the disease
(c) animal carriers of the organism
(d) all the above

3. Legionnaire's disease is transmitted by which method?
(a) water
(b) faecal–oral
(c) aerosol
(d) direct contact

4. Infections can be spread to humans by which of the following methods?
(a) vectors
(b) droplet spread
(c) computers
(d) direct contact

5. Infestation by helminths can occur in humans by which method(s)?
(a) active penetration of the skin by helminth larvae
(b) breathing in the larvae
(c) being bitten by an infected blood-sucking insect
(d) during sexual intercourse

6. Which three excretions contain important components of our innate immune system?
(a) breast milk
(b) urine
(c) semen
(d) sweat

7. Phagocytosis is:
(a) the production of cytokines
(b) the opsonisation of bacteria

(c) the movement of cells of the immune system to a site of infection

(d) the act of engulfing and destroying non-self matter

8. Which of these are cardinal signs of an inflammation?

(a) tiredness

(b) redness

(c) heat

(d) pallor

9. Which of these plasma protein systems are activated in inflammation?

(a) clotting

(b) creatinine

(c) complement

(d) coping

10. What causes the redness in inflammation?

(a) cellular infiltration

(b) vasodilation

(c) stimulation of nerve endings

(d) vascular permeability

Answers: 1.c, 2.d, 3.c, 4.a,b,d, 5.a,c, 6.a,c,d, 7.d, 8.b,c, 9.a,c, 10.b.

Test your knowledge

❓ What are the differences between a pathogenic microorganism and a commensal microorganism?

❓ How are the following infectious diseases transmitted?

   ❓ rabies

   ❓ HIV

   ❓ enteric fevers

   ❓ tuberculosis

   ❓ influenza

   ❓ tetanus

❓ Discuss the effectiveness of physical, chemical and mechanical barriers to infection and what they consist of.

❓ What are the organs of the lymphatic system?

❓ Briefly discuss the signs and symptoms of an inflammatory response and explain what causes them.

Glossary of terms

Antibodies: See immunoglobulins.

Antigen: Something that causes an antibody response, e.g. an infecting microorganism.

Asymptomatic: An infection in which the infected person shows no symptoms of infection (see symptomatic).

Autoimmunity: An overreaction of the immune system to an antigen which can lead to the immune system attacking the body's own cells.

Bacteria (single = bacterium): Single-cell microorganisms that can infect the body, but also may work with the body to the mutual benefit of both (symbiosis). *E. coli* is an example of a bacterium that can be both beneficial to the body and dangerous to it, depending upon the type of *E. coli* and where it is found within the body.

Bactericidal: Deadly to bacteria – kills them.

Chemotaxis: The movement of cells within the body to where they are needed.

Commensal: A microorganism that does not cause any problems to a human, and may even be beneficial (c.f. *E. coli*). The opposite of a pathogen.

Complement: A series of enzymatic proteins that work together to aid the immune system by means of being involved in the processes of opsonisation, chemotaxis and the death of bacterial cells.

Contaminated intermediate: Something that is itself contaminated and can contaminate something else. It acts as a 'go-between' for the infectious organism and the targeted potential host.

Cystitis: Inflammation of the urinary bladder – usually as a result of colonisation by an infectious microorganism.

Degranulation: The release of granules into the tissues from certain cells, particularly mast cells, eosinophils and basophils, which contain them. These granules contain, amongst other substances, serotonin and histamine, and these substances cause some of the signs and symptoms of inflammation.

Dilate: To widen – see vascular permeability.

Endocytosis: The general name for the various processes by which cells ingest foodstuffs and infectious microorganisms.

Endogenous: From inside of the body – in the case of infections, the infecting microorganism is already present in the body before becoming infectious.

Enteric fevers: Another name for typhoid or paratyphoid fever.

Enzymes: Molecules that speed up chemical reactions.

Exogenous: From outside of the body, i.e. an infectious organism that comes from outside of the body.

Fluke: A type of flattened worm (similar to helminths) that can infest humans and cause schistosomiasis or else liver fluke infestation.

Fomite: Non-living object that is contaminated by infectious microorganisms.

Fungi: Microorganisms that combine to form larger structures that can be seen by the naked eye. Include yeasts as well as fibrous forms.

Gut helminths: See helminths.

Helminths: Also known as intestinal worms. These worms exist as parasites in the human intestines, although other types of helminth can live in the blood, lymph system or the liver (some are even known to live in the eye).

Herd immunity: A natural population of people (the herd) who are immune to a particular infection. This can be achieved by the population having natural immunity to the infectious organism, or it may be induced by means of vaccination. This means that anyone within that population who may not be immune to the infection will still have only a low chance of becoming infected because there is so little of the infecting organism in existence within that population.

Histamine: See serotonin.

Histoplasmosis: A respiratory infection caused by inhaling the spores of the fungus *Histoplasma capsulatum* (found in soil contaminated with bird or bat droppings).

Hyphae: Tubular filament-like threads that make up certain fungi.

Immunodeficiencies: Deficiencies in the structure or functioning of the immune system – they can be either secondary (with an external cause) or primary (usually with a genetic cause).

Immunoglobulins: Another name for antibodies. Antibodies are opsonins that are manufactured by the B-cell lymphocytes and help the phagocytic cells to destroy invading microorganisms.

Kinin system: Kinins are proteins which play a role in inflammation. The primary kinin is bradykinin, which causes dilation of vessels, acts with prostaglandins to induce pain, increases vascular permeability, and may increase leucocyte chemotaxis.

Legionnaire's disease: A form of pneumonia caused by the bacterium *Legionella pneumophila*. It breeds in warm, moist conditions, such as central heating water, and is transmitted via water droplets, such as occur when taking a shower.

Leptospirosis: A disease that often affects the liver and kidneys and is caused by a bacterium found in the urine of rats. Also known as Weil's disease.

Microorganism: Any living self-contained organism that can only be seen when under a microscope, e.g. bacteria and viruses.

Mucosal membranes: The membranes containing mucus that cover all the passageways leading into or out of the body, e.g. the mouth, nose, bronchi and urethra.

Obligate intracellular parasites: Microorganisms that are obligated to reproduce inside cells.

Oedema: The abnormal collection of fluid in the tissues. It may be localised (following an injury = swelling) or it may be generalised (as in heart failure).

Opsonins: Factors found in plasma and other body fluids that can bind microorganisms to phagoctyes.

Opsonisation: The coating of microorganisms to make them more susceptible to phagocytosis.

Parasite: An organism living on or in another organism, and obtaining nourishment at the expense of the organism that is not parasitic.

Pathogen: A microorganism that causes problems – is 'infectious'.

Pelvic inflammatory disease: An inflammation of internal female reproductive organs.

Phagocytosis: The method by which some cells ingest large particles, including whole microorganisms.

Prostaglandins: Prostaglandins are produced by the mast cells. They cause increased vascular permeability, neutrophil chemotaxis and can induce pain.

Protozoa: The simplest and most primitive type of microorganism, although bigger than a bacterium. Examples of protozoa include those that cause malaria and sleeping sickness (see trypanosomiasis).

Puerperal fever: Also known as puerperal sepsis, this is an infection of the female genital tract. It occurs within 10 days of childbirth, a miscarriage or an abortion.

Pus: A thick green or cream-coloured fluid found at the site of a bacterial infections. It consists of millions of dead white blood cells of the immune system as well as dead bacteria.

Pyelonephritis: Inflammation of the kidney – usually as a result of bacterial infection.

Reservoir of infection: The place where infectious microorganisms reside before infecting people, e.g. human or animal carriers of the disease, or certain environments. For a disease to perpetuate itself there must be a continual source of the organisms that cause that disease.

Salbutamol: A bronchodilator drug used in the treatment of asthma – it widens the bronchial tubes to allow asthmatics to breathe more easily.

Schistosomiasis: A tropical disease caused by a fluke (schistosoma) and is contacted by bathing in a river infested by such schistosomes.

Serotonin: Serotonin is a substance that is released from platelets in response to injury, trauma or infection. Along with other substances, such as histamine, it causes temporary, rapid constriction of the smooth muscles of large blood vessel walls and dilation of the small veins (venules). This results in increased blood flow and increased vascular permeability.

Symptomatic: The infected person shows the signs and symptoms of the infection, such as a raised temperature and respirations (see asymptomatic).

Vascular permeability: The widening/dilating of blood vessels to allow fluid and other matter to pass through easily.

Vectors: An organism that houses parasites and transmits them from one host to another. A prime example of a vector is the mosquito that transfers the malaria parasite to humans.

Viruses: A group of very tiny microorganisms that are parasitic in that they can only multiply and survive within a cell that they have infected.

References

Ada, G.L. (2001). Vaccines and vaccination. *New England Journal of Medicine*, *345*(14), 1042–1053.

Ada, G.L. and Ramsey, A.J. (1997). *Vaccines, Vaccination and the Immune Response*. Philadelphia: Lippincott-Raven.

Davey, B., Halliday, T. and Hirst, M. (2001). *Human Biology and Health: An Evolutionary Approach*, 3rd edn. Buckingham: Open University Press.

Marieb, E.N. (2006). *Human Anatomy and Physiology*, 7th edn. San Francisco: Pearson Benjamin Cummings.

Mims, C., Dockrell, H.M., Goering, R.V. et al. (2004). *Medical Microbiology*, 3rd edn. Edinburgh: Elsevier Mosby.

Nairn, R. and Helbert, M. (2002). *Immunology for Medical Students*. Edinburgh: Mosby.

Re, V.L., III (2004). *Hot Topics: Infectious Diseases*. Philadelphia: Hanley & Belfus.

Roitt, I. and Rabson, A. (2000). *Really Essential Medical Immunology*. Oxford: Blackwell Science.

Traske, B.C., Rote, N.S. and Huether, S.E. (2006). Innate immunity: Inflammation. In: McCance, K.L. and Huether, S.E. (eds) *Pathophysiology: The Biologic Basis for Disease in Adults and Children*, 5th edn. St. Louis: Elsevier Mosby, pp. 175–210.

Tortora, G.J., Funke, B.R. and Case, C.L. (2004). *Microbiology: An Introduction*, 8th edn. San Francisco: Pearson Benjamin Cumming.

Chapter 4

Shock

Janet G. Migliozzi

KEY WORDS

- Anaphylactic shock
- Anaerobic metabolism
- Cardiac output
- Distributive shock
- Homeostasis
- Hypovolaemic shock
- Hypoperfusion
- Neurogenic shock
- Obstructive shock
- Peripheral vasodilatation
- Septic shock
- Toxic shock syndrome

Test your prior knowledge

- What does the cardiovascular system consist of?
- What is homeostasis?
- How is blood pressure maintained at a constant level?

Learning outcomes

On completion of this section, the reader will be able to:

■ Describe the different types of shock and their causative factors.

■ Describe the clinical presentation of different types of shock.

■ Describe the pathophysiology and three stages of shock.

■ Understand the nursing care of the patient in shock.

Introduction

The cardiovascular system consists of the heart, blood and a vascular network composed of arteries, veins, arterioles, venules and capillaries that work together to maintain tissue survival by ensuring that an adequate and constant supply of oxygen and nutrients reaches the cells and that metabolic waste products are removed.

Under normal circumstances, **homeostasis** is maintained by the four essential circulatory components, e.g. blood/interstitial fluid volume, blood flow, vascular resistance and the ability of the heart to contract (myocardial contractility). When one of these circulatory components fails, the others compensate. However, as compensatory mechanisms fail or if more than one of the circulatory components are affected, the cardiovascular system will fail to function, resulting in a state of circulatory shock (Sole *et al.*, 2005).

Types of shock

Any condition that leads to a reduction in cardiac output can lead to circulatory shock: consequently the effects of shock are not limited to one organ system and can be considered to be a general systemic reaction. However, shock is typically classified by its causative factors and includes the following.

Hypovolaemic shock

Hypovolaemic shock is the most common type of shock (Monahan *et al.*, 2007) and occurs as a result of fluid loss and includes both blood loss, plasma loss and/or loss of **interstitial fluid**. Blood can be lost from a bleeding organ or wound; however, the circulating volume can also be reduced as a result of plasma loss, e.g. from extensive burns or damaged tissues or excessive loss of fluid from either renal impairment or inadequate fluid intake, e.g. dehydration. This loss of fluid leads to a reduction in circulatory fluid in the blood vessels leading to insufficient quantities of blood returning to the heart. This poor venous return results in a decrease in cardiac output and subsequent decrease in blood pressure leading to a decrease in tissue perfusion, which results in impaired cellular metabolism and shock. Figure 4.1 outlines the physiological events leading to hypovolaemic shock.

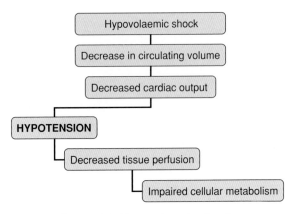

Figure 4.1 Hypovolaemic shock.

Cardiogenic and obstructive shock

Cardiogenic shock occurs when the heart 'fails' as a pump resulting in abnormal cardiac functioning. Obstructive shock occurs when a mechanical or physical obstruction impedes the flow of blood, e.g. a pulmonary embolism or tension pneumothorax.

Distributive shock

The next three types of shock (**anaphylactic**, **septic** and **neurogenic**) are collectively known as **distributive shock** (see Figure 4.2) in which (irrespective of the causative factors) widespread vasodilatation and decreased peripheral vascular resistance are a common feature (Peralta, 2006). This type of shock differs to hypovolaemic shock in that the circulating blood volume remains normal (Martini, 2001). However, cardiac output and blood pressure become impaired due to the blood vessels losing their vasomotor tone which leads to an increase in their diameter (vasodilatation). This leads to a decrease in peripheral vascular resistance resulting in the blood collecting or 'pooling' in the large veins causing circulating blood volume to be abnormally distributed. This results in blood pressure in the systemic

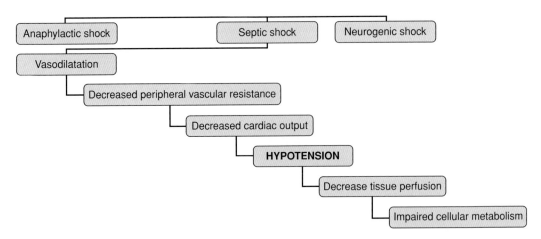

Figure 4.2 Distributive shock.

Box 4.1 Some common causes of anaphylaxis

■ Antibiotics (penicillins and cephalosporins)
■ Anaesthetic agents and muscle relaxants
■ Aspirin and non-steroidal anti-inflammatory drugs, e.g. ibuprofen
■ Blood products and plasma expanders
■ Intravenous radiocontrast media
■ Latex
■ Food allergies, e.g. shellfish, eggs, nuts and dairy products
■ Insect stings

Docherty and Hall (2002).

circulation falling to such a low point that venous return becomes so decreased that cardiac output becomes inadequate to perfuse the tissues adequately and shock ensues (see Figure 4.2).

Anaphylactic shock

This form of shock (also known as **anaphylaxis**) occurs following a widespread allergic or **hypersensitivity** reaction to the presence of an **allergen** or **antigen** that can lead to severe circulatory collapse within seconds (Resuscitation Council UK, 2005). Some common causes of anaphylaxis are summarised in Box 4.1.

Anaphylactic reactions can be either **immunoglobulin E** (IgE) mediated or non-IgE mediated and occurs as a result of repeated exposure to an **antigen** or **allergen** (to which the individual has previously produced an antibody response) which leads to an allergic response (Johnson and Peebles, 2004). The subsequent release of histamine causes **vasodilatation** of blood vessels, increases vascular permeability (which results in loss of intravascular fluid volume) and constricts respiratory smooth muscle (Smith and Bullock, 2000).

Signs and symptoms of anaphylactic shock can include:

■ sense of impending doom, anxiety and restlessness
■ altered levels of consciousness
■ severe air hunger
■ bronchospasm and dyspnoea
■ stridor caused by laryngeal oedema
■ urticaria (hives)
■ pruritus (itching)
■ rhinitis and conjunctivitis
■ abdominal pain, vomiting and diarrhoea
■ oedema of the lips, eyes, hands, neck and throat

Septic shock

Septic shock is the most common type of distributive shock (Smeltzer and Bare, 2000) and occurs as a result of widespread infection. This form of shock is most commonly associated with the release of Gram-negative and Gram-positive bacteria into the blood stream – a condition known as **bacteriaemia**

Type of shock	Common causative factors
Hypovolaemic shock	External and internal fluid volume loss
Anaphylactic shock	Repeated exposure to an antigen
Septic shock	Gram-negative bacteria Gram-positive bacteria
Neurogenic shock	Spinal cord injury Spinal anaesthetic Brain injury Vasomotor depression Drug overdose Severe pain
Cardiogenic shock	Myocardial infarction Cardiomyopathy Valvular disease Structural defects Cardiac arrhythmias
Obstructive shock	Cardiac tamponade Pulmonary embolism

Table 4.1 Types of shock and common causative factors

in which the pathogen's release of toxins into the blood stream results in massive vasodilatation and hypotension.

Toxic shock syndrome is a form of septic shock that can occur in women who use tampons during menstruation or in individuals who have body piercings and is caused by *Staphylococcus aureus.*

Neurogenic (vasogenic) shock

This is a rare form of shock which can occur following major brain or spinal trauma, emotional trauma, severe pain or following a drug overdose. The loss of sympathetic impulses causes a significant decrease in peripheral vascular resistance. This results in massive vasodilatation which affects venous return to the heart leading to a decrease in cardiac output, low blood pressure and a reduction in blood flow (see Table 4.1).

Pathophysiology of shock

Shock is a severe, life-threatening clinical syndrome that can result in death and is characterised by inadequate tissue perfusion that results in impaired cellular metabolism. Shock manifests itself as a syndrome within many diseases or traumatic injuries that may be life-threatening and is a state of insufficient oxygenation and perfusion to vital organs and tissues throughout the body. Therefore, whilst the causes of shock are varied and the individual's presentation may differ according to this (see

Manifestation	Hypovolaemic	Anaphylactic	Septic	Neurogenic
Heart rate	Tachycardia	Tachycardia	Tachycardia	Bradycardia
Respiratory rate	Tachypnoea	Tachypnoea and dyspnoea	Tachypnoea	
Blood pressure	Hypotension	Hypotension	Hypotension	Hypotension
Urine output	Decreased urine production	Decreased urine production	Increased initially then oliguria	Decreased urine production
Temperature	Temperature within normal range	Temperature within normal range	Temperature initially raised and then within normal range	Temperature regulation disrupted therefore may be experiencing hypo/hyperthermia
Skin	Cool, pale skin	Cyanosis, swollen oedematous face, hands	Skin is initially flushed and warm (warm shock) then cool and pale	Cool, pale skin
Mental state	Restless and anxious	Restless and anxious	Restless and anxious	May be unconscious due to fainting or head injury

Table 4.2 A summary of clinical presentation of different types of shock

Table 4.2), the end results (at a cellular level), e.g. cellular hypoxia/damage, are the same (Tortora and Grabowski, 2003).

Stages of shock

Although the patient's initial response to shock may vary as it is dependent on the individual's age and general state of health prior to the event leading to the shock state, three distinct stages of shock are recognised and occur regardless of the type of shock experienced (Sole *et al.*, 2005).

Stage 1
Compensatory (non-progressive) stage of shock
A sufficient blood pressure is essential to adequately perfuse cells with oxygen and nutrients. Shock begins when the blood pressure is unable to do this and the body then initiates a series of compensatory

mechanisms. Although the individual will be experiencing symptoms of shock during this stage he/she is not at imminent risk of death and shock may be reversed if appropriate interventions are initiated (Cummins, 2002). In the early stages of compensatory shock, a set of neural, hormonal and chemical compensatory mechanisms are initiated in an attempt to restore **homeostasis** and maintain blood flow to vital organs such as the heart, brain and kidneys.

Neural compensatory mechanisms

The sympathetic nervous system regulates blood flow and pressure through its ability to increase heart rate and total peripheral resistance. In the shock state, the baroreceptors and chemoreceptors located in the carotid sinus and aortic arch detect the reduction in blood pressure and impulses are relayed to the vasomotor centre in the medulla oblongata.

Hormonal compensatory mechanisms

Stimulation of the sympathetic nervous system causes the adrenal medullae to release the **catecholamines** (**epinephrine** and **norepinephrine**) which increase the heart rate and force of contractions to improve cardiac output. The coronary arteries vasodilate to increase blood flow to the heart and meet its increasing demands for oxygen. The rate and depth of respirations will also increase to try and increase gaseous exchange and oxygen levels in the blood (Sole *et al.*, 2005).

A fall in cardiac output will also impact on the renal system which detects a decrease in blood flow and pressure to the kidneys. This causes the kidneys to release **renin** which converts **angiotensinogen** into **angiotensin I** which is metabolised into **angiotensin II** – a powerful vasoconstrictor. The presence of angiotensin II leads to the release of the hormone **aldosterone** from the adrenal gland which causes the reabsorption of sodium from the renal tubule. This leads to the retention of water in the hope of increasing the falling blood volume (see Figure 4.3). Stimulation of the posterior pituitary gland causes the release of **antidiuretic hormone (ADH)** also known as **vasopressin hormone** which increases the amount of water reabsorbed by the kidney tubules; hence, the patient may produce small volumes of concentrated urine or in more severe cases, no urine (**anuria**).

Drop in BP $\longrightarrow$ drop in blood flow to kidneys $\longrightarrow$ release of rennin from cells of

kidney $\longrightarrow$ converts angiotensinogen to angiotensin I $\longrightarrow$ angiotensin II $\longrightarrow$ release

of aldosterone $\longrightarrow$ reabsorption of sodium and water $\longrightarrow$ restoration of blood volume

Figure 4.3 Renin angiotensin mechanism.

Chemical compensatory mechanisms

A reduction in cardiac output leads to a decrease in blood flow to the lungs which is detected by the chemoreceptors located in the aorta and carotid arteries. This leads to an increase in the rate and depth of respirations; however, this **hyperventilation** causes a reduction in carbon dioxide which impacts on blood flow and oxygen levels to the brain which can lead to confusion and restlessness. The individual will move to the next stage of shock if the physiological adaptations that the body has initiated to overcome shock start to fail.

Stage 2
Progressive (decompensated) stage of shock

Progressive shock occurs when the body's initial compensatory responses fail to restore an adequate blood pressure and tissue perfusion (Smith and Bullock, 2000). In the early stages of progressive shock, the individual's life can usually be saved if treatment is timely and appropriate. However, if the originating problem, e.g. haemorrhage, has not been corrected, the body's compensatory mechanisms can no longer cope with the continuing decreased cardiac output and blood pressure; consequently vital organs are not sufficiently perfused (**hypoperfusion**) and tissue damage can occur. The systemic circulation continues to vasoconstrict in the hope of shunting blood to vital organs; however, this is at the expense of the microcirculation resulting in **ischaemia** of the extremities. Impaired cellular metabolism occurs as a result of an inadequate supply of oxygen and nutrients and the decreased levels of oxygen causes the cells to switch from **aerobic metabolism** to **anaerobic metabolism** which results in the production of **lactic acid** and leads to **metabolic acidosis**.

Prolonged anaerobic metabolism results in a reduction in the production of adenotriphosphatase (**ATP**) which leads to failure of the sodium–potassium pump causing sodium ions to accumulate inside the cell, resulting in swelling and a deterioration in the cell's function.

As shock progresses, **histamine** and **bradykinin** (both of which have vasodilating properties) are released and decrease peripheral vascular resistance further resulting in a continued reduction in blood returning to the heart. This leads to a further decrease in cardiac output and blood pressure leading to cellular **hypoxia**.

Hypoxia can lead to depression of the vasomotor centre in the medulla and the sympathetic nervous system. Levels of consciousness decrease and the patient may become restless, disorientated and confused. Abdominal distension and paralytic ileus are common and the pancreas may become ischaemic (Smith and Bullock, 2000).

Stage 3
Irreversible (refractory) stage of shock

At this stage, the continued decrease in blood pressure and heart rate means that the inadequate tissue perfusion leads to the subsequent failure of the body to respond to any form of therapy which results in multiple organ failure and death within a matter of hours (Collins, 2000).

Table 4.3 summarises the stages of shock, the physiological changes that occur and how the individual may present clinically.

Care of the patient in shock

Because of the life-threatening nature of shock, it is essential that the condition is recognised and treated in a prompt manner if inadequate tissue perfusion and subsequent organ failure is to be avoided. Therefore, the shocked patient requires close and careful monitoring within an intensive care or high dependency unit. Common interventions include oxygen, fluid and/or drug therapy (Bench, 2004), and nursing care should be focused on the care of the patient whilst they are undergoing these restorative measures. Key nursing considerations include:

- Close monitoring of vital signs (blood pressure, pulse, temperature, respiratory rate) to ensure the early detection of any deterioration in the patient's condition. The frequency of monitoring will

Stage of shock	Physiological changes	Clinical presentation
1. Compensatory	Neural and hormonal compensation	Normal blood pressure
	Mild to moderate vasoconstriction	Increased pulse rate (tachycardia) and respiratory rate (tachypnoea)
	Some anaerobic metabolism	Increased thirst
		Decreased urinary output
		Altered level of consciousness/dilated pupils
2. Progressive	Overall aerobic metabolism	Low blood pressure (hypotension)
	Decrease oxygen levels (hypoxia) to vital organs	Raised pulse rate
	Little or no oxygen (anoxia) to non-vital organs	Tachydyspnoea
	Impaired blood flow (ischaemia) to tissues	Pulmonary oedema
	Failure of sodium–potassium pump	Peripheral oedema
		Decreased urinary output
		Altered level of consciousness
		Abdominal distension
		Paralytic ileus
		Cold, ashen skin
3. Irreversible	Severe tissue hypoxia, ischaemia and necrosis (tissue death)	Severe hypotension
	Build-up of toxic metabolites	Respiratory failure
		Acidosis
		Peripheral oedema
		Acute renal failure (oliguria)
		Alterations in the blood clotting cascade

Adapted from Sole *et al.* (2005).

Table 4.3 Physiological changes that occur at each stage of shock

be determined by the patient's progress; however, 1/2-hourly observations should be considered in the first instance unless the patient is at risk of deteriorating rapidly in which case, continuous monitoring should be instigated. Where there is a risk of neurological deterioration, e.g. if the patient is in neurogenic shock or experiencing fluctuations in levels of consciousness, then assessment of the patient's neurological status using the Glasgow Coma Scale (see Chapter 10) may also be required.

■ Administration of oxygen therapy as an imbalance between oxygen supply and tissue demand is fundamental to the nature of shock (Edwards, 2001). For patients who are conscious and able to breathe spontaneously, oxygen should be administered via a face mask or nasal cannulae. However, if the patient is unable to maintain their airway/sufficient oxygen levels in the blood, then they may have to be intubated and ventilated. The rate/percentage of oxygen required should be guided by regular measurements of pulse oximetry and blood gas analysis. As oxygen therapy is very drying to the mucosa, it should be humidified with sterile water and the patient should be given regular mouth care.

■ Administration of prescribed intravenous fluid to improve the patient's blood pressure and cardiac output as an adequate cardiac output and a systemic blood pressure that is sufficient to maintain perfusion of vital organs is essential to meet the body's metabolic requirements. Therefore, the patient will require intravenous fluid replacement to correct the decreased circulating volume (hypovolaemia). If the patient has lost blood, e.g. through a haemorrhage, then a blood transfusion is indicated to raise the haemoglobin level to a point that ensures that there is adequate oxygen-carrying capacity in the blood. Whilst the choice and volume of fluid given, e.g. blood, colloid or crystalloid infusion, is dependent on the type of shock the patient is experiencing, strict monitoring of fluid balance is required to ensure effectiveness of the fluid therapy and the early detection of complications related to fluid therapy, e.g. fluid overload. This will require the insertion of a urinary catheter and hourly monitoring of urine output to ensure an output of at least 30 mL of urine per hour is being produced and regular monitoring of vital signs (see above) for early detection of any adverse reactions.

■ Psychological care for the patient and their family. The patient in shock is a medical emergency and very frightening for both the patient and their family. Therefore, they should be kept fully informed about any changes/progress in the patient's condition, the purpose of any equipment used and any interventions given as this will help to reduce anxiety and alleviate fear.

■ Maintaining adequate nutrition as the patient in shock will have increased demand for energy to support metabolic processes. Additionally, the patient may be nil by mouth due to their need for

Drug	Action
Dopamine	Increase the heart's ability to contract
Dobutamine	Increase the heart's ability to contract
Amrinone	Increase the heart's ability to contract
Norepinephrine	Increase the heart's ability to contract
Epinephrine	Increases venous return to the heart by causing vasoconstriction
Norepinephrine	Increases venous return to the heart by causing vasoconstriction
Atropine	Increases heart rate and force of contraction
Isoporternol	Increases heart rate and force of contraction

Table 4.4 Common drugs used to manage shock

possible surgery or due to impairment in digestive function, e.g. paralytic ileus. Therefore, enteral or total parenteral feeding may be required depending on the patient's condition.

■ Ensuring the skin remains intact as due to poor tissue perfusion and immobility, the patient will be at increased risk of pressure sore formation. The patient will require regular pressure area care and should be nursed on a pressure-relieving mattress.

Pharmacological management of shock

In the shocked patient, drug therapy is primarily directed at enhancing the heart's ability to pump and to improve tissue perfusion (Monahan *et al.*, 2007) and common drugs used to manage the patient in shock are summarised in Table 4.4.

Table 4.5 provides additional measures that may be taken according to the type of shock being experienced.

Classification	Management
Hypovolaemic	Eliminate and treat cause of hypovolaemia
Distributive	
Anaphylactic	Antihistamines Steroids Bronchodilators
Septic	Establish and treat source of infection with appropriate antimicrobial agents
Neurogenic	Treat cause Adequate pain relief

Table 4.5 Additional management of shock according to type

Conclusion

Shock is a common threat to all patients and the causes and treatment of the patient in shock are varied and complex and represents a medical emergency. The overall aim of this chapter has been to explore the different types of shock and the resulting pathophysiology this creates. The prompt recognition of the signs and symptoms of shock are critical to the patient's prognosis and the nurse plays a central role in the early detection of any deterioration in the patient's condition.

Multiple choice questions

1. Causative factors for hypovolaemic shock include:

(a) dehydration

(b) extensive burns

(c) a perforated stomach ulcer

(d) all of the above

2. Neurogenic shock:

(a) is a form of distributive shock

(b) occurs only in patients who have had spinal surgery

(c) is the most common form of shock

(d) causes an increase in peripheral vascular resistance

3. A normal saline infusion:

(a) is useful in the treatment of hypovolaemic shock due to haemorrhage

(b) is a colloid solution

(c) is expensive to use

(d) replaces body fluid

4. Epinephrine:

(a) decreases venous return to the heart

(b) can be used to treat neurogenic shock

(c) causes vasodilatation

(d) increases the heart's ability to contract

5. An anaphylactic reaction:

(a) is always antibody mediated

(b) results in a low circulating blood volume

(c) has many diverse causes

(d) can occur on first exposure to an antigen

6. Toxic shock syndrome:

(a) is a form of distributive shock

(b) is caused by a virus

(c) occurs in women of all ages

(d) is a common cause of circulatory shock

7. The refractory stage of shock:

(a) is reversible

(b) results in multisystem organ failure

(c) causes an increase in cardiac output

(d) causes an increase in urine production

8. What causes hypotension to occur in anaphylactic shock?
(a) peripheral vasodilatation
(b) pulmonary oedema
(c) an increase in cardiac output
(d) all of the above

9. Raised levels of angiotensin II and anti-diuretic hormone will result in:
(a) an increase in venous return
(b) an increase in peripheral resistance
(c) an increase in peripheral blood flow
(d) a decrease in peripheral resistance

10. Which of the following is an indicator that treatment for hypovolaemic shock has been successful?
(a) warm, dry skin
(b) urine output of 20 mL an hour
(c) semiconscious state
(d) cool peripheries

Answers: 1.d, 2.a, 3.d, 4.b, 5.c, 6.a, 7.b, 8.a, 9.a, 10.a.

Test your knowledge

- Outline the mechanisms the body uses to regulate and maintain blood pressure.
- Compare and contrast the signs and symptoms of hypovolaemic and distributive shock.
- Describe the mode of action of three pharmaceutical agents used in the treatment of circulatory shock.
- Outline a plan of care for the patient in circulatory shock.
- Which patients are at most risk of developing septic shock and why? Describe how these risks can be prevented.

Glossary of terms

Aerobic: Requiring the presence of oxygen.

Anaerobic: Without oxygen.

Allergen: A compound that produces a hypersensitivity response.

Anaphylaxis: A sudden, acute allergic reaction to a material, e.g. food, environment, drug or biological substance.

Antibody: A substance in the blood which destroys or neutralises various toxins.

Antigen: A substance which causes the formation of antibodies.

Anuria: A condition in which no urine is produced.

Bacteriaemia: The presence of bacteria in the bloodstream.

Bradykinin: A substance derived from plasma proteins – its prime action is in producing dilatation of arteries and veins.

Dyspnoea: Difficulty in breathing.

Histamine: A substance that causes constriction of smooth muscle, dilates arterioles and capillaries and stimulates gastric juices.

Homeostasis: Maintenance of relatively constant conditions within the body's internal environment.

Hypersensitivity reaction: An overreaction to an allergen that results in inflammation and tissue damage.

Hyperventilation: Abnormally deep and prolonged breathing.

Hypoperfusion: Abnormally low blood flow through a tissue.

Hypoxia: A low tissue oxygen concentration.

Immunoglobulin: A protein in the blood that carries the antibody activity of the blood against infectious microorganisms.

Interstitial fluid: The fluid in the tissues that fills the spaces between cells.

Ischaemia: Lack of blood to a part of the body due to constriction or blockage of the artery.

Peripheral vascular resistance: Refers to the resistance blood encounters at it flows through the systemic circulation.

Vasoconstriction: A decrease in the diameter of a blood vessel due to relaxation of smooth muscle in the vessel wall which may occur as a result of hormones or after stimulation of the vasomotor centre leading to increased peripheral resistance.

Vasodilatation: An increase in the diameter of a blood vessel due to relaxation of smooth muscle in the vessel wall which may occur as a result of hormones or after decreased stimulation of the vasomotor centre leading to decreased peripheral resistance.

References

Bench, S. (2004). Clinical skills: Assessing and treating shock. A nursing perspective. *British Journal of Nursing*, *13*(12), 715–721.

Collins, T. (2000). Understanding shock. *Nursing Standard*, *14*(49), 35–39.

Cummins, R. (2002). *Textbook for Advanced Cardiovascular Life Support*. Texas: American Heart Association.

Docherty, B. and Hall, S. (2002). Anaphylaxis in adults. *Professional Nurse*, *18*, 73–74.

Edwards, S. (2001). Shock: Types, classifications and explorations of their physiological effects. *Emergency Nurse*, *9*(2), 29–38.

Johnson, R.F. and Peebles, R.S. (2004). Anaphylactic shock: Pathophysiology, recognition, and treatment. *Seminars in Respiratory Critical Care Medicine*, 25(6), 695–703.

Martini, F. (2001). *Fundamentals of Anatomy and Physiology*, 5th edn. London: Prentice Hall.

Monahan, F.D., Neighbors, M., Sands, J.K. and Marek, J.F. (2007). *Phipps' Medical and Surgical Nursing – Health and Illness Perspectives*, 8th edn. St. Louis: Mosby.

Peralta, R. (2006). *Shock, Distributive*. Available at www.emedicine.com/med/topic2114.htm. Accessed on 11 July 2007.

Resuscitation Council UK (2005). *The Emergency Medical Treatment of Anaphylactic Reactions for First Medical Responders and for Community Nurses*. London: Resuscitation Council (UK).

Smeltzer, S. and Bare, B. (2000). *Brunner and Suddarth's Textbook of Medical-Surgical Nursing*, 9th edn. Philadelphia: Lippincott.

Smith, M.A. and Bullock, B.L. (2000). Shock. In: Bullock, B.L. and Henze, R.L. (eds) *Focus on Pathophysiology*. Philadelphia: Lippincott.

Sole, M.L., Klein, D.G. and Moseley, M.J. (eds) (2005). *Introduction to Critical Care Nursing*, 4th edn. St. Louis: Elsevier Saunders.

Tortora, G. and Grabowski, S. (2003). *Principles of Anatomy and Physiology*, 10th edn. New York: John Wiley and Sons.

Chapter 5

The heart and associated disorders

Muralitharan Nair

Test your prior knowledge

- ❖ What are the layers of the heart called?
- ❖ How many chambers does the heart have and what are they called?
- ❖ Can you trace the blood flow through the heart?

> **Learning outcomes**
>
> On completion of this section, the reader will be able to:
> - Describe the structure and functions of the heart.
> - Outline the conduction system(s) of the heart.
> - Describe the blood flow through the heart.
> - Trace the systemic and pulmonary circulations.

Introduction

In order for water to flow through a pipe, it must be under pressure or a force pushing the water though the pipe. When the pressure is increased water will flow with greater force and when the pressure drops the flow is decreased. The same principle can be applied to the heart and blood flow. In the human body, the heart is the muscular pump that provides the pressure necessary to propel the blood throughout the body. It must continue its cycle of contraction and relaxation, otherwise blood will stop flowing and the cells in the body will be unable to obtain nutrients from food sources and get rid of waste such as carbon dioxide and other products. Thus, a healthy and efficient heart is essential for cellular function. This chapter discusses the structure and functions of the heart, the conducting system and the blood flow through the heart. It also includes cardiac dysfunctions such as myocardial infarction, heart failure (left and right heart failure), cardiogenic shock and angina and their related nursing management.

Location of the heart

The heart is a muscular organ that rests on the diaphragm near the midline of the thoracic cavity in the **mediastinum** (Jenkins *et al.*, 2007), which is the space in the middle of the thorax between the right and the left lung. It lies more to the left than the right side of the chest and the base of the heart is over its apex (see Figure 5.1). It is about the size of the owner's closed fist and is approximately 12 cm long and 9 cm wide. In men, it weighs approximately 250–390 g and in women, it is 200–275 g (Marieb and Hoehn, 2007).

Structures of the heart

The heart is composed of specialised cardiac muscle and is surrounded by a membrane called the **pericardium**. The pericardium is divided into parietal and visceral pericardium. The parietal pericardium, which is the outer layer, is a fibrous sac. The inner layer called the visceral pericardium or the epicardium is a serous membrane, which is close to the heart (see Figure 5.2). The two layers are separated by a thin film of serous fluid which allows the heart to move freely. The cardiac muscle is called the **myocardium** and is only found in the heart. The fibres of the myocardium branch and join with each other (see Figure 5.2). The **endocardium** lines the chambers and the valves of the heart. It is a thin,

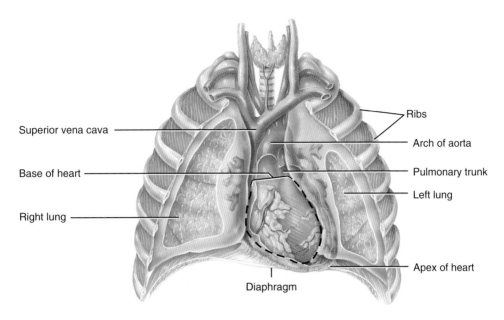

Figure 5.1 Location of the heart.

smooth and shiny membrane which allows the smooth flow of blood (Waugh and Grant, 2006). Thus, the heart can be described as having three layers:

■ The pericardium – the outer layer
■ The myocardium – the middle layer
■ The endocardium – the inner layer

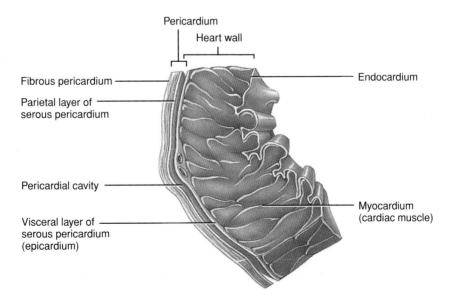

Figure 5.2 The cardiac muscle.

Chambers of the heart

The heart is divided into two sides, right and left, and is separated by a muscle called the **septum**. The septum ensures that the oxygen-rich blood from the left side of the heart does not mix with the oxygen-poor blood on the right side (Tortora and Derrickson, 2006). Each side of the heart is divided into two chambers. The upper chambers are called the **atria** (right and left) (singular atrium) and the lower chambers are called the **ventricles** (right and left) (see Figure 5.3). The walls of the atria are much thinner compared to the walls of the ventricles.

Valves of the heart

The valves between the atria and the ventricles are called the **atrioventricular valves**. The right atrioventricular valve is known as the **tricuspid valve** because it has three cusps and the left has two cusps and is also known as bicuspid **(mitral) valve** (McCance and Huether, 2006). These valves will only allow the flow of blood from the atria to the ventricles and prevent the blood from flowing in the opposite direction. Similarly, there are valves in the aorta and pulmonary artery and they are known as **semilunar valves** (see Figure 5.3).

Vessels of the heart

Blood flows in and out of the heart through several large vessels. The right atrium receives venous blood through the **superior** and **inferior venae cavae**. Oxygen-poor blood from the right ventricle is carried to the lungs by the **pulmonary artery** and the **pulmonary veins** return oxygen-rich blood from the lungs to the left atrium. The **aorta** transports oxygenated blood from the left ventricle to the whole body (McCance and Huether, 2006). However, the heart has its own blood supply and this is delivered by the coronary arteries and the coronary veins return oxygen-poor blood from the heart tissue to the right atrium (see Figure 5.4). See Table 5.1 for the summary of the vessels and their functions.

Blood flow through the heart

The right atrium receives oxygen-poor blood via the superior and inferior venae cavae and the coronary sinus. The right atrium then empties the blood into the right ventricle via the tricuspid valve. The right ventricle then pumps the blood to the lungs via the pulmonary arteries (right and left) by the opening of the pulmonary semilunar valve. In the lungs, carbon dioxide is exchanged for oxygen molecules. The blood returning to the lungs has a higher content of carbon dioxide, which diffuses out of the lung capillaries into the **alveolar sac** and is disposed of during expiration. During inspiration, oxygen diffuses from the alveolar sac into lung capillaries where it attaches itself to the haemoglobin **molecules** in the red blood cells. The red blood cells rich in oxygen are then transported in the blood to the left atrium by four sets of pulmonary veins. The short circulation from the right ventricle to the lungs and from the lungs to the left atrium is called the **pulmonary circulation** (Marieb and Hoehn, 2007).

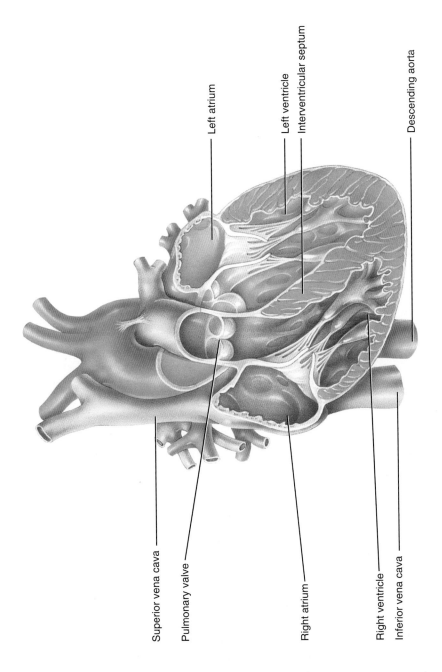

Figure 5.3 The chambers of the heart.

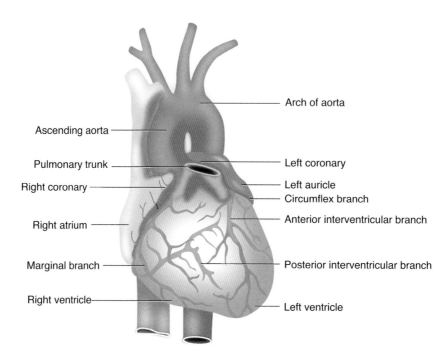

Figure 5.4 Vessels of the heart.

Superior vena cava	Returns oxygen-poor blood to the right atrium from the thoracic organs, head, neck and both arms
Inferior vena cava	Returns oxygen-poor blood to the right atrium from the rest of the body
Pulmonary artery (divides into right and left pulmonary artery)	Takes oxygen-poor blood from the right ventricle to the lungs
Pulmonary veins (two from the right lung and two from the left lung)	Returns oxygen-rich blood from the lungs to the left atrium
Aorta	Takes oxygen-rich blood from the left ventricle to the whole body
Coronary arteries	Takes oxygen-rich blood to the heart tissues
Coronary veins	Returns oxygen-poor blood from the heart tissues to the right atrium via the coronary sinus

Table 5.1 Summary of the vessels and their functions

From the left atrium, the blood is then pumped into the left ventricle via the bicuspid (mitral) valve. From the left ventricle, the blood is then pumped to the whole body via the aorta through the aortic semilunar valve (see Figure 5.5). The aorta and its branches then transport the oxygen-rich blood to all parts of the body. The blood is then returned to the right atrium via the venae cavae. This loop is called the **systemic circulation** (Marieb and Hoehn, 2007). The role of the systemic circulation is to transport oxygen and nutrients and to remove waste products, for example carbon dioxide from the tissues.

Conducting system of the heart

The heart has a built-in regulatory mechanism which produces a coordinated myocardial contraction of the four chambers. This is achieved by the cardiac conducting system which is composed of:

- the **sinoatrial** (SA) **node**
- the atrioventricular (AV) node
- the bundle of His
- the right and left bundle branches
- the Purkinje fibres

See Figure 5.6 for the conducting system.

The SA node

The SA node is situated in the right atrium just below the opening of the superior vena cava. It is also known as the **pacemaker**, so called because it initiates impulses much faster than other groups of neuromuscular cells (Waugh and Grant, 2006). Impulses from the SA node cause the atria to contract.

The AV node

The AV node is situated at the base of the right atrium. This is the last region of the atria to be stimulated, thus allowing time for the atria to empty the blood into the ventricles before the ventricles start to contract again. This ensures that the blood will flow in one direction only.

Bundle of His

This is a set of fibres that originate from the AV node.

Right and left bundle branches

From the bundle of His the nerve fibres split into the right and left bundle branches (see Figure 5.6).

Purkinje fibres

These tiny nerve fibres innervate both the right and left ventricular myocardial cells.

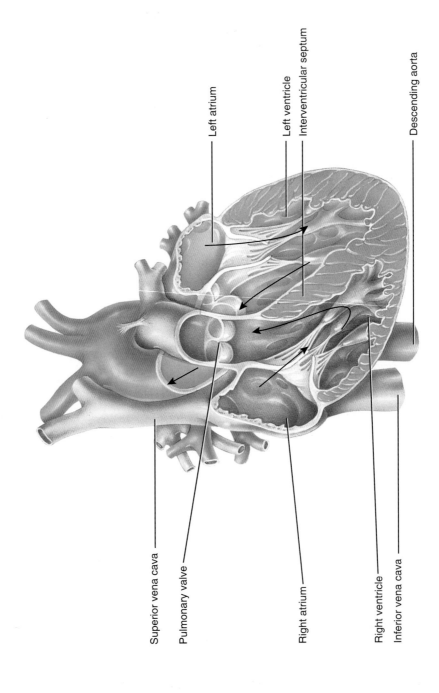

Left atrium

Left ventricle

Interventricular septum

Descending aorta

Superior vena cava

Pulmonary valve

Right atrium

Right ventricle

Inferior vena cava

Figure 5.5 Blood flow through the heart. The arrows indicate the pathway of blood flow.

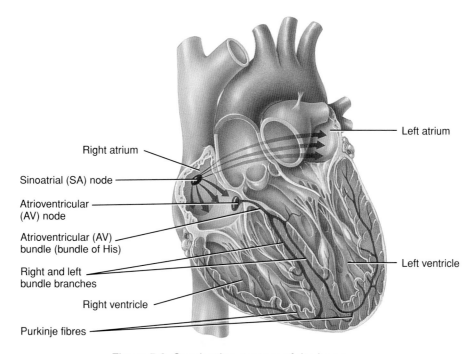

Figure 5.6 Conducting system of the heart.

Nerve supply of the heart

The pumping action of the heart is rhythmic. In other words, the cardiac muscle has the inherent power of automatic rhythmic contraction, independent of its nerve supply. However, the rate of contraction is influenced by the nerve supply to the heart. The nerve supply originates from the cardio-regulatory centre in the **medulla oblongata** which is situated in the brainstem (see Figure 5.7). These nerves are a branch of the autonomic nervous system and they are called the **sympathetic** and **parasympathetic nerves** (Waugh and Grant, 2006).

The sympathetic nerve increases heart rate; it innervates the SA node, AV node, and the myocardium of the atria and ventricles. The parasympathetic (vagus) nerve slows down the heart rate and it supplies the SA and AV nodes, and the atria muscles. See Box 5.1 for factors affecting heart rate.

Diseases of the heart

Learning outcomes

On completion of this section, the reader will be able to:

- List some of the common heart diseases.
- Describe the pathophysiology of the common heart diseases.
- Outline the nursing management of the conditions described in this section.

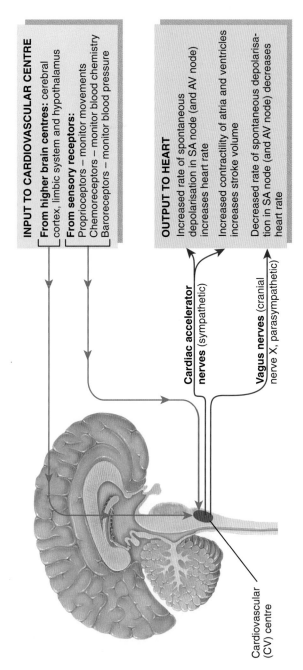

INPUT TO CARDIOVASCULAR CENTRE

From higher brain centres: cerebral cortex, limbic system and hypothalamus

From sensory receptors:
Proprioceptors – monitor movements
Chemoreceptors – monitor blood chemistry
Baroreceptors – monitor blood pressure

OUTPUT TO HEART

Increased rate of spontaneous depolarisation in SA node (and AV node) increases heart rate

Increased contractility of atria and ventricles increases stroke volume

Decreased rate of spontaneous depolarisation in SA node (and AV node) decreases heart rate

Cardiac accelerator nerves (sympathetic)

Vagus nerves (cranial nerve X, parasympathetic)

Cardiovascular (CV) centre

Figure 5.7 Cardio-regulatory centre.

Box 5.1 Factors affecting heart rate

■ Hormones such as adrenaline, steroids
■ Stress
■ Age of the individual
■ Drugs such as propranolol, dopamine
■ Body temperature
■ Autonomic nervous system
■ Circulating volume of blood
■ Electrolyte imbalance
■ Levels of oxygen and carbon dioxide in the blood

Adapted from Waugh and Grant (2006).

Myocardial infarction

The term **myocardial infarction** (MI) is commonly referred to as 'heart attack' which results from oxygen starvation of the myocardium (see Figure 5.8). When the coronary blood flow is occluded as a result of a blood clot or fatty deposits (**atheromatous plaque**) over a period of time, death of the myocardium will take place (McCance and Huether, 2006) resulting in MI. Porth (2005) states that MI occurs more frequently in the early morning hours (between 0600 and 1200) than during the evening.

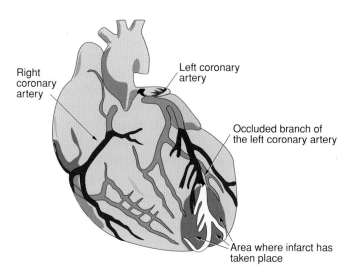

Figure 5.8 Myocardial infarction.

Aetiology of MI

MI is a medical emergency that needs quick intervention; it is the main cause of death for both men and women (Bullock and Henze, 2000). Individuals at risk include:

- People who have a medical history of vascular disease such as **atherosclerosis**, a condition where fatty deposits build up in the arteries causing them to become narrow and restrict the blood flow to the tissue.
- Previous heart attack or stroke.
- Older age group (men over the age of 40 years and women over the age of 50 years).
- Smokers are more susceptible to MI because of the nicotine content in cigarettes which could cause narrowing of the arteries.
- People who drink excessive amounts of alcohol are more prone because a high intake of alcohol increases the level of low-density lipoproteins (LDL).
- People with familial history.
- The misuse of drugs such as cocaine.
- Diabetics with or without insulin resistance are also prone to MI.
- People with hyperlipidaemia and obesity are at risk.

Investigations

The following investigations may be carried out to confirm diagnosis:

- chest X-ray
- blood chemistry (urea and electrolytes, cardiac enzymes, for example creatine kinase, full blood count)
- electrocardiogram (ECG) to detect any abnormal changes in the rhythm
- angiogram

Pathophysiology

Myocardial ischaemia results in a lack of oxygen to the myocardial cells due to an occluded coronary artery. If the heart tissue is deprived of oxygen for a prolonged period of time, approximately 20–45 minutes, this could lead to cell death (necrosis) distal to the occlusion (see Figure 5.8) (Hogan and Hill, 2004). The extent of the ischaemia depends on the location, extent of occlusion, amount of heart tissue supplied by the blood vessel and duration of the occlusion. It may affect the three layers of the heart (pericardium, myocardium and endocardium) or a combination of these layers (Porth, 2005).

Where the infarct has taken place, a **collagen** scar forms in its place and the damaged muscle does not contract efficiently. Collagen is a bundle of inelastic fibres that do not stretch nor contract effectively. Damaged heart tissue conducts electrical signals much more slowly than normal heart tissue, which could result in inefficient contraction of the myocardium. This could result in:

- Decreased volume of blood ejected by the left ventricle with each heartbeat.
- Decreased cardiac output (volume of blood pumped out by the left ventricle each minute).
- Decreased blood pressure.
- Decreased tissue perfusion.

Box 5.2 Summary of symptoms of myocardial infarction

- Severe pain radiating to arms and neck
- Pain may last for more than 20 minutes
- Shortness of breath
- Nausea and vomiting
- Cyanosis
- Excessive sweating
- Irregular heart rate
- Signs of shock
- Hypotension

Signs and symptoms of MI

- Central chest pain which radiates down the left arm and also to the lower jaw, neck, back and right arm. The pain may be described by the patient as crushing or tightness in the chest.
- Rapid, irregular pulse, hypotension and dyspnoea (shortness of breath) may all present as symptoms.
- Diaphoresis (excessive sweating), nausea, vomiting, palpitations, loss of consciousness and even sudden death could all occur in MI.
- McSweeney *et al.* (2003) suggest that women often experience markedly different symptoms compared to men. Symptoms such as dyspnoea, fatigue, sleep disturbances and weakness are more common in women than men. See Box 5.2 for summary of symptoms of MI.

Nursing management

When symptoms of MI occur, it is a medical emergency and prompt action is needed because time is an important factor in the prevention of extended damage to the heart muscle (Elton, 2003). Key nursing considerations are:

- The patient must be kept pain free as it presents myocardial ischaemia. Accurate pain assessment should be carried out using pain assessment tools such as the Numerical Rating Scale or the Verbal Rating Scale (Alexander *et al.*, 2006). Patients should be encouraged to report their pain as it happens.
- Bed rest for the first 24 hours is important to reduce the effort and strain on the heart.
- Administer prescribed oxygen to treat tissue hypoxia, which helps to reduce ischaemia and pain (Lemone and Burke, 2004).
- Monitoring of all the vital signs (heart rate, blood pressure, temperature and respirations) is important to detect early complications or changes in the patient's condition. This is normally carried out 1–2 hourly depending on the patient's condition.
- Observe for signs of shock such as lethargy, bradycardia or tachycardia, cyanosis, hypotension and excessive sweating (diaphoresis).
- Document any care given to the patient in accordance with the Nursing and Midwifery Council (NMC) guidance on record keeping (Nursing and Midwifery Council, 2005).

Pharmacological and non-pharmacological treatment of MI

Some of the pharmacological and non-pharmacological interventions are as follows:

■ Drugs to dissolve clots such as reteplase or streptokinase is administered within 2 hours of developing MI to limit tissue damage.

■ A continuous ECG monitoring is carried out to detect abnormal cardiac rhythms to take prompt action.

■ A urinary catheter may be inserted to monitor urine output.

■ Drugs such as morphine or morphine derivatives are administered to control pain in heart attack. Sublingual or intravenous nitrates such as GTN are also considered (Adams *et al.*, 2008).

■ Anticoagulant such as heparin is commenced to minimise the risk of a thrombus developing.

■ In some patients, an emergency coronary angioplasty may be required to increase blood flow to the coronary arteries. This involves insertion of a catheter into the obstructed coronary artery under local anaesthesia. The balloon in the catheter is then inflated for 15 seconds to 2 or 3 minutes (Porth, 2005) which dilates the artery.

Heart failure/congestive heart failure

Heart failure (HF) is a general term used to describe several types of cardiac disease which lead to poor perfusion of tissues. Congestive heart failure is a progressive and debilitating disease that is accompanied by congestion of body tissues. Heart failure may affect either side of the heart; however, as all the chambers are part of the heart structure, if one side fails then it affects the other side (Waugh and Grant, 2006). Nevertheless, left heart failure (LHF) is more common than right heart failure (RHF).

Aetiology of heart failure

Heart failure may be caused by a variety of conditions and they include:

■ acute MI where there is a loss of myocardial muscle which could lead to poor contraction
■ hypertension
■ valvular heart disease
■ inadequate emptying from the left ventricle due to poor contraction of the myocardium
■ anaemia resulting from reduced red blood cells

Pathophysiology

The onset of HF may be acute or chronic. It is often associated with systolic and diastolic congestion and with myocardial weakness. This weakness impairs the ability of the heart to pump efficiently. In acute HF, there is a sudden decrease in the amount of blood pumped out from both ventricles which leads to a reduction in oxygen supply to the tissues. However, in chronic HF the progression of the disease is gradual and in the early stages there may be no symptoms of heart failure.

Investigations

The following investigations may be carried out to confirm diagnosis:

■ electrocardiogram
■ chest X-ray
■ full blood chemistry and cardiac enzymes

- physical examination
- echocardiogram

Pathophysiology of right heart failure

RHF is associated with the right ventricle being unable to pump the blood into the pulmonary artery leading into the lungs. This leads to an increase in volume of the right ventricle during the end-diastolic phase, which causes an increase in volume of the right atria (Bullock and Henze, 2000). This in turn increases the volume of blood and pressure in the systemic venous system. There is accumulation of blood in some of the major organs and they include the liver, the kidneys and the spleen (Nowak and Handford, 1999) resulting in enlargement of these organs and their eventual destruction.

Signs and symptoms of right heart failure

- Pitting oedema may be observed in the sacrum of a patient confined to bed as well as the feet and legs when the patient is sitting. This is due to the impaired pumping ability of the heart and as a result fluid accumulates in the tissues.
- Enlargement of the organs such as the liver (hepatomegaly) and the spleen (splenomegaly) can cause pressure on the surrounding organs such as the stomach.
- Pleural effusion may occur due to the increased capillary pressure.
- Distended jugular veins are a visible sign in patients who suffer from right heart failure.
- Patients have difficulty in breathing due to ascites.

See Box 5.3 for summary of signs and symptoms of RHF.

Pathophysiology of left heart failure

LHF results from the damage of the left ventricular myocardium. The contraction of the left ventricle is ineffective and cannot pump out all the blood it receives from the left atrium (Hogan and Hill, 2004). This results in pooling of blood in the left atrium and raised pressure in the pulmonary veins, which leads to **pulmonary oedema**. Patients with pulmonary oedema may experience symptoms such as **dyspnoea**, **orthopnea**, productive cough, frothy sputum and pallor. Failure of the left ventricle also results in poor cardiac output. As the cardiac output decreases, perfusion to the tissues also diminishes resulting in poor delivery of oxygen and nutrients to the tissues (McCance and Huether, 2006).

Box 5.3 Summary of signs and symptoms of right heart failure

- Oedema of sacrum and feet
- Ascites
- Enlarged liver
- Enlarged spleen
- Jugular venous distension
- Fatigue
- Difficulty in breathing
- Pleural effusion
- Jaundice and coagulation problem may be present due to liver damage

Left heart failure (backward effects)

- Emptying of left ventricle is diminished.
- There is an increase in volume and end-diastolic pressure of the left ventricle.
- Pressure in the left atrium increases.
- Volume and pressure in the pulmonary veins increase.
- Volume of fluid in the pulmonary capillary bed increases.
- Movement of fluid from lung capillaries to interstitial space of alveoli.
- Rapid filling of alveoli spaces with fluid leading to pulmonary oedema.

Left heart failure (forward effects)

- Cardiac output decreases.
- Perfusion to tissues of the body decreases.
- Blood flow to the kidneys and other organs decrease.
- This leads to reabsorption of sodium and water by the kidneys to increase circulating fluid volume.

Signs and symptoms of left heart failure

- Patients with LHF may develop dyspnoea in the early stages due to fluid accumulation in the pulmonary capillary bed resulting in poor exchange of gases (oxygen and carbon dioxide) in the lungs.
- The patient may complain of dizziness, fatigue and weakness due to poor oxygenation of body tissues resulting from low cardiac output and oxygen saturation. The dizziness is the result of low oxygen to the brain which may result in disorientation, confusion and unconsciousness.
- The patient may experience orthopnoea. This is a term used to describe when the patient is unable to breath in a supine position.
- The patient may present with cyanosis. Cyanosis is the bluish discolouration of the mucous membranes around the lips and in the nail bed.
- The patient may experience wheezing due to **bronchospasm**.
- The patient may have crackles at lung bases due to pulmonary oedema.

See Box 5.4 for summary of signs and symptoms of LHF.

Box 5.4 Summary of signs and symptoms of left heart failure

- Dyspnoea
- Orthopnea
- Productive cough
- Frothy sputum
- Tachycardia
- Fatigue
- Dizziness
- Wheezing
- Cyanosis
- Pulmonary crackles

Nursing management of patients with heart failure

In order to provide high-quality care, nurses need to undertake a full and accurate nursing assessment and devise a care plan for all the actual problems identified. Vital signs are monitored hourly until they are stable. Early detection in changes in vital signs and prompt treatment may save the patient's life. Key nursing considerations are:

- Patients with heart failure may experience breathing problems such as breathlessness especially on exertion. Prescribed oxygen should be administered to improve oxygenation of the blood.
- Patients with LHF may expectorate large amounts of frothy sputum due to pulmonary oedema and therefore they will need a sputum mug/carton to expectorate and be provided with tissues and a waste receptacle to put the used tissues in.
- The patient should be nursed in the upright position in the bed supported by pillows to assist breathing unless contraindicated.
- Accurate monitoring of daily fluid intake and output is important in patients with HF. Output should be in excess of 30 mL/hour (Kozier *et al.*, 2004) and this should be recorded hourly (if urinary catheter is in situ) and any changes in output reported immediately.
- The patient should be encouraged to reduce salt intake in the diet as salt promotes fluid retention.
- The nurse should provide assistance when bathing or showering.
- The nurse must ensure that all treatment and care is explained to the patient in a way that the patient will understand.
- Patients may need laxatives to avoid straining when defaecating.

Pharmacological and non-pharmacological treatment of HF

The treatment of HF focuses on treating the signs and symptoms and improving the quality of life. Such measures include:

- Moderate physical activity when symptoms are mild or moderate.
- Weight reduction is important through physical activity and healthy eating, as obesity is a risk factor for heart disease.
- Reduction in salt intake is essential as excessive intake of salt can cause fluid retention and lead to an exacerbation of cardiac problems.
- Patients with HF will need their fluid intake monitored carefully to prevent fluid overload.

The pharmacological interventions for HF include:

- Anti-hypertensive drugs, for example quinapril 2.5–5 mg daily or captopril 6.25 mg three times per day should be prescribed for patients with heart failure (National Institute for Health and Clinical Excellence, 2003).
- Diuretic such as furosemide (maximum recommended dose is 250–500 mg) or matolazone (maximum dose 10 mg) are used to decrease fluid load in patients with HF (National Institute for Health and Clinical Excellence, 2003).
- Beta-blockers are also used in the treatment of HF. Bisoprolol 10 mg daily is used to improve left ventricular function (National Institute for Health and Clinical Excellence, 2003).

Box 5.5 Summary of other causes of cardiogenic shock

■ Acute pulmonary embolism
■ Myocarditis
■ Acute mitral regurgitation
■ Right ventricular infarction
■ Septic shock
■ Mitral stenosis
■ Complications of cardiac surgery
■ Valvular heart disease

Cardiogenic shock

Cardiogenic shock is a physiological state in which inadequate **tissue perfusion** occurs from cardiac failure mainly caused by acute MI (Hollenberg *et al.*, 1999). It can occur relatively quickly due to the effect of infarction on the myocardial tissue. It is a medical emergency and if not treated quickly the patient will die.

Aetiology of cardiogenic shock

There are numerous causes of cardiogenic shock but the most common cause is acute MI. The severity of the shock is associated with myocardial damage. Low cardiac output due to cardiogenic shock also impairs perfusion of the coronary arteries and the myocardium, thus further increasing myocardial damage. Although MI is the most common cause of cardiogenic shock, several other factors may be implicated. See Box 5.5 for summary of causes of cardiogenic shock.

Investigations

The following investigations may be carried out to confirm diagnosis:

■ chest X-ray
■ electrocardiogram to confirm diagnosis and to rule out other causes and diseases
■ arterial blood gas analysis
■ full blood chemistry
■ cardiac enzymes, for example troponins

Pathophysiology

Cardiogenic shock results from the diminished ability of the heart to function effectively. In MI, cardiogenic shock usually develops when approximately 40% of the myocardium is damaged. This leads to decreased blood pressure, poor cardiac output and inadequate perfusion to the tissues (Alexander *et al.*, 2006). As a result of this, the sympathetic nervous system's response is to increase the heart rate and induce **vasoconstriction**. This causes unwanted stress on the heart, which results in further damage to the cardiac muscle leading to poor cardiac output and hypotension, and it becomes a vicious cycle of cardiogenic shock (see Figure 5.9). Poor cardiac output reduces blood flow to essential body

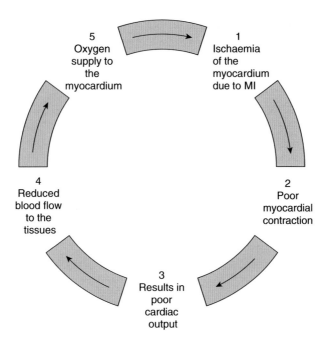

Figure 5.9 Vicious cycle of cardiogenic shock.

organs, thus affecting their functions. The sympathetic stimulation also causes decreased renal blood flow which could lead to acute renal failure.

As the perfusion to the tissues is reduced, the peripheral cells utilise **anaerobic metabolism** to produce energy. Anaerobic metabolism is the process in which cells use carbohydrates to produce energy in the absence of oxygen. The effect of this energy production is to keep the cells functioning; however, the production of **lactic acid** leads to metabolic acidosis, which in turn depresses cardiac function.

Signs and symptoms

Signs and symptoms of cardiogenic shock include the following:

- pulmonary oedema
- severe hypotension
- oliguria/anuria
- pale and cold skin
- raised jugular venous pressure
- chest pain
- nausea and vomiting
- dyspnoea
- profuse sweating
- confusion/disorientation

Nursing management of cardiogenic shock

Patients in cardiogenic shock will require precise and immediate nursing management and if the condition is not treated immediately, it could lead to severe complications and the death of the patient. The priority in the management of cardiogenic shock is to prevent further damage to the myocardium.

- Maintaining a clear airway and monitoring respiration is important in patients with cardiogenic shock. The nurse should observe the patient for signs of restlessness, breathlessness, dyspnoea and confusion. Oxygen must be administered as prescribed either by nasal cannula or ventimask.
- Patients in cardiogenic shock and their relatives are very anxious and frightened. They will need support and reassurance both from nurses and doctors.
- Vital signs must be monitored hourly and they include heart rate, blood pressure and respiratory rate. Any changes in the vital signs must be reported immediately in order to take prompt action.
- The nurse must observe and report any side effects of the drugs administered.

Pharmacological interventions for cardiogenic shock

Some of the medications include:

- analgesia for pain relief
- anti-hypertensive drugs to treat hypertension and decrease effort on the heart
- diuretics to decrease fluid load

Angina

Angina is chest pain that occurs when the heart muscle does not receive enough oxygenated blood. It is also described as a crushing pain in the chest. The term is derived from a Latin word meaning to choke. The pain can radiate through to the back and shoulder, or down one or both arms or into the neck and jaw. However, not all patients present with such extensive pain.

Investigations

These include:

- physical examination
- medical history
- electrocardiogram
- full blood analysis
- stress test

Pathophysiology of angina

Angina pain closely resembles the signs and symptoms of MI; thus it is vital that nurse are able to differentiate the two conditions, as the treatment differs in both cases. If a patient has angina pain, this is usually relived by vasodilators, for example glycerine trinitrate (GTN), but the angina pain is rarely fatal.

Angina results from a blockage in the coronary arteries resulting in diminished blood supply to the affected part of the heart muscle (see Figure 5.10). At rest the blood supply may be sufficient to provide nutrients and oxygen to the heart muscle; however, during activity, for example, walking or running,

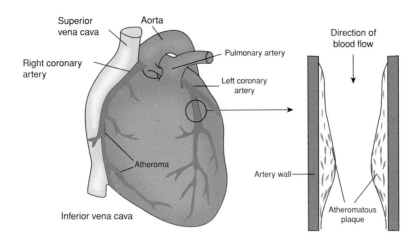

Figure 5.10 Blockage of the coronary arteries.

the heart rate increases which puts more effort on the heart. During exertion, if the blood flow to the heart muscle is inadequate, the oxygen supply is also diminished leading to severe pain. The patient may present with pallor, dyspnoea, cyanosis, diaphoresis and tachycardia (Adams *et al.*, 2008).

Types of angina

There are three types of angina and they include:

■ stable angina
■ unstable angina
■ variant angina

Stable angina is the most common type and it occurs when there is a greater demand on the heart than usual. It is estimated that over 1.2 million people in the UK suffer from angina. Stable angina is mainly caused by myocardial ischaemia. The pain usually lasts about 3–5 minutes. If the blood flow is restored by immediate treatment, no permanent damage results (McCance and Huether, 2006).

Unstable angina (also known as crescendo angina) is characterised by a change in frequency, intensity and duration of pain. It is more serious than stable angina and is unpredictable. It can also occur when the person is at rest and is not relieved by rest or medication. Patients who develop unstable angina are at risk of having an MI (Hogan and Hill, 2004).

Variant angina is a rare form of angina. It is thought to occur as a result of coronary artery vasospasm resulting in diminished blood flow. Variant angina is very painful and occurs from midnight to early morning. It usually occurs at rest and the same time each day (Hogan and Hill, 2004).

Signs and symptoms of angina

■ crushing pain in the chest
■ pain radiates to arms, jaw, neck and back
■ shortness of breath on exercise
■ sweating

- light headedness
- hypotension
- irregular pulse
- indigestion

Nursing management of angina

Nurses play a crucial role in the management of patients with angina. An accurate assessment of the patient must be carried out to ascertain the location, duration and the intensity of the pain. Risk factors must be identified to provide high-quality care. The care will include:

- controlling pain
- reducing anxiety in patient
- advising the patient on the possible risks and preventative measures
- providing health promotion where appropriate

Non-pharmacological interventions in the treatment of angina

- Advise the patient to eat a healthy diet and avoid saturated fat. This will help lower cholesterol as high cholesterol could lead to vascular complications.
- Encourage the patient to take up leisure pursuits such as walking and swimming as physical activity aids circulation and improves cardiac function unless contraindicated.
- Patients, who are overweight, should be encouraged to loose weight through individual programmed activity unless contraindicated.
- Advice in the consumption of excessive alcohol and smoking should be offered as these are risk factors associated with cardiac problems.
- Patients should be advised to have their blood pressure monitored regularly by the practice nurse.

Pharmacological intervention in the treatment of angina

The following medications could be prescribed for angina; it is the nurse's responsibility in the safe administration of these medicines to recognise and advise patients on the side effects of these drugs (Nursing and Midwifery Council, 2004).

- GTN is administered as tablets (sublingual) or sprays and it is quick-acting drug which dilates blood vessels and improves blood flow.
- A statin group of drugs such as simvastatin may be prescribed to lower blood cholesterol (Scottish Intercollegiate Guidelines Network, 2007).
- Aspirin may be prescribed to reduce platelet aggregation (sticking together).
- Beta-blocker drugs may be prescribed to decrease heart rate and to reduce the workload of the heart (Scottish Intercollegiate Guidelines Network, 2007).

Other treatments such as bypass surgery and balloon angioplasty may be performed if the medications are ineffective in controlling the angina or if the conditions get progressively worse.

Conclusion

The overall aim of this chapter was to provide the reader with insight into some related problems of the heart. In order to help patients with cardiac problems, nurses need an in-depth knowledge about the normal anatomy and physiology of the heart in order for them to recognise the related dysfunctions and to provide the appropriate nursing care. There are numerous dysfunctions associated with the heart and it is not the remit of this chapter to address all of these dysfunctions. Some of the common conditions are discussed with their associated nursing management. Nurses are often in the forefront in delivering high-quality care for patients with cardiac problems, and it is their duty to ensure that have a sound knowledge base and they are confident in delivering safe and effective individualised care. Nurses care for patient with cardiac problems in both hospital and community settings. Nurses need to recognise various signs and symptoms quickly and take immediate action to prevent any further complications arising from the illness. Ongoing assessment and evaluation of nursing interventions are important in order to respond to the changing need of the patient, which may have implications for patient outcome.

Multiple choice questions

1. Which of the following sequences is correct to describe the blood flow through the heart?
(a) right atrium → left atrium → left ventricle → right ventricle
(b) right atrium → right ventricle → left atrium → left ventricle
(c) left atrium → right ventricle → left ventricle → right atrium
(d) left ventricle → right ventricle → right atrium → left atrium

2. After mowing the lawn a patient complains of severe chest pain. This is the result of:
(a) pericardial effusion
(b) pulmonary emboli
(c) myocardial ischaemia
(d) pulmonary oedema

3. In planning the care for the client with acute MI, which of the following is of the highest priority of care?
(a) to stabilise oxygen saturation level
(b) to relieve anxiety of the patient
(c) to give immediate pain relief
(d) to record his vital signs

4. If the cardiac muscle is deprived of its normal blood supply, damage would primarily result from:
(a) an inadequate supply of carbon dioxide
(b) an inadequate supply of oxygen
(c) an inadequate supply of nutrients
(d) an inadequate supply of vitamins

5. How long can cardiac muscle cells withstand ischaemic conditions before cellular death takes place?
(a) about 20 minutes
(b) about 1 hour
(c) about 30 seconds
(d) about 5 minutes

6. The backward effect of left ventricular failure leads to:
(a) systemic oedema
(b) ascites
(c) pulmonary oedema
(d) increased cardiac output

7. Cardiac output depends on:
(a) atrial and brain natriuretic peptides
(b) cytokines and vasopressin
(c) decreased end-diastolic pressure and decreased afterload
(d) heart rate and stroke volume

8. To produce energy in cardiogenic shock, cells utilise:
(a) aerobic metabolism
(b) anaerobic metabolism
(c) cellular transport
(d) simple diffusion

9. The objective in the management of cardiogenic shock is to:
(a) protect the myocardial tissue from further damage
(b) increase the fluid load
(c) increase the oxygen demand of the myocardium
(d) increase the heart rate

10. Angina pectoris is chest pain caused by:
(a) myocardial ischaemia
(b) infection of the blood
(c) platelet adhesions
(d) hypertrophy of the myocardial cells

Answers: 1.b, 2.d, 3.c, 4.b, 5.a, 6.c, 7.d, 8.b, 9.a, 10.a.

Test your knowledge

❷ How does the heart rate affect the cardiac output?

❷ Explain the differences between ischaemia and infarction.

❷ Explain how the backward effect causes pulmonary oedema.

❷ Define cardiongenic shock and list the possible causes.

❷ What advice would you give a patient with congestive heart failure?

Glossary of terms

Aetiology: The cause of a disease.

Alveolar sac: A small sac structure in the lungs where gas exchange takes place.

Anaerobic metabolism: Metabolism by the body cells in the absence of oxygen.

Antidiuretic hormone: A protein hormone which is produced in the hypothalamus, stored in the posterior pituitary gland and aids reabsorption of water by the kidneys.

Arteries: Blood vessels that carry blood away from the heart.

Atherosclerosis: A condition where cholesterol and lipid deposits accumulate on the inner layer of the medium and large blood vessels leading to narrowing of these vessels.

Athromatous plaque: Collection of lipids and cholesterol that accumulate in large- and medium-sized vessels.

Ascites: Accumulation of fluid in the peritoneal cavity.

Atria: The upper chambers of the heart.

Atrioventricular valve: A heart valve made up of membranous flaps that allow blood to flow in one direction only, also known as bicuspid valve.

Bicuspid valve: As its name suggests it contains two cusps, also know as atrioventricular valve.

Bronchospasm: Constriction of the walls of the bronchi.

Collagens: A protein that is the main organic component of connective tissues.

Dyspnoea: Shortness of breath; laboured breathing.

Endocardium: Endothelial membrane that lines the inner surface of the heart.

Inferior vena cava: The large vein that returns oxygen-poor blood all parts of the body below the diaphragm to the right atrium.

Interstitial space: The space between the cells.

Intracellular space: The space found within the cell.

Lactic acid: Product of anaerobic metabolism, especially in the muscle.

Mediastinum: A subdivision of the thoracic cavity.

Medulla oblongata: Lowest portion of the brain, concerned with control of internal organs.

Mitral valve: The left atrioventricular valve.

Molecules: Particles containing two or more atoms joined together by chemical bonds.

Myocardial infarction: Gross necrosis of myocardial tissue due to interruption of blood supply to the affected area.

Myocardium: The middle layer of the heart.

Oliguria: Deficient secretion of urine, less than 30 mL/hour.

Orthopnea: Difficulty in breathing unless in an upright position.

Pacemaker: The sinoatrial node.

Parasympathetic nerve: A division of the autonomic nervous system.

Parietal: Pertaining to the walls of a cavity.

Pericardium: Double-layered sac that encloses the heart.

Pulmonary artery: The vessel that takes oxygen-poor blood from the right ventricle to the lungs.

Pulmonary circulation: The flow of blood from the right ventricle to the lungs.

Pulmonary oedema: Abnormal collection of fluid in the tissue space and the alveolar sac.

Pulmonary vein: The vessel that returns oxygenated blood from the lungs to the left atrium.

Semilunar valve: Valves that prevent the backflow of blood to the ventricles after contraction.

Septum: A wall dividing the two cavities.

Sinoatrial node: Also known as the pacemaker of the heart.

Superior vena cava: The large vein that returns oxygen-poor blood superior to the diaphragm to the right atrium.

Sympathetic nerve: A division of the autonomic nervous system.

Systemic circulation: The flow of blood from the left ventricle to all parts of the body.

Tissue perfusion: Blood flow through body tissues and organs.

Tricuspid valve: The right atrioventricular valve.

Vasoconstriction: Narrowing of the blood vessel.

Ventricles: The two larger lower cavities of the heart.

References

Adams, M.P., Holland, L.N. and Bostwick, P.M. (2008). *Pharmacology for Nurses: A Pathophysiologic Approach*, 2nd edn. New Jersey: Pearson Prentice Hall.

Alexander, M.F., Fawcett, J. and Runciman, P.J. (2006). *Nursing Practice – Hospitals and Home*, 3rd edn. Edinburgh: Churchill Livingstone.

Bullock, B.A. and Henze, R.L. (2000). *Focus on Pathophysiology*. Philadelphia: Lippincott.

Elton, J. (2003). *Care Deliver: The Needs of the Mature Adult*. London: Arnold.

Hogan, M.A. and Hill, K. (2004). *Pathophysiology – Reviews and Rationales*. New Jersey: Prentice Hall.

Hollenberg, S.M., Kavinsky, C.J. and Parrillo, J.E. (1999). Cardiogenic shock. *Annual International Medicine*, *131*(1), 47–59.

Jenkins, G.W., Kemnitz, C.P. and Tortora, G.J. (2007). *Anatomy and Physiology*. New Jersey: John Wiley & Sons.

Kozier, B., Erb, G., Berman, A. and Snyder, S.J. (2004). *Fundamentals of Nursing*. New Jersey: Pearson Prentice Hall.

Lemone, P. and Burke, B. (2004). *Medical and Surgical Nursing – Critical Thinking in Client Care*. New Jersey: Pearson Education.

Marieb, E.N. and Hoehn, K. (2007). *Human Anatomy and Physiology*, 7th edn. San Francisco: Pearson Benjamin Cummings.

McCance, K.L. and Huether, S.E. (2006). *Pathophysiology: The Biological Basis for Disease in Adults and Children*, 5th edn. St Lewis: Mosby.

McSweeney, J.C., Marisue, C., O'Sullivan, P., Elberson, K., Moser, D.K. and Garvin, B.J. (2003). Women's early warning symptoms of acute myocardial infarction. *Cirulcation*, *108*, 2619–2623.

National Institute for Health and Clinical Excellence (2003). *Chronic Heart Failure*. National Clinical Guidelines for diagnosis and management in primary and secondary care. Guideline No 5. London: NICE.

Nowak, T.J. and Handford, A.G. (1999). *Essentials of Pathophysiology: Concepts and Applications for Health Care Professionals*, 2nd edn. Boston: McGraw-Hill.

Nursing and Midwifery Council (2004). *Guidelines for Administration of Medicines*. London: NMC.

Nursing and Midwifery Council (2005). *Guideline for Record and Record Keeping*. London: NMC.

Porth, C.M. (2005). *Pathophysiology: Concepts of Altered Health States*, 7th edn. Philadelphia: Lippincott Williams & Wilkins.

Scottish Intercollegiate Guidelines Network (SIGN) (2007). *Management of Stable Angina*. Edinburgh: Scottish Intercollegiate Guidelines Network.

Tortora, G.J. and Derrickson, B. (2006). *Principles of Anatomy and Physiology*. New Jersey: John Wiley & Sons.

Waugh, A. and Grant, A. (2006). *Ross and Wilson: Anatomy and Physiology in Health and Illness*, 10th edn. Edinburgh: Churchill Livingstone.

Chapter 6

The vascular system and associated disorders

Muralitharan Nair

KEY WORDS

- Arteries
- Arterioles
- Tunica media
- Vasodilatation

- Veins
- Venules
- Tunica intima
- Vasoconstriction

- Capillaries
- Tunica externa
- Aorta

Test your prior knowledge

- List three differences between arteries and veins.
- Can you name the arteries that transport oxygen-poor blood and the veins that transport oxygen-rich blood?
- Between the arteries or veins, which one has a greater volume of blood?

Learning outcomes

On completion of this section, the reader will be able to:

■ Describe the structures of the arteries, veins and capillaries.

■ List some of the differences between an artery and a vein.

■ How do venous valves function?

■ Describe the factors controlling blood vessel diameter.

■ Explain the microcirculation of the blood.

Introduction

Although the heart is the principle organ that pumps blood to the whole body, it is the blood vessels that transport blood throughout the system (see Figure 6.1). As the blood flows through the arterial system, it transports nutrients and other substances essential for cellular metabolism and for homeostatic regulation. The waste products of metabolism are transported by the venous system for removal by the kidneys, lungs and the skin. This chapter discusses the structure and functions of the blood vessels, factors affecting blood pressure, vascular disorders and their related care. Where appropriate, the arteries and veins are collectively called blood vessels.

Overview of blood vessels

In the human body there are several kinds of blood vessels. They are **arteries** and **arterioles** and these vessels convey blood away from the heart. They transport oxygen-rich (oxygenated) blood except the pulmonary artery which carries oxygen-poor blood. **Veins** and **venules** carry blood towards the heart and transports oxygen-poor (deoxygenated) blood, except the pulmonary veins which carries oxygenated blood. **Capillaries** are minute blood vessels where arteries terminate and veins begin. They form a delicate network of vessels and are in proximity to most parts of the body tissues. Blood vessels can dilate, constrict, pulsate and form a closed delivery system for the blood which begins and ends at the heart.

Structure of the blood vessels

Blood vessels are composed of three distinct layers except the capillaries (Marieb and Hoehn, 2007) and a central **lumen** through which blood flows (see Figure 6.2). These layers are named **tunica externa**, formally known as tunica adventitia. It is largely composed of **collagen fibres** that protect, supports the blood vessels and secures them to surrounding tissues. The tunica externa is supplied with sympathetic nerve fibres, lymphatic vessels and the larger veins are also supplied with elastic fibres (Jenkins *et al.*, 2007). The **tunica media** is the middle layer and it contains smooth muscles and elastic tissue. The sympathetic nervous system (SNS) also innervates the smooth muscle layer and controls the diameter of the blood vessel (Marieb, 2006). As the blood vessels constrict or dilate the blood pressure increases

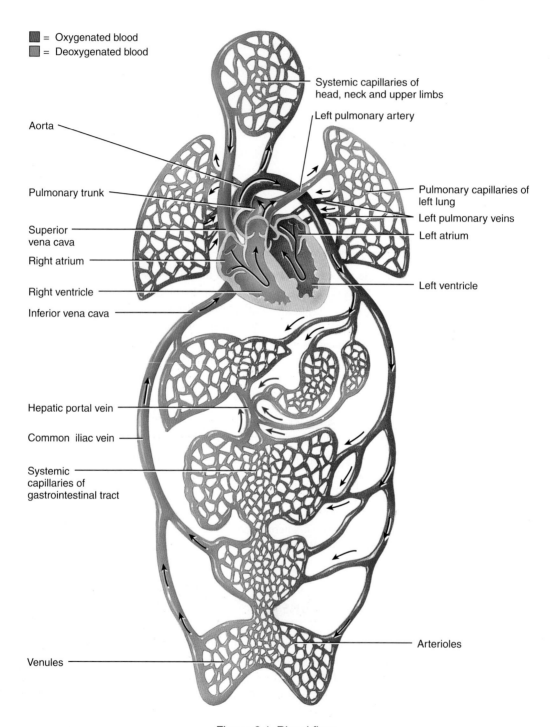

Figure 6.1 Blood flow.

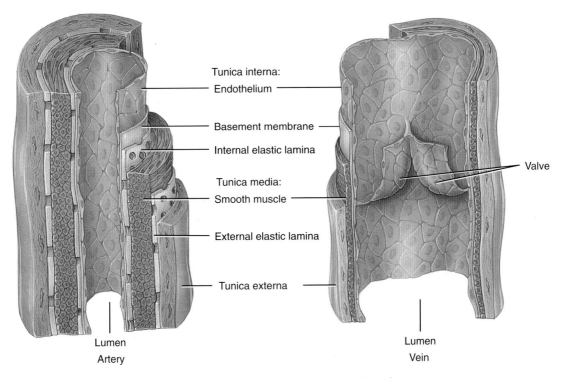

Figure 6.2 Structures of an artery and a vein.

or decreases, respectively. The inner layer is called **tunica interna** and it is lined with **endothelium**. This lining makes the inner surface smooth, thus minimising friction as the blood flows through the vessel.

Although the role of the blood vessels is to transport blood, the tunica externa of the large blood vessels receive their blood supply via a network of blood vessels called vasa vasorum. They provide nutrients to this part of the blood vessels. Vessels with thin walls receive oxygen and nutrients by diffusion from the blood passing through the lumen.

Arteries

Arteries can be subdivided into three groups, namely elastic arteries, muscular arteries and arterioles. Elastic arteries are thick-walled vessels found near the heart of which the **aorta** is the main artery. These vessels contain a high proportion of elastic fibres in the tunica media. Their larger lumen provides low resistance to blood flow, thus propelling blood onward (see Figure 6.3). This ensures that the blood is moving forward even though the left ventricle is relaxed. As these arteries conduct blood from the left ventricle to small arteries, they are sometimes referred to as conducting arteries.

From the elastic arteries the blood flows into the medium-sized arteries called the muscular arteries. They contain more smooth muscles and fewer elastic fibres; therefore, they are capable of greater **vasoconstriction** and **vasodilatation**. Muscular arteries are also called distributing arteries because they distribute blood to specific organs and parts of the body. They include axillary, brachial, radial, splenic, femoral, popliteal and tibial arteries.

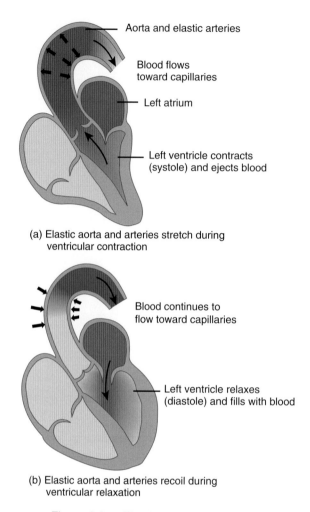

(a) Elastic aorta and arteries stretch during
ventricular contraction

(b) Elastic aorta and arteries recoil during
ventricular relaxation

Figure 6.3   Elastic recoil of the aorta.

The muscular arteries then divide into smaller arteries called the arterioles and they play an important role in determining the amount of blood flowing into organs and tissues. Arterioles will branch into smaller arteries and direct the flow of blood into the capillaries (see Figure 6.4). Larger arterioles have all the three layers but the tunica media mainly consists of smooth muscle with a few elastic fibres, whilst the arterioles near the capillary end are composed of endothelial cells and incomplete layer of smooth muscle (Jenkins *et al.*, 2007). Arterioles regulate the blood flow into the capillaries by altering the diameter of the capillaries. When they constrict, blood flow is diverted from organs or tissue they supply. On the other hand, blood flow increases dramatically when the arterioles dilate.

Capillaries

Capillaries are the smallest network of blood vessels with walls mostly one cell thick and they connect the arteriole to the venule (see Figure 6.1). The thin walls of the capillaries allow water, nutrients, gases and waste products of metabolism to move in and out of the blood and to nearby cells (Jenkins

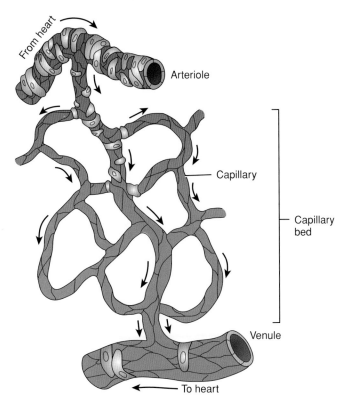

Figure 6.4 Capillaries.

et al., 2007). Capillaries are composed of a single layer of tunica intima and they are found throughout the body except the epidermis of the skin and the cornea of the eye. Capillaries merge to form venules (see Figure 6.4).

Venules

Blood flows from the capillaries to the venules (see Figure 6.4). The smallest venules are mainly composed of endothelium and a few **fibroblast cells**. The venules are extremely porous and therefore will allow substance such as water, solutes and white blood cells to move in and out of the vessel into the **extracellular fluid**.

Veins

Venules unite to form veins and they contain the same three layers as the arteries. The walls of the veins, compared to the arteries, are thinner and contain less elastic and collagenous tissues and smooth muscles. The lumen of the veins are larger compared to the lumen of the arteries. Veins become larger and less branched as they move away from the capillaries and towards the heart. Some veins, most commonly in the lower extremities, contain paired semilunar bicuspid valves (see Figure 6.5) that allow blood flow towards the heart. Like arteries, veins receive their nourishment from tiny blood vessels called vasa vasorum (McCance and Huether, 2006).

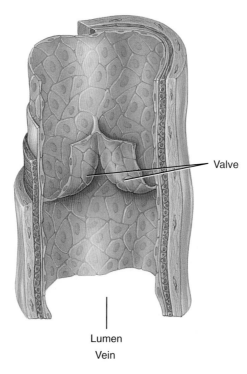

Figure 6.5   Bicuspid valves of a vein.

Blood pressure

Blood pressure (BP) refers to the force exerted by the circulating blood on the walls of the blood vessel. As the blood moves through the arteries, arterioles, capillaries, venules and veins the blood pressure drops and thus the term *blood pressure* refers to arterial blood pressure and it is usually measured in the larger arteries. BP fluctuates during the day and it depends on the state of the health of the individual. The blood pressure is low when the person is sleeping at night and increases as the person is awake in the morning. There are three main factors that regulate blood pressure and they include:

- neuronal regulation
- hormonal regulation
- autoregulation of blood pressure

The neuronal regulation of BP is via a negative feedback system which includes **baroreceptors** and the **chemoreceptors**. The baroreceptors are located in the carotid sinus and the aortic arch and they are sensitive to arterial blood pressure changes. The chemoreceptors are located in the aortic and carotid bodies. These bodies detect changes in the oxygen, carbon dioxide and hydrogen ion concentrations. There are several hormones involved in the regulation of BP and they include rennin–angiotensin system, adrenaline and noradrenaline, antidirutic hormone and atrial natriuretic peptide.

Factors that can affect blood pressure

Several factors affect blood pressure and they include:

■ cardiac output
■ circulating volume
■ peripheral resistance
■ blood viscosity
■ hydrostatic pressure

Other factors that can affect BP include age, gender, stress, hormones and drugs.

Diseases of the blood vessels

Learning outcomes

On completion of this section, the reader will be able to:

■ List some of the common diseases of the blood vessels and the risk factors associated with these diseases.
■ Describe the pathophysiological responses associated with specific vascular health problems.
■ Outline the nursing management and interventions of the disorders.

Atherosclerosis/arteriosclerosis

Arteriosclerosis is a term describing arterial disorders in which degenerative changes result in decreased blood flow (Paradiso, 1999). **Atherosclerosis** is the most common form of arteriosclerosis where there is thickening and hardening of the vessel walls due to lipid accumulation. This condition is found mainly in the large- and medium-sized arteries such as the aorta and its branches, the coronary arteries and the arteries that supply the brain whereas arteriosclerosis mainly affects arterioles (Nowak and Handford, 1999).

Aetiology

The real cause of atherosclerosis is not known, but certain risk factors have been identified and they include:

■ hypertension
■ cigarette smoking (nicotine has a vasoconstricting effect)
■ high lipid levels in the blood
■ familial history
■ obesity
■ diabetes mellitus (high serum glucose levels cause vascular damage)
■ life style
■ alcohol
■ men are at a higher risk than women

Investigations

The following investigations may be done to confirm diagnosis.

- full blood chemistry
- Doppler ultrasound
- electrocardiogram
- arteriogram

Pathophysiology of atherosclerosis

Atherosclerosis is a form of arteriosclerosis where the walls of the arteries are hard, thick and narrow as a result of lipid accumulation within the arterial walls. Lipids (low-density lipoproteins) are deposited on the tunica intima of the damaged blood vessel where **oxidation** of low-density lipoproteins (LDL) takes place. The oxidised LDL then enters into the tunica intima of the arterial wall (Jowett and Thompson, 2003) where they are ingested by **macrophages**. The lipid-filled macrophages then become foam cells.

Once the foam cells accumulate in significant numbers, they form a lesion called fatty streak which over time causes a bulge in the lumen of the vessel which restricts blood flow. Affected blood vessels become hard, loose their elasticity, restrict blood flow and eventually occlude the artery (see Figure 6.6). Greater blood pressure is needed to push the blood through these narrow blood vessels, which leads to **hypertension**. Although atherosclerosis can affect any organ or tissue, the arteries supplying the heart, brain, small intestines, kidneys and the lower extremities are mostly affected. See Table 6.1 for the effected sites.

Signs and symptoms of atherosclerosis

- diminished or absent pulses
- skin is pallor or cyanosed
- pain
- muscle weakness

Nursing management

A full nursing history is essential in order to provide high-quality care for patients with atherosclerosis. The nursing assessment must include identifying risk factors and symptoms of any cardiovascular disease. The nursing management includes:

- Health promotion in relation to preventing the disease must include advice on a healthy diet and regulating the lipid levels within normal range (Dyson, 2002). Regular physical examination with their GP in order to monitor their blood pressure and cholesterol levels should be encouraged.
- Advice on the cessation of smoking and alcohol consumption should be offered as they are identified risk factors in atherosclerosis.
- Patients should be advised to loose weight if obesity is a problem (Caterson, 2005).
- Encourage patient to undertake programmed exercise under the supervision of the practice nurse. This would help in lowering their weight, lowering their cholesterol level, reducing their blood pressure and reducing their stress.

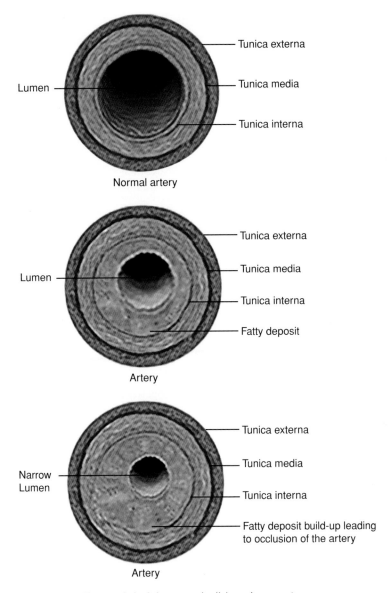

Figure 6.6 Atheroma build-up in an artery.

Pharmacological interventions for atherosclerosis

The aim of medications in the treatment of atherosclerosis is to restore blood flow and preventing the disease. The medications include:

- antihypertensives such as beta-blockers
- anticoagulant therapy with heparin
- lipid-lowering drugs such as simvastatin
- antiplatelet drugs

Site	Effects
Abdominal aorta	Gangrene of toes and feet Aneurysms
Aortoiliac and femoral arteries	Intermittent claudication Gangrene of toes and feet Aneurysms of iliac arteries
Coronary arteries	Myocardial infarction Angina pectoris
Carotid and vertebral arteries	Cerebrovascular accident Transient ischaemic attack
Renal artery	Hypertension, renal ischaemia
Mesenteric arteries	Intestinal ischaemia
Adapted from Bullock and Henze (2000).	

Table 6.1 Effects of atherosclerosis on different sites

In some patients, surgical procedures such as balloon angioplasty may be indicated to improve the blood flow through the vessel.

Hypertension

Hypertension refers to sustained elevation in systemic arterial blood pressure (McCance and Huether, 2006). The elevation may be in either systolic or diastolic pressure or in both pressures. A normal upper limit for an adult is 130–139/85–89 mm Hg (Alexander *et al.*, 2006) and any readings consistently above this is considered as hypertension. There are many classifications of hypertension and some are classified according to their severity, for example mild or moderate. Some of the types include:

- Primary or essential hypertension.
- Secondary hypertension where there is an underlying cause such as renal diseases or tumour of the adrenal medulla.
- Malignant hypertension occurs in the younger age groups with renal and collagen disease.
- Isolated systolic hypertension mainly occurs from a combination of factors seen in the elderly due to increases in cardiac output, increased peripheral resistance and renal vascular resistance. Other possible causes include **Paget's disease** of the bone and beriberi (McCance and Huether, 2006).

NOTE

Blood pressure = cardiac output × peripheral vascular resistance
(BP = CO × PVR)

Aetiology of hypertension

Although the cause or causes of primary hypertension is unknown, several risk factors have been identified for its development such as:

- obesity
- stress
- cigarette smoking and alcohol consumption
- excessive intake of sodium causing fluid retention
- family history

Secondary hypertension results from underlying causes such as:

- renal diseases
- Cushing's syndrome
- hypo/hyperthyroidism
- oral contraceptives
- excessive alcohol consumption
- coarctation (narrowing) of the aorta

Investigations

These include:

- full blood chemistry
- physical examination
- electrocardiogram
- assessment of risk factors

Common presenting symptoms

Many patients are unaware that they have hypertension and go untreated. They ignore symptoms such as headache, dizziness, nosebleed and fatigue. It is frequently identified through blood pressure screening or as a result of other diseases. Some patients have reported blurred visions and tinnitus, but usually when symptoms of hypertension do occur the disease is in advance stage (Bullock and Henze, 2000).

Pathophysiology of hypertension

Primary hypertension

Primary hypertension results from a combination of genetic and environmental factors which have an effect on renal and vascular functions and it accounts for 95% of the cases. One of the possible causes of primary hypertension includes the deficiency in the kidney's ability to excrete sodium which increases extracellular fluid volume and cardiac output resulting in an increase in blood flow to the tissues. The increased blood flow to the tissues results in arteriolar constriction and an increase in peripheral vascular resistance (PVR) and blood pressure (Nowak and Handford, 1999).

Secondary hypertension

Secondary hypertension accounts for 5% of the cases and is caused by diseases of the organs resulting in raised PVR and increased cardiac output. In most cases, the focus is on kidney diseases or excessive levels of hormones such as aldosterone and cortisol. These hormones stimulate the retention of sodium and water resulting in increased blood volume and blood pressure. Once the underlying cause is treated such as the removal of the deceased organ, the blood pressure returns to normal.

Malignant hypertension

This is a rapidly progressive hypertension where the diastolic pressure is in excess of 120 mm Hg (Waugh and Grant, 2006) which could result in encephalopathy, cerebral oedema and loss of consciousness. Malignant hypertension does not indicate that there is cellular injury, but because it is life-threatening, it is considered as an emergency. If untreated, cerebral oedema and cerebral dysfunction occurs leading to death of the individual. Malignant hypertension can cause a variety of complications, for example **papilloedema**, cardiac failure, cerebrovascular accident and retinopathy.

Isolated systolic hypertension

This is caused by an increase in cardiac output or PVR and has a higher incidence in the old age group. The rigidity of the vessels is often caused by atherosclerosis. The ageing process leads to hardening of the arteries, increased PVR and decreased baroreceptor sensitivity. In isolated systolic hypertension, the systolic blood pressure of over 140 mm Hg and a diastolic pressure of less than 90 mm Hg (Hogan and Hill, 2004). It is recognised as an important risk factor for cerebrovascular accident and cardiac failure and thus should be treated as a medical emergency.

Nursing management of hypertension

Non-pharmacological interventions of hypertension

- A single recording of raised blood pressure does not indicate that the patient is suffering from hypertension. To confirm it requires at least three recordings of raised blood pressure at different intervals to indicate hypertension. Some doctors will monitor patient's blood pressure using a 24-hour ambulatory monitoring device. This measurement is much more accurate than the blood pressure measurements done in the clinic (Wilkinson *et al.*, 2002).
- Advice the patient to restrict sodium intake as it promotes water retention resulting in increased circulating volume and increased cardiac output which leads to hypertension.
- Nurses need to advise the patient on the cessation of cigarette smoking and excessive alcohol consumption. Both are identified as risk factors for hypertension.
- Weight reduction through exercise, in obese patients, should be encouraged as exercise helps in the reduction of weight (BMI should be less than 25), in lowering cholesterol levels and the control of any underlying problems such as diabetes mellitus (National Institute for Clinical Excellence, 2002). Encourage patients to have their weights checked weekly.
- Dietary advice should be offered to the patient. A diet rich in fruits and vegetables and low in saturated fats can help in the reduction of blood pressure. Reduction of salt in cooking should be encouraged as excessive intake of salt promotes fluid retention thus increasing circulating volume.
- Encourage patient to reduce their stress levels because relaxation aids in the reduction of blood pressure by decreasing the workload of the heart. Listening to music, gardening and or even going for walks have all been identified in the reduction of blood pressure.

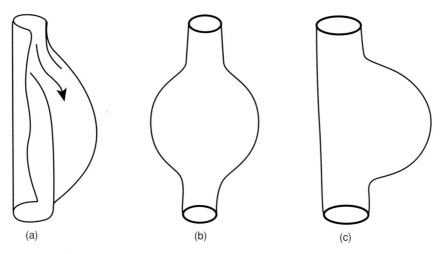

Figure 6.7 (a) A dissecting aneurysm; (b) a fusiform aneurysm; and (c) a saccular aneurysm.

Pharmacological interventions in hypertension

In some patients, non-pharmacological interventions are sufficient in controlling their blood pressure while in others, combinations of both pharmacological and non-pharmacological methods are used in the treatment of hypertension. The medications include:

■ Diuretics are prescribed to reduce fluid load which leads to reduction in cardiac output, thus helping to reduce blood pressure.
■ Medications, for example beta-blockers, calcium channel-blockers and ACE inhibitor drugs are indicted for the treatment of hypertension (Jackson *et al.*, 2005).

Aneurysm

An **aneurysm** is a permanent dilatation of an artery or a chamber of the heart. Although it can occur in both arteries and veins, the aorta and the arteries at the base of the brain are the vessels most susceptible to aneurysms. It can occur in a localised part of the aorta or all along the vessel (Alexander *et al.*, 2006) because it is under constant pressure. The commonest cause of an aneurysm is atherosclerosis because the fatty deposits erodes and weaken the vessel wall. Aneurysms can be classified according to their shape (see Figures 6.7(a)–6.7(c)) and they include:

■ Fusiform – involves the entire circumference of the vessel.
■ Saccular – appears only on one part or side.
■ Dissecting – is a false aneurysm resulting from a tear in the tunica intima.

Aetiology of aneurysm

There are several causes and they include:

■ Atherosclerosis – main cause of an aneurysm affecting the descending aorta.
■ Infection – mainly due to syphilis affecting the ascending aorta.
■ Hypertension – due to constant pressure weakening of the vessel wall can occur in the elderly.

■ Cystic medial degeneration – it mainly affects thoracic aorta by a disorder called Marfan's syndrome. It affects the elastic fibres of the tunica media.

Investigations

These include:

■ full blood chemistry
■ angiography
■ ultrasound
■ chest X-ray

Symptoms related to aneurysms

Most aortic aneurysms are asymptomatic until they start to leak or rapture and the symptoms vary depending on the affected vessel. Symptoms may include:

■ pain in the abdominal region or in the extremities due to comprehension of neighbouring organs
■ dyspnoea (breathlessness) due to pressure on internal organs
■ dysphagia (difficulty in swallowing)
■ signs and symptoms of cerebrovascular accident occur if the cerebral arteries are affected

Nursing management

The main treatment for an aneurysm is surgery, and therefore it is vital that a full assessment of the patient is obtained. The surgery may include insertion of a graft (see Figure 6.8). It is the nurse's duty in the safe preparation of the patient for theatre to ensure all the relevant protocols of the individual hospital and the Nursing and Midwifery guidelines are adhered to. All care given is documented in accordance with the Nursing and Midwifery Council (2005).

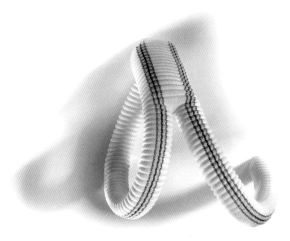

Figure 6.8 Dacron graft for an abdominal aortic aneurysm. Synthetic graft used for surgery, reproduced with permission from Vascutek.

Postoperatively nurses should monitor the following:

- ABC – airway, breathing and circulation
- fluid and nutritional management
- elimination
- pain management
- wound management
- detect early signs of postoperative complications of chest infection, deep vein thrombosis and wound infection
- communication
- documentation
- safe preparation of the patient for discharge

Pharmacological interventions for an aneurysm

The following medications may be prescribed for a patient with an aneurysm.

- antihypertensive
- anticoagulants
- antibiotics
- analgesics

Peripheral vascular disease

Peripheral vascular disease (PVD) is a condition where the blood flow is affected in both arteries and veins. The disorders include arterial occlusions due to arterial and venous insufficiency, varicose veins and Raynaud's disease.

Aetiology of PVD

The causes of PVD include:

- cardiovascular disease
- thrombi
- pulmonary disease
- prolonged standing

Investigations

These include:

- Doppler ultrasound
- arteriogram/venogram
- full blood chemistry
- physical examinations
- electrocardiogram

	Arterial	Venous
Pain	Sudden severe pain, rest pain, intermittent claudication	Aching and cramp relieved by elevating the foot
Pulse	Diminished or absent	Present
Ulcer characteristics	Mainly in the toes, feet or other areas of the skin	Mainly over the inner or outer ankle
Skin characteristics	Shiny, cool or cold temperature; mild oedema if present	Thick and tough; skin normal colour; may have oedema, warm to touch
Complications	Gangrene	Poor healing
Blood flow	Doppler pressure readings lower below blockage	Normal pressure reading

Adapted from Hogan and Hill (2004).

Table 6.2 Comparison between an arterial and venous insufficiency

Pathophysiology of PVD

Arterial insufficiency

Any occlusions of the artery due to a thrombus or atherosclerosis results in diminished blood flow through that vessel. As the blood flows with reduced pressure, it could lead to complications such as formation of a thrombus which could occlude the flow of blood in the vessel. The lower limbs are most susceptible to arterial occlusion. The affected limbs are prone to arterial ulcers as a result of tissue hypoxia. A more severe blockage could lead to the development of gangrene usually in the toe (Stubbling and Chesworth, 2003). Venous insufficiency may occur as the result of an obstruction in the veins by a thrombus or incompetent valves, which could lead to the formation of a venous ulcer as a result of poor circulation. There are distinct differences between an arterial and a venous insufficiency (see Table 6.2).

Signs and symptoms of arterial insufficiency
- intermittent claudication
- white, pale colour when legs are elevated
- ulcers on the leg (see Table 6.2)
- absent pedal pulses
- numbness and cold extremity
- thickened toenails

Nursing management of arterial insufficiency

Pain control is paramount in patients with arterial insufficiency. If pain is caused by exercise such as walking long distances, then they should be advised against it (Gibson and Kenrick, 1998). However, light exercise which they can tolerate should be encouraged as it helps to improve circulation. Patients should be advised to keep themselves warm if they are affected by cold weather, but they should avoid the following:

- Avoid tight fitting clothing as it restricts arterial blood flow.
- Avoid cigarette smoking as it may cause vasoconstriction.
- Avoid very clod temperatures as it may cause vasoconstriction.
- Avoid having hot baths or sitting near fires because of the risk of burns with decreased sensation to the limbs.
- Avoid cutting their toenails as soft tissue damage may take place which may be difficult to heal because of poor peripheral circulation. Toenails should be cut by a chiropodist.
- Avoid sitting cross-legged for too long as it will restrict blood flow to the lower limbs.

A well-balanced healthy diet high in fruits, fibre and vegetables and low in saturated fat should be encouraged. Fluid intake of 2.5–3 L should be encouraged as dehydration causes increased viscosity of the blood which increases the risk of clot formation.

Some patients may require bypass surgery to treat the condition, which would involve using a vein or Dacron graft (see Figure 6.9) (Donohue, 1997). It is the nurse's duty in the safe preparation of the patient for theatre and their postoperative recovery. Postoperative complications should be reported and treated immediately to prevent undue harm to the patient.

Pharmacological interventions of PVD

Patients with PVD may have the following medications:

- vasodilators
- anticoagulants
- antiplatelet drugs

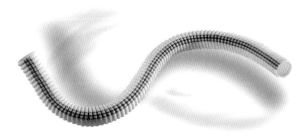

Figure 6.9 Dacron graft for PVD. Synthetic graft used for surgery, reproduced with permission from Vascutek.

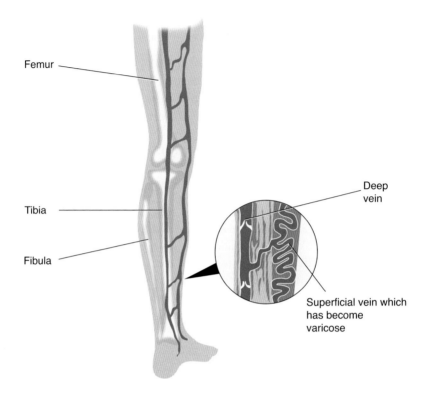

Figure 6.10 Varicose veins.

Venous insufficiency/varicose veins

Varicose veins are vessels that have become dilated and tortuous due to incompetent valves resulting in pooling of blood in the veins. This mainly happens in the saphenous veins of the leg, deep communicating veins and superficial veins (see Figure 6.10). Varicosity in these vessels is caused by damaged valves which allow back flow and pooling of blood to take place. One possible cause of venous distension is prolonged standing which diminishes the action of the calf-muscle pump (see Figure 6.11) (Vowden and Vowden, 2003). The calf-muscle pump aids venous return to the heart.

People who are susceptible to varicose veins are pregnant women, people who are obese, those who have to stand for a long period because of the nature of the occupation, for example theatre nurses, and the older age group. There is no conclusive evidence to suggest that varicosity is hereditary.

Veins affected with varicosity

Any vein in the leg can develop varicosity (see Figure 6.12); however, the common veins are:

- long saphenous veins
- short saphenous veins
- perforating veins

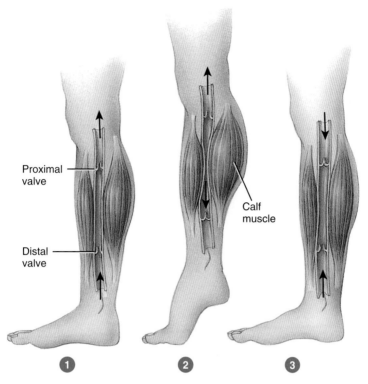

Figure 6.11 Calf-muscle pump.

Signs and symptoms of varicose veins

■ swelling of the lower extremities
■ distended and tortuous veins
■ dull aching in the leg
■ ulcers are rare
■ leg fatigue and heaviness

Complications of varicose veins

Complications such as venous ulcers, venous eczema, lipodermatosclerosis and skin pigmentation (see Figures 6.13(a)–6.13(c)) are seen in some patients with varicose veins. Untreated tissue necrosis and infection can occur.

Nursing management of varicose veins

In the UK, stripping and ligation of varicose veins are not routinely undertaken in the National Health Service unless it is a health risk; however, it can be treated privately. After surgery most patients return to normal routine within 1–3 weeks. Postoperative care includes applying pressure bandage for about 6 weeks, elevating the foot and gradually increasing ambulation (Lemone and Burke, 2004). The surgical

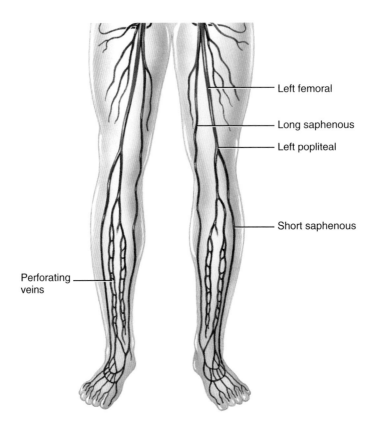

Left femoral

Long saphenous

Left popliteal

Short saphenous

Perforating veins

Figure 6.12 Veins of the leg susceptible to varicosity.

treatment is successful; however, 20–30% of the patients may require repeat surgery (London and Nash, 2000).

Pain should be managed by bed rest and elevation of the feet which improves venous return. Prolonged standing in one position should be discouraged and walking should be encouraged to activate calf-muscle pump which helps in venous flow (see Figure 6.10) and to reduce oedema. Supportive anti-embolism stockings should be worn to reduce swelling in the leg and to provide support to the veins. Patients who have had surgery should be encouraged to walk 2–3 miles/day to prevent complications such as DVT and should avoid standing in one position for a long period of time.

■ Encourage patients to stop smoking as the nicotine may cause vascular damage.
■ Encourage adequate fluid intake of 2–3 L and a healthy diet for tissue healing.
■ Avoid unnecessary trauma to the feet.
■ Inform patients not to cross their leg when seated as it restricts blood return.
■ Educating patients the benefits of regular exercise.
■ Encourage all patients to maintain normal weight for their height.

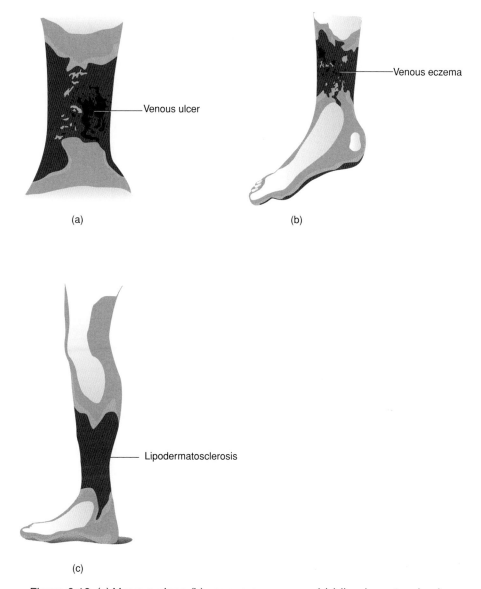

Figure 6.13 (a) Venous ulcer; (b) venous eczema; and (c) lipodermatosclerois.

Deep vein thrombosis

Deep vein thrombosis (DVT) is formation of a thrombus (clot) in the veins when the flow of blood is reduced. It primarily occurs in the veins of the lower extremity (see Figure 6.14) such as the femoral, popliteal and the deep veins of the pelvis (Porth, 2005).

Aetiology of DVT

DVT is associated with:

■ Stasis of blood in the veins which could result from immobility after surgery.

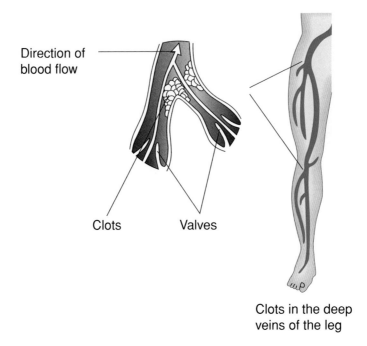

Clots in the deep
veins of the leg

Figure 6.14 Formation of thrombosis.

■ Obstruction to the flow of blood in the veins as a result of trauma.
■ Hypercoagulability of blood due to dehydration, hormone replacement therapy and oral contraceptive pills.
■ An increase in use of intravenous cannula may cause damage to the tunica intima resulting in the formation of clots.

Other factors include age (people over the age of 40 are at greater risk), obesity, pregnancy, varicose veins and smoking.

Pathophysiology of DVT

A thrombus can develop in the superficial or deep veins of the legs. The blood flow is sluggish in the affected vessels and **clotting cascade** takes place. Platelets aggregate at the site of injury to the vessel wall or where there is venous stasis (Lemone and Burke, 2004). Platelet aggregation occurs because platelets are exposed to collagen (a protein in the connective tissue which is found in the inner surface of the blood vessel). When platelets come into contact with the exposed collage, they release **adenosine diphosphate** and **thromboxane**. These substances make the surface of the platelets become sticky and as they adhere to each other a platelet plug is formed (see Figure 6.15). Other cells such as the red blood cells are trapped in the fibrin meshwork (see Figure 6.16) and the thrombus grows.

The thrombus triggers the inflammatory response causing tenderness, swelling and **erythema** at the affected site. Initially the thrombus stays within the affected area; however, fragments of the thrombus

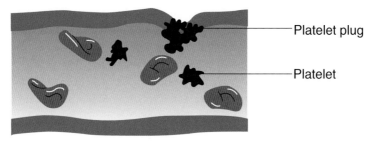

Formation of a platelet plug

Figure 6.15 Platelet plug.

may become loose and travel through the circulation as an emboli (Tiernay *et al.*, 2001) which may lodge in the lungs and cause a pulmonary embolism.

Signs and symptoms of DVT
The signs and symptoms of DVT are as follows:

- usually asymptomatic
- dull aching pain in the affected limb especially when walking
- oedema of the affected leg
- cyanosis of the affected leg
- redness and warmth on the affected part
- dilatation of the surface vein

Nursing management of DVT
- Maintain the patient on bed rest until mobilisation is encouraged.
- The nurse must monitor the vital signs (temperature, pulse, respiration and blood pressure) of the patient hourly to 2 hourly to prevent complications such as pulmonary embolism.

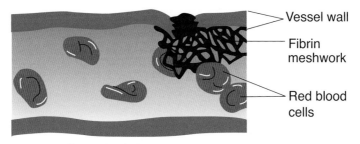

Formation of a clot

Figure 6.16 Fibrin meshwork.

■ Observe the calf muscle for swelling. Measure the circumference 10–20 cm above and below the knee. An accurate record of the measurements should be maintained in order to detect changes in the measurements for prompt interventions (Paradiso, 1999).

■ Elevate the foot to promote venous return and to reduce oedema.

■ The patient should be advised not to massage the affected calf muscle so as not to dislodge the clot.

■ The assessment of pain includes using Homan's sign which involves the patient lying flat with their legs straight and dorsiflexing the foot quickly (Alexander *et al.*, 2006). The test is positive if the patient complaints of pain in the calf.

■ Check with the patient every 4 hours for pain or any discomfort in the affected leg.

■ The patient should be advised to maintain fluid intake of 2–2.5 L/day to prevent dehydration.

■ Check to ensure that compression stockings are fitted correctly.

Pharmacological interventions for DVT

The following medications may be prescribed for the patient with DVT.

■ anticoagulants such as low-molecular-weight heparin
■ antiplatelet drugs
■ anti-inflammatory drugs
■ thrombolytic drugs

Conclusion

The overall aim of this chapter was to provide the learner an understanding into the vascular system and its related disorders. In order to care for the patient with vascular dysfunction, nurses need to understand the normal physiology of the vascular system. There are numerous diseases related to vascular system; however, it is not the remit of this chapter to cover all the disorders. Some of the main diseases are discussed with their related nursing management. The key role of the nurse is to provide comfort, offer advice and prevent complications that could be detrimental to the patient's health. Caring for patients with vascular disorders requires skilled nursing management which incorporates ongoing assessment, implementing and evaluating the care.

Multiple choice questions

1. Which of the following tissue contains connective tissue and smooth muscle cells?
(a) tunica intima
(b) tunica externa
(c) tunica media
(d) a and b

2. Which factor(s) influence(s) the resistance of blood flow?
(a) radius of the lumen
(b) length of the vessel
(c) blood viscosity
(d) a, b and c

3. The pathophysiology of hypertension is related to:
(a) baroreceptors
(b) endocrine system
(c) circulating fluid volume
(d) chemoreceptors

4. Low-density lipoproteins (LDLs) are known as bad cholesterol because:
(a) it contains equal amounts of protein and cholesterol
(b) it contains more cholesterol than proteins
(c) it contains more proteins than cholesterol
(d) none of the above

5. Fatty streak is the result of the accumulation of:
(a) red blood cells
(b) foam cells
(c) phagocytes
(d) lymphocytes

6. The commonest cause of an aneurysm in the descending aorta is:
(a) atherosclerosis
(b) diabetes mellitus
(c) Paget's disease
(d) syphilis

7. When assessing a patient with arterial disease the nurse must be aware that the risk factors may include:
(a) low-fat diet

(b) genetic predispositions

(c) high-carbohydrate diet

(d) high-protein diet

8. Nursing management of the patient with arteriosclerosis obliterans includes:

(a) elevation of the extremity

(b) administration of diuretics

(c) limit activity

(d) encourage activity

9. Priority teaching for a patient with Buerger's disease would include:

(a) wearing gloves if the extremities are cold and painful

(b) avoid wearing flat-heeled shoes

(c) cessation of smoking

(d) taking opioid analgesia for pain

10. Varicosity is caused by:

(a) incompetent valves

(b) lack of exercise

(c) poor left ventricular contraction

(d) mitral stenosis

11. The commonest cause of a thrombus is:

(a) arterial stasis, hypocoagulability and arterial wall injury

(b) myocardial infarction, failing heart and prolonged bed rest

(c) venous stasis, hypercoagulability and venous wall injury

(d) left ventricular failure arterial wall injury

Answers: 1.c, 2.d, 3.c, 4.b, 5.b, 6.a, 7.b, 8.d, 9.c, 10.a, 11.c.

Test your knowledge

❷ Describe the process of atherosclerotic occlusion of a vessel.

❷ List the possible causes of PVD.

❷ Describe the pathophysiology of hypertension.

❷ Briefly describe the pathophysiology of an aneurysm.

❷ Discuss the nursing management of the patient with varicose veins.

Glossary of terms

Adenosine diphosphate: A product of the hydrolysis of adenosine triphosphate.

Aneurysm: A localised dilatation of a blood vessel usually found in the aorta and the arteries at the base of the brain.

Atherosclerosis: It is a condition where cholesterol and lipid deposits accumulate on the inner layer of the medium- and large-sized blood vessels leading to narrowing of these vessels.

Aorta: The biggest artery that emerges from the left ventricle.

Arteries: These are blood vessels that carry blood away from the heart.

Arterioles: These are small arteries.

Arteriosclerosis: A condition in which there is thickening, hardening, loss of elasticity of the vessel wall leading to narrowing of the artery.

Baroreceptor: Neurone sensing changes in fluid, air and blood pressures.

Blood pressure: Force exerted by the blood against the walls of the blood vessel due to the contraction of the heart.

Capillaries: These are small blood vessels where exchanges between blood and tissue cells take place.

Chemoreceptor: Sensory receptor that detects the presence of specific chemical.

Clotting cascade: A series of steps in the clotting process of the blood.

Collagen fibres: The most abundant of the three fibres found in the connective tissues.

Endothelium: Single layer of simple squamous cells found in the heart, blood vessels and lymphatic vessels.

Erythema: A superficial redness of the skin.

Extracellular fluid: Fluid that surrounds and bathes body cells.

Fibroblast cells: The most common connective tissue cells and only found in the tendons.

Hypertension: Raised blood pressure.

Lumen: Cavity inside a blood vessel or a hollow organ.

Macrophages: Phagocytes produced from monocytes and is important in cellular initiation of the inflammatory response.

Oxidation: Chemical reaction where electrons are lost.

Padget disease: Disorder of the bone. Excessive remodelling of the bone causes enlarged and deformed bones and weakening of the bones leading to bone pain and fractures.

Papilloedema: Swelling of the optic disk in the eye.

Thromboxane: A compound synthesised in platelets from prostaglandin. It acts to aggregate platelet.

Tunica externa: Membranous outer layer of the blood vessel.

Tunica intima: The inner lining of a blood vessel.

Tunica media: Middle muscle layer of the blood vessel.

Vasoconstriction: Narrowing of blood vessel.

Vasodilatation: Dilatation of blood vessel due to smooth muscle relaxation.

Veins: These are blood vessels that carry blood to the heart.

Venules: These are small veins.

References

Alexander, M.F., Fawcett, J. and Runciman, P.J. (2006). *Nursing Practice – Hospitals and Home*. Edinburgh: Churchill Livingstone.

Bullock, B.A. and Henze, R.L. (2000). *Focus on Pathophysiology*. Philadelphia: Lippincott.

Caterson, I.D. (2005). Obesity in 2005 and in DOM. *Diabetes, Obesity and Metabolism*, *7*(3), 209–210.

Donohue, S.J. (1997). Lower limb amputation 3. The role of the nurse. *British Journal of Nursing*, *6*, 1171–1174, 1187–1191.

Dyson, P. (2002). Nutrition and diabetes control: Advice for non-diabetics. *British Journal of Community Nursing*, *7*(8), 414–419.

Gibson, J.M.E. and Kenrick, M. (1998). Pain and the powerlessness: The experience of living with peripheral vascular disease. *Journal of Advanced Nursing*, *27*(4), 737–745.

Hogan, M.A. and Hill, K. (2004). *Pathophysiology – Reviews and Rationales*. New Jersey: Prentice Hall.

Jackson, S., Bereznicki, L. and Peterson, G. (2005). Under-use of ACE-inhibitor and beta blocker therapies in congestive heart failure. *Australian Pharmacist*, *24*(12), 936.

Jenkins, G.W., Kemnitz, C.P. and Tortora, G.J. (2007). *Anatomy and Physiology*. New Jersey: John Wiley & Sons.

Jowett, N.I. and Thompson, D.R. (2003). *Comprehensive Coronary Care*, 3rd edn. London: Baillere Tindall.

Lemone, P. and Burke, K. (2004). *Medical – Surgical Nursing: Critical Thinking in Client Care*. New Jersey: Pearson Education

London, N.J.M. and Nash, R. (2000). ABC of arterial and venous disease – vevicose veins. *BMJ*, *320*, 1391–1394.

Marieb, E.N. (2006). *Essentials of Human Anatomy and Physiology*, 8th edn. San Francisco: Pearson Benjamin Cummings.

Marieb, E.N. and Hoehn, K. (2007). *Human Anatomy and Physiology*, 7th edn. San Francisco: Pearson Benjamin Cummings.

McCance, K.L. and Huether, S.E. (2006). *Pathophysiology: The Biological Basis for Disease in Adults and Children*, 5th edn. St. Lewis: Mosby.

National Institute for Clinical Excellence (2002). *Management of Type 2 Diabetes: Management of Blood Glucose*. London: NICE.

Nowak, T.J. and Handford, A.G. (1999). *Essentials of Pathophysiology: Concepts and Applications for Health Care Professionals*. Boston: McGraw-Hill.

Nursing and Midwifery Council (2005). *Guidelines for Record and Record Keeping*. London: NMC.

Paradiso, C. (1999). *Pathophysiology*, 2nd edn. Philadelphia: Lippincott.

Porth, C.M. (2005). *Pathophysiology: Concepts of Altered Health States*, 7th edn. Philadelphia: Lippincott Williams & Wilkins.

Stubbling, N. and Chesworth, J. (2003). Assessment of patients with vascular disease. In: Murray, S. (ed) *Vascular Disease: Nursing and Management*. London: Whurr.

Tiernay, L.M., McPhee, S.J. and Papadakis, M.A. (2001). *Current Medical Diagnosis and Treatment*, 40th edn. New York: McGraw Hill.

Vowden, K. and Vowden, P. (2003). Venous disorder. In: Murray, S. (ed) *Vascular Disease: Nursing and Management*. London: Whurr.

Waugh, A. and Grant, A. (2006). *Ross and Wilson: Anatomy and Physiology in Health and Illness*, 10th edn. Edinburgh: Churchill Livingstone.

Wilkinson, I.B., Waring, W.S. and Cockcroft, J. (2002). *Hypertension: Your Questions Answered*. Edinburgh: Churchill Livingstone.

Chapter 7

The blood and associated disorders

Muralitharan Nair

KEY WORDS

- Erythrocytes
- Platelets
- Haemostasis
- Antigens

- Plasma
- Haemoglobin
- Coagulation
- Agglutination

- White blood cells
- Erythropoietin
- Blood groups
- Haematocrit

Test your prior knowledge

- ❓ What is the function of the red blood cell?
- ❓ How many types of white blood cells are there? Can you name them?
- ❓ Why does the arterial blood look bright red?
- ❓ What do you understand by the term blood doping?

Introduction

Blood is a type of **connective tissue** consisting of cells and cell fragments. It does not connect or give mechanical support. It is called a connective tissue because it develops from **mesenchyme** and consists of blood cells which are surrounded by non-living fluid called **plasma**. The cells and the cell fragments are formed elements of the blood and the liquid part is called the plasma. The formed elements are made up of red blood cells (**erythrocytes**) which accounts for 45% of the blood and plasma makes up 55% of the total blood volume (Seeley *et al.*, 2006). The remaining 1% consists of white blood cells and **platelets** (see Figure 7.1). The percentage of the formed elements constitutes the **haematocrit** or packed cell volume. The volume of blood is constant in a healthy person unless the person has physiological problems. This chapter focuses on the composition, structure and functions of various blood cells and their related disorders.

Composition of blood

Blood is composed of plasma, a yellowish liquid-containing nutrients, hormones, minerals and various cells mainly red blood cells, **white blood cells** and platelets (see Figure 7.2). Both the formed elements and the plasma play an important role in **homeostasis**.

Properties of blood

In a healthy person, blood forms about 7–9% of total body weight. A man has 5–6 L of blood while a woman has 4–5 L (Wynsberghe *et al.*, 1995). Blood is thicker, denser and flows much slower than water due to the red blood cells and proteins such as albumin and fibrinogen. It has a high viscosity which offers resistance to blood flow. The red blood cells and proteins contribute to the viscosity of the blood which ranges from 3.5 to 5.5 compared with 1.000 for water. The more red blood cells and plasma proteins in blood, the higher the viscosity and the slower the flow of blood. The specific gravity (density) of blood is 1.045–1.065 compared with 1.000 for water and the pH of blood ranges from 7.35 to 7.45.

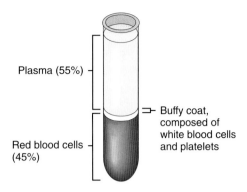

Figure 7.1 Components of blood.

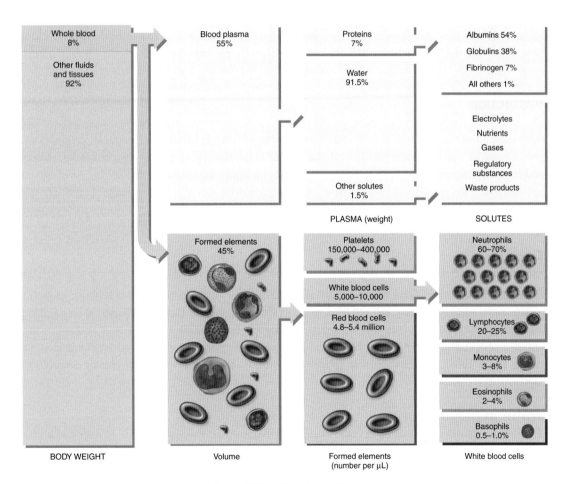

Figure 7.2 Cells of the blood.

Function of blood

Overall the functions of the blood can be classified into three sections and they are as follows:

- transportation
- regulation
- protection

Transportation

Red blood cells in the blood transports oxygen from the lungs to body tissues and waste products of cellular metabolism from the body tissues to the kidneys, liver, lungs and sweat glands for elimination from the body. Blood also transports nutrients, hormones, clotting factors and enzymes throughout the body to maintain homeostasis.

Regulation

Blood regulates blood clotting to stop bleeding, body temperature by increasing or decreasing blood flow to the skin for heat exchange and acid–base balance to maintain the pH of blood within a normal range (7.35–7.45). It also regulates fluid and electrolyte balance through renal function.

Protection

Blood defends the body against bacteria and viruses (**pathogens**) in several ways. Some white blood cells such as the neutrophils engulf and destroy pathogens while others, for example lymphocytes, produce and secrete **antibodies** into blood. Antibodies in the blood play a vital role in the inflammatory and immune response. They prevent blood loss after an injury by initiating the clotting mechanisms without which the person will bleed to death. Clotting involves platelets, the plasma protein fibrinogen and the clotting factors.

Plasma

Plasma is the liquid part of the blood and is composed of water (91%), protein (8%) (albumin, globulin, prothrombin and fibrinogen), salts (0.9%) (sodium chloride, sodium bicarbonate and others) and the remaining 0.1% is made up of organic materials, for example fats, glucose, urea, uric acid, cholesterol and amino acids (Mader, 2005). The blood cells are composed of erythrocytes (red blood cells), leucocytes (white blood cells) and thrombocytes (platelets). These substances give plasma greater density and viscosity than water.

Water in plasma

The water in plasma is available to cells, tissues and extracellular fluid of the body to maintain homeostasis. It is a solvent where chemical reactions between intracellular and extracellular reactions occur. Water-contains solutes, for example electrolytes whose concentrations change to meet body needs.

Plasma proteins

Plasma contains three principal types of proteins and they are:

- albumins
- globulins
- fibrinogen

Plasma proteins make up 7% of the plasma and these proteins stay in the blood vessel as they are too large to diffuse through capillaries and are responsible for creating the osmotic pressure of blood. When plasma proteins are lost in patients who suffer from burns, fluid moves into tissues causing oedema by a process called **osmosis**.

Albumin
Albumin is the most abundant plasma protein (about 60%). It is synthesised in the liver and its main function is to maintain plasma osmotic pressure. Albumins also act as carrier **molecules** for other substances such as hormones and lipids (Waugh and Grant, 2006).

Globulins
The next most abundant plasma proteins are globulins (about 36%). They are synthesised from the liver and **B lymphocytes**. They are divided into three groups based on their structure and function, they are:

- alpha globulin
- beta globulin
- gamma globulin

The alpha and beta globulins are produced by the liver and they transport lipids and fat-soluble vitamins. Gamma globulins are **immunoglobulins** which are complex proteins produced by lymphocytes that have a vital role in **immunity**. They prevent diseases such as measles and tetanus (Waugh and Grant, 2006).

Fibrinogen
Fibrinogen forms approximately 4% of the plasma proteins which is essential for blood clotting and it is synthesised in the liver. When fibrinogen and several other proteins involved in clotting are removed, the remaining fluid is called serum.

Plasma electrolytes
Electrolytes are inorganic molecules that separate into ions when dissolved in water. They are involved in muscle contraction and transmission of nerve impulses, and play a role in maintaining the pH of blood. The ions are either positively charged (cations) or negatively charged (anions). The principal plasma cation is sodium (Na^+) and the principal anion is chloride (Cl^-) (Wynsberghe et al., 1995).

Gases
Oxygen, carbon dioxide and nitrogen are the principal gases dissolved in plasma. Oxygen is transported by **haemoglobin** in red blood cells and some are dissolved in plasma. Most of the carbon dioxide is transported by bicarbonate ions in plasma.

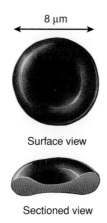

8 μm

Surface view

Sectioned view

Figure 7.3 Red blood cell.

Nutrients and waste products of metabolism

Nutrients such as amino acids, fatty acids and glycerol are obtained from the digestion of food sources in the gastrointestinal tract. They are vital in cellular function. Waste products of protein metabolism such as urea, creatinine and uric acid are transported in the blood to the kidneys for elimination (Mader, 2005).

Formed elements of blood

The formed elements of the blood consist of:

- red blood cells
- white blood cells
- platelets

Red blood cells

Red blood cells are also known as erythrocytes and are small biconcave disks (see Figure 7.3). The biconcave shape is maintained by a network of proteins called spectrin. This network of protein will allow the red blood cells to change shape as they are transported through the blood vessel. There are approximately 4–5.5 million red blood cells in each cubic millimetre of blood (Marieb and Hoehn, 2007). They are a pale buff colour that appears lighter in the centre. Young red blood cells contain a nucleus; however, the nucleus is absent in a mature red blood cell and without any **organelles** such as **mitochondria**.

The main function of the red blood cell is to transport respiratory gases oxygen and carbon dioxide (approximately 20%). As red blood cells lack mitochondria to produce energy (**adenosine triphosphate**), they utilise anaerobic respiration to produce energy and do not use any of the oxygen they are transporting.

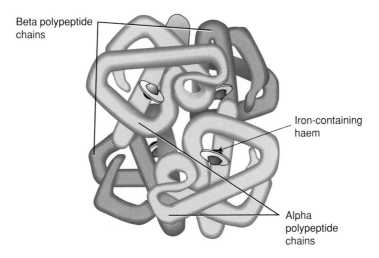

Beta polypeptide chains

Iron-containing haem

Alpha polypeptide chains

Figure 7.4 Haemoglobin molecule.

Haemoglobin

Haemoglobin is composed of the protein called globin bound to the iron-containing pigments called haem. Each globin molecule has four **polypeptide** chains consisting of two alpha and two beta chains (see Figure 7.4). Each haemoglobin molecule has four atoms of iron and each atom of iron will transport one molecule of oxygen; therefore, one molecule of haemoglobin will transport four molecules of oxygen. There are approximately 250 million haemoglobin molecules in one red blood cell and therefore one red blood cell will transport 1 billion molecules of oxygen.

Formation of red blood cells

Red blood cells are formed from the stem cells in the red bone marrow. In the bone marrow, the multipotent stem cells divide to produce myeloid stem cells which divide to produce erythroblasts (see Figure 7.5). Erythroblasts undergo development in the red bone marrow to form red blood cells. During maturation, red blood cells loose their **nucleus** and organelles and gain more haemoglobin molecules, thus increasing the amount of oxygen they transport. As mature red blood cells do not have a nucleus, the lifespan of a red blood cell is approximately 120 days. It is estimated that approximately 2 million red blood cells are destroyed per second (Mader, 2005); however, an equal number is replaced each time to maintain the balance.

The production of red blood cells is controlled by the hormone **erythropoietin** (Marieb and Hoehn, 2007) and the essential components for the synthesis of red blood cells are:

- iron
- folic acid
- vitamin B_{12}

Transport of respiratory gases

The major role of red blood cells is to transport oxygen from the lungs to the tissues. The oxygen in the alveoli (air sac) of the lungs combines with iron molecules in the haemoglobin to form oxyhaemoglobin.

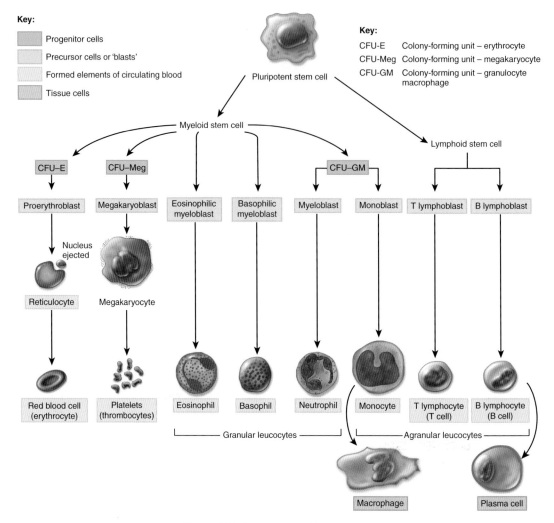

Key:

- Progenitor cells
- Precursor cells or 'blasts'
- Formed elements of circulating blood
- Tissue cells

Key:

CFU-E   Colony-forming unit – erythrocyte
CFU-Meg Colony-forming unit – megakaryocyte
CFU-GM   Colony-forming unit – granulocyte
         macrophage

Pluripotent stem cell

Myeloid stem cell

Lymphoid stem cell

CFU–E   CFU–Meg   CFU–GM

Proerythroblast Megakaryoblast Eosinophilic   Basophilic   Myeloblast Monoblast T lymphoblast B lymphoblast
                                 myeloblast   myeloblast

Nucleus ejected

Reticulocyte   Megakaryocyte

Red blood cell Platelets   Eosinophil   Basophil   Neutrophil Monocyte   T lymphocyte   B lymphocyte
(erythrocyte)   (thrombocytes)   (T cell)   (B cell)

└──── Granular leucocytes ────┘   └──── Agranular leucocytes ────┘

Macrophage   Plasma cell

Figure 7.5 Formation of blood cells.

This is then transported by the blood to the tissues. As the oxygen level in the red blood cell increases, it becomes bright red, and when the level of oxygen content drops the colour changes to dark bluish red (Waugh and Grant, 2006).

In addition to transporting oxygen from the lungs to the body tissues, red blood cells transport carbon dioxide from the tissues to the lungs. Carbon dioxide is transported in three ways:

1. 10% of the carbon dioxide is dissolved in the plasma.
2. 20% of the carbon dioxide combines with haemoglobin of the red blood cell to form carbamino-haemoglobin.
3. 70% of the carbon dioxide reacts with water to form carbonic acid which is converted to bicarbonate and hydrogen ions (see equation).

$$CO_2 + H_2O \overset{\text{carbonic anhydrase}}{\longleftrightarrow} \underset{\text{carbonic acid}}{H_2CO_3} \leftrightarrow \underset{\text{bicarbonate ion}}{HCO_3^-} + \underset{\text{hydrogen ion}}{H^+}$$

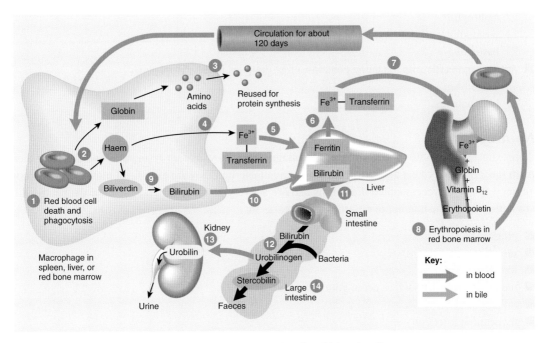

Figure 7.6 Haemolysis of red blood cell.

The reaction occurs primarily in red blood cells which contain large amounts of carbonic anhydrase (an enzyme that facilitates the reaction). Once the bicarbonate ions are formed, they move out of the red blood cells into the plasma.

Destruction of red blood cells

Haemolysis (breakdown) is carried out by macrophages in the spleen, liver and the bone marrow (see Figure 7.6). As red blood cells age, they are susceptible to haemolysis; haem and globin are separated. The globin is broken down into amino acids and used for protein synthesis. Iron is separated from haem and is stored in the muscle and the liver and reused in the bone marrow to manufacture new red blood cells. Haem is portion of the haemoglobin that is converted to bilirubin and is transported by plasma albumin to the liver and eventually secreted in **bile**.

White blood cells

White blood cells are also known as leucocytes. There are approximately 5000–10 000 white blood cells in every cubic millimetre of blood. The number may increase in infections to approximately 25 000 per cubic millimetre of blood. An increase in white blood cells is called leucocytosis and an abnormally low level of white blood cell is called leucopenia. Unlike red blood cells, white blood cells do have nuclei and they are able to move out of blood vessel walls into the tissues. White blood cells are able to produce a continuous supply of energy, unlike the red blood cells. They are able to synthesise proteins and thus their lifespan can be from a few days to years. There are two main types of white blood cells and they are:

■ granulocytes (contains granules in the cytoplasm)

- ☐ neutrophils
- ☐ eosinophils
- ☐ basophils
- ■ agranulocytes (despite the name contains a few granules in the cytoplasm)
  - ☐ monocytes
  - ☐ lymphocytes

Neutrophils

Approximately, 60–65% of granulocytes are **phagocytes**. They contain **lysozymes** and therefore their main function is to protect the body from any foreign material. They are capable of moving out of blood vessel walls by a process called diapedesis and are actively phagocytic. The nuclei of the neutrophils are multi-lobed. The number of neutrophils increases in:

- ■ pregnancy
- ■ infection
- ■ leukaemia
- ■ metabolic disorder such as acute gout
- ■ inflammation
- ■ myocardial infection

Eosinophils

These form approximately 2–4% of granulocytes and have B-shaped nuclei. Like neutrophils, they too migrate from blood vessels. They are phagocytes; however, they are not as active as neutrophils. They contain lysosomal enzymes and peroxidase in their granules, which are toxic to parasites resulting in the destruction of the organism. Numbers increase in allergy such as hay fever and asthma and parasitic infection, for example tapeworm infection.

Basophils

Basophils account for approximately 1% of granulocytes and contain elongated lobed nuclei. In inflamed tissue they become mast cells and secrete granules containing heparin, histamine and other proteins that promote inflammation. Basophils play an important role in providing immunity against parasites.

Monocytes

Monocytes account for 5% of the agranulocytes and they are circulating leucocytes. Monocytes develop in the bone marrow. Some of the monocytes migrate into the tissue where they develop into macrophages and engulf pathogens or foreign proteins. Macrophages play a vital role in immunity and inflammation by destroying specific **antigens**.

Lymphocytes

Lymphocytes account for 25% of the leucocytes and most are found in the lymphatic tissue such as the lymph nodes and the spleen. They get their name from the lymph, the fluid that transports them. They can leave and re-enter the circulatory system, the lifespan of the lymphocytes ranges from a few hours to years. The main difference between lymphocytes and other white blood cells is that lymphocytes are not phagocytes (Wynsberghe *et al.*, 1995). Two types of lymphocytes are identified and they are T and

B lymphocytes. T lymphocytes originate from the thymus gland hence the name, while B lymphocytes originate in the bone marrow. T lymphocytes mediate cellular immune response which is part of the body's own defence. The B lymphocytes, on the other hand, become large plasma cells and produce antibodies which attach to antigen.

Platelets

Platelets are small blood cells consisting of some cytoplasm surrounded by a plasma membrane. They are produced in the bone marrow from megakaryocytes (see Figure 7.5) and fragments of megakaryocytes break off to form platelets. The lifespan is approximately 5–9 days (Seeley *et al.*, 2006). The surface of platelets contains proteins and glycoproteins that allow them to adhere to other proteins such as collagen in the connective tissues. Platelets play a vital role in blood loss by the formation of platelet plugs (see Chapter 6, Figure 6.15) which seal the holes in the blood vessels.

Haemostasis

Haemostasis plays an important part in maintaining homeostasis and it consists of three main components. They are:

- vasoconstriction
- platelet aggregation
- coagulation

Vasoconstriction
- results from contraction of the smooth muscle of the vessel wall
- constriction blocks small blood vessels thus preventing blood flow through them
- the action of the sympathetic nervous system is to cause vasoconstriction
- platelets release thromboxanes

Platelet aggregation
- platelets contain contractile proteins called actin and myosin
- platelet adhesion occurs when they are exposed to collagen in the blood vessels
- platelets release adenosine diphosphate, thromboxane and other chemicals

Coagulation

If blood vessel damage is so extensive that platelet **aggregation** and vasoconstriction cannot stop the bleeding, the complicated process of **coagulation** (blood clotting) will begin to take place. The clotting phase involves several clotting factors (see Table 7.1). Most of the clotting factors are synthesised in the liver.

The simplified clotting stages involve the following:

1. Thromboplastinogenase is an enzyme released by the blood platelets and combines with antihaemophilic factor to convert the plasma protein thromboplastinogen into thromboplastin.
2. Thromboplastin combines with calcium ions to convert the inactive plasma protein prothrombin into thrombin.

I	Fibrinogen
II	Prothrombin
III	Thromboplastin
IV	Calcium
V	Proaccelerin, labile factor
VII	Serum prothrombin conversion accelerator
VIII	Antihaemophilic factor
IX	Christmas factor, plasma thromboplastin component
X	Stuart–Power factor
XI	Plasma thromboplastin antecedent
XII	Hageman factor
XIII	Fibrin-stabilising factor

Table 7.1 Blood clotting factors

3. Thrombin acts as a catalyst to convert the soluble plasma protein fibrinogen into insoluble plasma protein fibrin.
4. The fibrin threads trap blood cells to form a clot.
5. Once the clot is formed, the healing of the damaged blood vessel takes place which restores the integrity of the blood vessel.

Two pathways were identified in triggering a blood clot and they include the intrinsic and extrinsic pathways. The extrinsic pathway is a rapid clotting system activated when the blood vessels are ruptured and tissue damage takes place. The intrinsic pathway is slower than the extrinsic pathway and it is activated when the inner walls of the blood vessels are damaged.

Blood groups

The surface of the red blood cell contains molecules called antigen and in the plasma there are molecules called antibodies. The antibodies are specific to certain antigens. When the antibodies combine with the specific antigen on the red blood cell, they form a link to connect other red blood cells to it. As a result, clumping or **agglutination** of the red blood cells occurs.

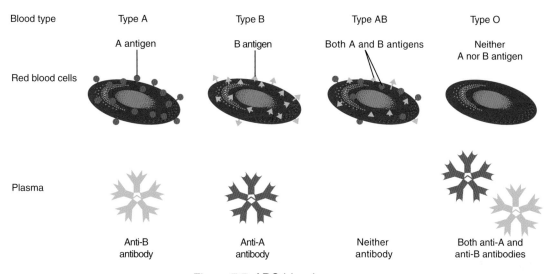

Figure 7.7 ABO blood groups.

The antigens on the red blood cells have been categorised into **blood groups**. Although numerous blood groups have been identified, ABO (see Figure 7.7) and Rh blood groups are the most important in blood transfusion.

Type A blood group has type A antigen on its surface and anti-B antibody in the plasma, type B blood group has type B antigen on its surface and anti-A antibody in the plasma, type AB blood group has both antigens A and B on its surface but do not contain either antibodies in the plasma and type O blood group has neither antigens A nor B on its surface but contains both anti-A and anti-B antibodies in the plasma. About 45% of the population in the UK are blood group O and 55% of the population are either blood group A, B or AB (Waugh and Grant, 2006). People with blood group O are known as universal donors as their red blood cells do not have either A or B antigen on its surface. Conversely, people with blood group AB are known as universal recipient as their red blood cells contain antigens A and B on its surface (see Table 7.2).

Blood type	Antigens	Antibodies	Can donate blood to	Can receive blood from
A	Antigen A	Anti-B	A, AB	A, O
B	Antigen B	Anti-A	B, AB	B, O
AB	Antigen A Antigen B	None	AB	A, B, AB, O
O	None	Anti-A Anti-B	A, B, AB, O	O

Table 7.2 Blood groups

Rhesus factor

The rhesus factor (Rh) is another important antigen identified on the surface of red blood cells. The rhesus factor is so called because it was first identified in rhesus monkeys. In the UK, approximately 85% of the population are rhesus positive, that is they possess factor D on their red blood cells. The remaining 15% of the population are rhesus negative as their red blood cells do not have factor D. It is important to consider the rhesus factor when cross-matching and transfusing blood to patients to avoid unnecessary complications such as agglutination.

Diseases of the blood

Learning outcomes

On completion of this section, the reader will be able to:

■ List some of the common diseases of blood and identify risk factors associated with the diseases.

■ Describe the pathophysiological processes related to specific blood disorders.

■ Outline the nursing management and interventions related to the disorders described.

Anaemia

Anaemia from the Greek word meaning 'without blood' refers to a reduction in red blood cells and/or haemoglobin. This results in a reduced ability of the blood to transport oxygen to the tissues, causing hypoxia. The normal level of haemoglobin in an adult male is approximately 13–17 g/100 mL of blood and in an adult female it is approximately 12–16 g/100 mL of blood (Porth, 2005). Anaemia can result from:

■ excessive loss of blood through haemorrhage
■ destruction of red blood cells (haemolysis)
■ deficient red blood cell production due to red bone marrow failure
■ infections such as malaria
■ lack of intake of iron, folic acid and vitamin B_{12}
■ pregnancy

There are three major types of anaemia and they include:

■ microcytic anaemia (small red blood cells)
■ macrocytic anaemia (large blood cells)
■ normocytic anaemia (normal-sized red blood cells)

Microcytic anaemia

Microcytic anaemia is characterised by small red blood cells. There are several types of microcytic anaemia of which iron deficiency anaemia is the most common cause of anaemia in the UK. Iron is essential for the production of young red blood cells. As iron is a component of haem, a deficiency of iron leads to decreased haemoglobin synthesis resulting in impairment of oxygen transport. In iron deficiency anaemia, the red blood cells are small (microcytic) and pale (hypochromic).

Aetiology of iron deficiency anaemia

Iron deficiency anaemia results from:

- dietary deficiency of iron
- loss of iron through haemorrhage
- poor absorption of iron from the gastrointestinal tract after **gastrectomy**
- increased demands such as growth and pregnancy

Investigations

The following investigations may be carried out to confirm diagnosis:

- full blood count (red blood cells, white blood cells, haemoglobin concentration, mean corpuscular volume, haematrocrit)
- test for levels of ferritin, serum iron, transferring, folate, vitamin B_{12}
- bone marrow examination
- physical examination

Pathophysiology of iron deficiency anaemia

Iron deficiency anaemia is present when the demand for iron in the body exceeds supply; anaemia develops slowly in three stages and they are:

1. The body's iron stores are depleted; however, erythropoiesis continues normally.
2. Iron transportation to bone marrow is diminished resulting in deficiency in red cell production.
3. The numbers of microcytic red blood cells increases in circulation replacing the normal mature red blood cells.

Iron is constantly used in the production of young red blood cells. Iron is obtained from food sources and absorbed from the gastrointestinal tract. Excess iron is stored in the liver and muscle cells and is readily available for the production of red blood cells. Some inflammatory disorders such as Crohn's disease will affect the absorption of iron from the gastrointestinal tract affecting the synthesis of red bloods cells.

In some instances, substantial segments of bowel are surgically removed, due to carcinoma of the bowel, affecting the absorption of iron from the gastrointestinal tract. Inadequate dietary intake also contributes to iron deficiency anaemia in the older adult. Access to transportation may limit the patient from eating a healthy diet rich in meat, fruits and vegetables. Iron deficiency can produce significant gastrointestinal abnormalities such as angular stomatitis and glossitis. Other diseases include peptic ulcer where the condition produces gastrointestinal bleeding and iron deficiency. The organs affected are the stomach and the duodenum where there is inflammation and erosion of the membrane.

Signs and symptoms of iron deficiency anaemia

Patients suffering from iron deficiency anaemia may experience:

- brittle nails
- spoon-shaped nails (koilonychias)
- atrophy of the papillae of the tongue
- brittle hair
- cheilosis (cracks at the corners of the mouth)
- dizziness – due to lack of oxygen supply to the brain
- hypoxia
- pica (craving to eat unusual substances such as clay, starch and coal)
- breathlessness – physiological compensation resulting from the lack of oxygen
- loss of appetite may be due to sore mouth

Nursing management of iron deficiency anaemia

The nursing management of the patient with iron deficiency anaemia will include a full nursing assessment including a comprehensive risk assessment to prevent injuries from falls before planning the appropriate care. The care planned should consider a holistic approach which includes physical, psychological and social aspects of care.

Patients with iron deficiency anaemia may require blood transfusion. It is the nurse's duty to ensure that the transfusion is administered without complications from transfusion such as reactions from incompatible blood and hypertension. The patient's vital signs, for example temperature, blood pressure, heart rate and respirations should be monitored every 15 minutes for the first hour as transfusion reactions are likely to occur in the first 15 minutes. Any change in the vital signs should be reported immediately to the nurse in charge and documented in the nursing notes in accordance with the Nursing and Midwifery Council (2005) guidelines and local policies.

Patients receiving blood transfusion may be concerned about the risk of contracting HIV or hepatitis C through blood transfusion, and therefore it is the nurse's duty to explain the screening procedures on donor's blood (Alexander et al., 2006) and the low risk associated with blood transfusion.

Dietary advice on foods rich in iron such as red meat, liver and vegetables should be encouraged as iron is an essential component for the production of red blood cells.

Advice on oral hygiene should include on the use of soft-toothed toothbrush, care of dentures and the use of suitable ointments to prevent cracked lips (Jamieson et al., 2002).

Anaemic patients should be advised not to change position suddenly, for example standing up quickly from a sitting position, to avoid falling down and injuring themselves as a result of dizziness.

Pharmacological interventions of iron deficiency anaemia

Patients with iron deficiency anaemia may be prescribed an iron supplement, for example ferrous sulphate. Patients should be advised about the side effects, which include constipation, nausea and in some patients even diarrhoea. They should be advised to drink 2–3 L of fluid per day to prevent constipation.

Macrocytic anaemia

Macrocytic anaemia is also termed megaloblastic anaemia. It is characterised by defective deoxyribonucleic acid (DNA) synthesis resulting in the production of unusually large stem cells (macrocytes) in circulation. In addition to an increase in diameter, the thickness and volume of the cell also increases.

Aetiology of macrocytic anaemia

- folate deficiency
- vitamin B_{12} deficiency

Both these **coenzymes** are essential for DNA maturation. Vegans and vegetarians are at risk of developing macrocytic anaemia due to the lack of vitamin B_{12} which is found in most meat products.

Folate deficiency

Folic acid (folate) is an essential vitamin for the production and maturation of red blood cells. Folate is obtained from diet and is absorbed from the jejunum and is stored in the liver. It is found in leafy vegetables, fruit, cereals, meat and most of the vitamins are lost in cooking.

Aetiology of folate deficiency

Deficiency in folate could result from:

- malnutrition
- malabsorption from the jejunum caused by diseases such as coeliac disease
- medications that inhibit absorption from the jejunum, for example oral contraceptives and anticonvulsants such as phenytoin
- alcohol abuse – alcohol interferes with folate metabolism in the liver
- anorexia

Symptoms of folate deficiency

- fatigue
- palpitations
- shortness of breath
- diarrhoea
- progressive weakness
- pallor

Vitamin B_{12} deficiency

The most common type of megaloblastic anaemia is pernicious anaemia (PA) resulting from vitamin B_{12} deficiency. Vitamin B_{12} is essential for the synthesis of DNA and a deficiency impairs cellular division and maturation especially in rapidly proliferating red blood cells. The absorption of vitamin B_{12} in the intestine requires the presence of **intrinsic factor** (IF), which is produced by the gastric mucosa. IF binds to vitamin B_{12} in food and protects it for gastrointestinal enzymes and facilitates its absorption. Lack of vitamin B_{12} alters the structure and disrupts the function of the peripheral nerves, spinal cord and brain.

Aetiology of vitamin B_{12} deficiency

Deficiency in vitamin B_{12} can result from:

- total gastrectomy, partial gastrectomy or gastrojejunostomy
- gastric lesions
- carcinoma of the stomach
- alcohol abuse
- malabsorption due inflammatory disease such as Crohn's disease

Symptoms of vitamin B₁₂ deficiency

- pallor
- slight jaundice
- smooth sore tongue
- diarrhoea
- paresthesias – numbness and tingling in the extremities
- impaired proprioception (ability to identify one's position in space)
- problems with balance

Nursing management of macrocytic anaemia

Nursing management of the patient with macrocytic anaemia would be the similar as described for microcytic anaemia. A full nursing assessment is essential for planning high-quality care. Most patients with folate deficiency are cared for in the community in their general practice. Patients with folate deficiency anaemia will need dietary advice on which food contains folic acid and how to avoid destroying it in cooking preparation (Alexander *et al.*, 2006). Advice on folic acid supplement and how to take them should be offered to patients.

Some patients with vitamin B₁₂ deficiency may be admitted to hospital for their treatment. The treatment includes the administration of cyanocobalamin by injection monthly for those patients who are lacking in the IF. Initially, the treatment is carried out weekly until vitamin B₁₂ deficiency is corrected. Patients should be advised to eat food that contains vitamin B₁₂ such as eggs, meat and diary products. PA as a result of vitamin B₁₂ deficiency cannot be cured, so the treatment is lifelong. Some patients may need a blood transfusion if they develop complications such as heart failure.

Normocytic anaemia

Normocytic anaemia is characterised by red blood cells that are relatively normal in size and in haemoglobin content but insufficient in number. It is less common than microcytic and macrocytic anaemias. Normocytic anaemias include:

- aplastic anaemia
- haemolytic anaemia
- sickle cell anaemia

Aplastic anaemia

Aplastic anaemia (AA) is a serious condition affecting the bone marrow. It is characterised by a reduction of all the blood cells, that is, the red blood cells, white blood cells and platelets. When all three types of blood cells are low the condition is termed pancytopenia.

Aetiology of aplastic anaemia

The condition is **idiopathic**; however, the condition has been associated with:

- viral diseases, for example hepatitis and HIV
- ionising radiation
- metastases of the bone

- cytotoxic drugs
- chemical compounds, for example benzene

Pathophysiology of aplastic anaemia

AA occurs as a result of reduced bone marrow function resulting in low numbers of blood cells. Fat cells proliferate to replace stem cells. The formed red blood cells are immature and the transportation of oxygen is affected. As a result of shortened lifespan of platelets and white blood cells, patients are prone to infections and bleeding. The most common causes of death are severe haemorrhage, infections and septic shock (Bullock and Henze, 2000). In severe cases, mortality can be high and thus requires prompt intervention.

Symptoms of aplastic anaemia

The initially presenting symptoms include:

- weakness
- fatigue
- pallor caused by anaemia
- petechiae – small haemorrhages under the skin
- ecchymoses – bruises on the skin
- bleeding from mucous membranes of the nose, gums, vagina and gastrointestinal tract may occur as a result of decreased platelet level
- prone to infections as a result of low neutrophil count

Nursing management of aplastic anaemia

AA could result in life-threatening complications, such as septic shock, which requires prompt intervention. Specific therapy is determined by the underlying cause of the disorder. The nursing management will include treatment with medications, dietary modifications and blood transfusion if necessary. The role of the nurse will include:

- early detection and treatment of the disease
- prevention of infections and providing nursing care for septic patients
- early detection and management of bleeding

Blood transfusion may be indicated to replace the blood lost and discontinued as soon as the bone marrow commences the synthesis of blood cells. Nurses need to be aware of blood transfusion complications such as:

- hypertension as a result of fluid overload from transfusion
- transfusion reaction such as rashes and bronchial wheezing
- electrolyte imbalance
- incompatibility between patient's blood and donor's blood, for example back pain, dyspnoea, cyanosis and tachycardia

As the risk of adverse reaction is high when the blood is transfused, patient's vital signs must be monitored every 15 minutes for the first hour as many reactions are evident within 30 minutes of transfusion (Kozier *et al.*, 2004).

Nursing management in the prevention of AA includes teaching good dietary habits such as diet high in iron, folate and vitamin B_{12} as these food sources are essential in the synthesis of red blood cells. Patients, who are vegetarian, should be encouraged to take foodstuff rich in vitamin C as it enhances the absorption of iron from grains and other sources.

Pharmacological interventions of aplastic anaemia

Patients with AA may be prescribed:

- iron supplement
- folic acid supplement
- vitamin B_{12} supplement

Haemolytic anaemia

Haemolytic anaemia results from the premature destruction of red blood cells resulting in the retention of iron and other products of red blood cell destruction. This condition is either acquired or inherited and is a rare condition. In haemolytic anaemia, the bone marrow increases the synthesis of red blood cells to match the number of red blood cells destroyed.

Aetiology of haemolytic anaemia

The causes of haemolytic anaemia can be either inherited or acquired and they include:

- spherocytosis – fragility of the red blood cell membrane
- haemoglobin defects – thalassaemia and sickle cell disease
- mismatched blood transfusion
- direct cell injury from drugs, for example sodium chlorate
- disseminated intravascular coagulation
- haemoglobinpathies – abnormalities in haemoglobin structure

Pathophysiology of haemolytic anaemia

The lifespan of red blood cells in haemolytic anaemia is much shorter than the normal lifespan of 120 days. The cell membrane is fragile, resulting in the excessive destruction of the red blood cells; this in turn causes a reduction in the number of red blood cells available for the transportation of oxygen which leads to hypoxia in the tissues. The bone marrow in response to the excessive destruction becomes hyperactive and produces more red blood cells by erythropoiesis. In haemolytic anaemia, red blood cell destruction can occur in the vascular system or by phagocytosis by the reticuloendothelial system (Porth, 2005). As a result of increased destruction of the red blood cells, there is an increased level of **bilirubin** and **urobilinogen**.

Signs and symptoms of haemolytic anaemia

The presence of signs and symptoms depends on the severity of the disease. Some of the clinical manifestations are:

- jaundice, if red blood cell destruction exceeds the liver's ability to conjugate and excrete bilirubin
- fatigue

■ hypoxia from impaired oxygen transport
■ dyspnoea
■ spleen may become enlarged in patients with congenital haemolytic disorders

Nursing management of haemolytic anaemia

Nursing management of the patient with haemolytic anaemia will include advice on diet as for other forms of anaemia, relieving anxiety in patients and their relatives, management of blood transfusion and administration of prescribed medication (see aplastic anaemia). If patients are breathless, they must be nursed upright supported by pillows and oxygen administered as prescribed.

Sickle cell anaemia

Sickle cell anaemia is a hereditary, chronic haemolytic anaemia characterised by the presence of an abnormal haemoglobin (HbS) molecule (see Figure 7.8). This abnormality is formed by genetic mutation in which one amino acid (valine) replaces another amino acid (glutamic acid). The haemoglobin forms a sickle shape when the oxygen content is removed from the haemoglobin (Mehta and Hoffbrand, 2000).

In heterozygous twins, the child inherits the abnormal haemoglobin gene from one parent and a normal haemoglobin (HbA) from the other parent. The child develops the sickle cell trait and is unaware until exposed to hypoxic conditions. The trait is passed on to any child. In homozygous twins, the child inherits the abnormal gene from both parents and will suffer from sickle cell anaemia.

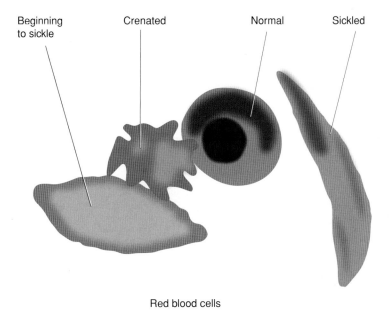

Red blood cells

Figure 7.8 Sickled red blood cell.

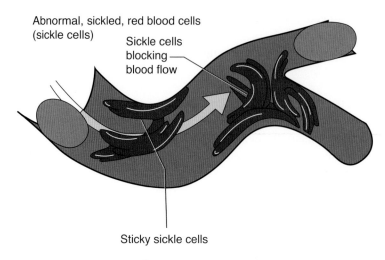

Figure 7.9 Sickle cell in microcirculation.

Pathophysiology of sickle cell anaemia

The possible cause of the sickle shape is the deoxgenation of the haemoglobin. When the haemoglobin is fully saturated with oxygen, the red blood cell is in normal shape but changes into sickle shape as the oxygen content is reduced. Sickled red blood cells are stiff and cannot change shape as normal red blood cells when they pass through capillaries (see Figure 7.9). As a result, the sickled red blood cells obstruct blood flow causing vascular obstruction, pain and tissue ischaemia.

Sickling is not permanent; most sickled red blood cells regain their normal shape once they are saturated with oxygen. However, repeated sickling causes loss of elasticity of the cell membrane and the cells fail to return to normal shape when oxygen concentration increases. The weakened red blood cells are haemolysed and removed from circulation.

Symptoms of sickle cell anaemia

Common presenting symptoms include:

- pain and swelling caused by occluded blood vessels affecting hands and feet
- priapism – persistent painful erection of the penis
- abdominal pain if the abdominal blood vessels are occluded
- increased incidence of infection such as osteomyelitis
- pulmonary hypertension
- tachycardia
- may present with haematuria (blood in the urine)
- may develop stasis ulcers of hand, ankles and feet
- often white blood cells and platelets that are elevated thus contributing to vaso-occlusion

Nursing management of sickle cell anaemia

There is no known cure for sickle cell anaemia. Nursing management of the patient will include alleviation of symptoms and promoting a good quality of life. The care will include:

■ Pain management – patients with sickle cell disease may have intensely painful episodes called vaso-occlusive crises. Pain management will require opioid analgesia until pain has settled. For patients with milder pain level, non-steroidal anti-inflammatory drugs such as diclofenac could be the drug of choice. For more severe pain crises most patients will require admission to the hospital for intravenous opioids or patient-controlled analgesia to control their pain level. Patients experiencing pain crises, their treatment includes rest, oxygen therapy, analgesia and hydration.
■ Patients will need advice on the avoidance of situations that may trigger a crisis. Risk factors include emotional stress, extreme fatigue and infection. Early treatment of infection with antibiotics is important to prevent a crisis occurring.
■ Blood transfusion is indicated for patients who are breathless as a result of severe hypoxia.
■ Patients' vital signs should be monitored 2–4 hourly to detect infection in order to commence treatment with antibiotics.
■ Genetic counselling should be offered to patients and their families to inform them about the disorder and its consequences.
■ During a crisis, fluid therapy is essential to improve blood flow, reduce pain, prevent renal damage and prevent dehydration.

Leukaemia

Leukaemia is a malignant disorder where there is an abnormal or excessive proliferation of immature white blood cells. In the UK, leukaemia is the twelfth most common cancer in adults affecting more men than women. There are two principal types and they are acute and chronic leukaemia. Each of these is further subdivided into:

■ acute myeloid leukaemia (AML)
■ acute lymphoblastic leukaemia (ALL)
■ chronic myeloid leukaemia (CML)
■ chronic lymphoblastic leukaemia (CLL)

Aetiology of acute and chronic leukaemia

The risk factors include:

■ exposure to radiation
■ exposure to benzene (one of the chemicals used in petrol and a solvent used in the rubber and plastic industry)
■ certain genetic conditions such as Down's syndrome
■ smoking
■ age – chronic leukaemia is more common over the age of 40
■ previous cancer treatments
■ diseases that affect the immune system such as HIV

Pathophysiology of leukaemia

White blood cells are produced by the bone marrow. They then pass from the bone marrow into the blood stream and the lymphatic system. White blood cells are involved in various functions of the body's immune system which protects the body against infections.

Acute leukaemia is more aggressive and develops rapidly. It is more common in the younger age group and the symptoms develop quickly and if untreated it becomes life-threatening. Leukaemic cells are immature and poorly differentiated; they proliferate rapidly, have a long lifespan and do not function normally. AML is overproduction of immature myeloid white blood cells and ALL is the overproduction of immature myeloid lymphocytes called lymphoblasts. In acute leukaemia, the cells reproduce very quickly, and do not become mature enough to carry out their role in the immune system.

CLL is more common in men and occurs frequently between the ages of 50 and 70 years. In CLL, abnormal lymphocytes proliferate, accumulate in the blood and spread to the lymphatic tissue. Patients affected may live with symptoms for several years. CML has a gradual onset occurring primarily between the ages 30 and 50 years and the incidence is slightly higher in men. In CML, there is uncontrolled production of myeloid cells. These cells are abnormal and are not able to carry out the normal functions of white blood cells, such as fighting infections. Their lifespan is long, so over a period of time they replace normal functioning cells (red, white and platelets) in the bone marrow (Blows, 2005). This is a slow process and progressively gets worse over time.

Symptoms of leukaemia

Common presenting symptoms include:

- tiredness, breathlessness and pale skin (due to anaemia and reduction in red blood cells)
- abnormal bleeding from the gums and **epistaxis**
- bone pain
- abdominal pain due to enlarged spleen and/or liver
- swollen lymph glands in the groin, neck and under the arms
- weight loss

Nursing management of leukaemia

Patients suffering from leukaemia will need an accurate and full assessment of pain level, activity tolerance, vital signs, nutrition, signs of bleeding or infection in order to plan high-quality care.

- Advice of preventative measures for bleeding should be offered, that is the use of soft-bristle toothbrush, safety in the use razors and measures in the prevention of falls.
- Patients will need advice on the measures of maintaining hydration and nutrition. Weight is monitored weekly in order to assess weight loss.
- Encourage patients and their relatives to discuss concerns and fears (which may include bone marrow and stem cell transplants.
- Stomatitis (inflammation of the mouth) is a common occurrence and therefore daily oral hygiene should be encouraged.

- Fatigue as a result of anaemia may be problem and therefore patients should be advised to take frequent rest periods and not to over-exert themselves.
- Protect patient from infections such as washing hands before and after attending to the patient and discourage unnecessary visitation by relatives.

Pharmacological and non-pharmacological interventions of leukaemia

Medications and other treatments of leukaemia include:

- chemotherapy (use of cytotoxic drugs) treatment
- radiotherapy treatment
- stem cell and bone marrow transplants
- monoclonal antibodies
- ATRA (all trans-retinoic acid) is given alongside chemotherapy
- opioid drugs to control pain

Thrombocytopenia

Thrombocytopenia is the term for a reduced platelet count. It occurs when platelets are lost from circulation faster than they are produced in the bone marrow. Haemorrhage from trauma or spontaneous bleeding may occur when the platelet count is below 20 000 per cubic millimetre of blood (Hogan and Hill, 2004).

Aetiology of thrombocytopenia

Many disease processes can cause thrombocytopenia and they include:

- anaemia as a result of vitamin B_{12} or folic acid deficiency
- systemic lupus erythematous
- sepsis, systemic viral or bacterial infections
- chemotherapy
- radiation
- heparin-induced thrombocytopenia (white clot syndrome)
- HIV

Pathophysiology of thrombocytopenia

The pathophysiology is related to three basic mechanisms:

- accelerated platelet destruction
- defective platelet production
- disordered platelet distribution

Three distinct types identified:

- idiopathic thrombocytopenic purpura (acute and chronic) (ITP)
- thrombotic thrombocytopenic purpura (TTP)
- haemolytic–uremic syndrome (HUS)

ITP is a disease in which antibodies form and destroy the body's platelets. As the destruction is believed to be caused by the body's immune system, it is therefore classified as an autoimmune disorder. Although the bone marrow increases the synthesis of platelets, it cannot keep up with the demand. Acute ITP is more common in children, while chronic ITP is more common in adults. Platelets become coated with antibodies as a result of autoimmune response mediated by B lymphocytes. Although the platelets function normally, the spleen identifies them as foreign protein and destroys them.

TTP is a rare disease in which small blood clots form suddenly throughout the body. The numerous amounts of blood clots result in a high level of platelet usage in clotting which leads to a reduction in platelets.

HUS is a rare disorder related to TTP in which the number of platelets decreases and there is reduction in the number of red blood cells. HUS can also occur with intestinal infections with *Escherichia coli* and with the use of some drugs such as cyclosporine.

Signs and symptoms of thrombocytopenia

Patients with thrombocytopenia may experience:

- unexpected bruising
- petechia (small red spots under the skin)
- bleeding from the gastrointestinal tract
- epistaxis (bleeding from the nose)
- pain in joints and muscles
- heavier than usual menstrual period for women

Nursing management of thrombocytopenia

As a result of a low level of platelets, the patient is at risk for bleeding especially from the gums. Early identification of bleeding is important in order to prevent blood loss.

- Nurses need to monitor vital signs, heart, respiratory rates and blood pressure every 4 hours. Observe for bleeding from other parts of the body such as in the urine (haematuria), gastrointestinal tract, nasal membrane and vaginal bleeding.
- Observe the skin for petechiae.
- Advise the patient about the use of safety measures to minimise the risk of bleeding such as a soft-bristle toothbrush and the use of electric razor for shaving. Hard bristles may abrade the oral mucosa, causing bleeding, and increase the risk of infection.
- Encourage the patient to rinse the mouth with salt solution 2–4 hours to maintain oral hygiene.
- Advise patient to take 2–2.5 L of fluid over 24 hours to prevent dehydration and infection.
- The patient should be advised to avoid medications that interfere with platelet function such as aspirin.
- A healthy diet high in fibre should be encouraged to prevent constipation. Straining to have a bowel movement could increase the risk in internal bleeding from the gastrointestinal tract.

Pharmacological and other intervention of thrombocytopenia

- platelet transfusion may be required to treat acute bleeding
- oral glucocorticoids such a prednisolone may be prescribed to suppress the autoimmune response
- splenectomy may be performed in patients with ITP

Conclusion

This chapter has discussed some of the common disorders of blood the learner might encounter. Nurses need to have a good knowledge about the physiology of blood in order to understand the pathophysiology of blood disorders and to provide appropriate nursing care. Patients are often frightened when they informed that they have a certain blood disorder. It is nurses' duty to ensure that the patients receive accurate information relating to their disease and provide the necessary care.

Multiple choice questions

1. Red blood cells are also known as:
(a) white blood cells
(b) erythrocytes
(c) lymphocytes
(d) basophils

2. Haematocrit is also known as:
(a) packed cell volume
(b) plasma
(c) platelet
(d) neutrophil

3. Which of these is not a component of plasma?
(a) nitrogen
(b) water
(c) platelets
(d) urea

4. Mature red blood cells do not have:
(a) a nucleus
(b) haemoglobin
(c) haem
(d) iron molecules

5. A person with type O blood:
(a) is a universal recipient
(b) is a universal donor
(c) can receive blood type A
(d) can receive blood type B

6. Thrombocytopenia is a term for:
(a) reduced white blood cells
(b) reduced red blood cells
(c) reduced platelets
(d) reduced lymphocytes

7. Destruction of red blood cells is called:
(a) haemolysis
(b) leukaemia
(c) osteomyelitis
(d) phagocytosis

8. Epistaxis is:

(a) bleeding from the gums

(b) bleeding from the rectum

(c) bleeding from the lungs

(d) bleeding the nose

9. Stomatitis is:

(a) inflammation of the lungs

(b) inflammation of the mouth

(c) inflammation of the lymph glands

(d) inflammation of the gums

10. Haematuria is:

(a) blood in the stool

(b) blood in the urine

(c) bleeding from the kidneys

(d) bleeding from the stomach

Answers: 1.b, 2.a, 3.c, 4.a, 5.b, 6.c, 7.a, 8.d, 9.b, 10.b.

Test your knowledge

❓ List the functions of blood?

❓ Explain the clotting process.

❓ Explain what would happen if the patient received mismatched blood.

❓ Where is most of the body's blood found?

❓ If the blood in the veins is dark red, why do they appear bright red when the vein is cut and bleeding?

Glossary of terms

Adenosine triphosphate: Organic molecule that stores and releases chemical energy for use in body cells.

Agglutination: Process by which red blood cells adhere to one another.

Aggregation: Clumping together.

Antibodies: Protein produced in response to the presence of some foreign substances.

Antigens: Foreign proteins against which antibodies are produced.

Bile: An alkaline fluid secreted by the liver and aids digestion of lipids.

Bilirubin: A pigment found in bile resulting from the destruction of red blood cells.

Blood groups: Classification of blood based on the type of antigen found on the surface of the red blood cell.

B lymphocytes: A type of lymphocytes that produces specific antibodies.

Coagulation: Changing from liquid to solid; formation of a blood clot.

Coenzymes: Organic compounds or metals required for enzyme function.

Connective tissue: A primary tissue characterised by cells separated by a matrix.

Epistaxis: Bleeding from the nose.

Erythrocytes: Another name for red blood cells.

Erythropoietin: Hormone that stimulates the production of red blood cells.

Gastrectomy: Excision of part or whole of the stomach.

Haematocrit: Percentage of blood volume occupied by erythrocytes.

Haemoglobin: An iron-containing protein found in red blood cells and it transports oxygen.

Haemostasis: The stoppage of bleeding.

Homeostasis: A state of inner balance in the body which remains relatively constant despite external environment changes.

Idiopathic: Without a known cause.

Immunity: A protective mechanism that forms antibodies to help protect the body against foreign substances.

Immunoglobulin: An antibody in the globulin group of proteins involved with immune response.

Intrinsic factor: A protein secreted by the parietal cells of the gastric glands and essential for the absorption of vitamin B_{12}.

Lysozymes: Enzymes that digest and breakdown microorganisms.

Mesenchyme: Embryonic mesoderm that develops into connective tissue.

Mitochondria: Cytoplasmic organelles responsible for ATP production.

Molecule: The chemical combination of two or more atoms.

Nucleus: A large organelle that contains genetic information and acts as the control centre of the cell.

Organelles: Small cellular proteins that perform specific metabolic functions.

Osmosis: Passive movement of water from an area of high concentration to an area of low concentration through a selective permeable membrane.

Pathogens: Disease causing foreign substances.

Phagocytes: Are white blood cells that engulf and destroy microorganism.

Plasma: Fluid portion of blood.

Platelet: A type of blood cell important in blood clotting.

Polypeptide: A chain of amino acids.

Urobilinogen: A product of bilirubin breakdown.

White blood cells: These are leucocytes.

References

Alexander, M.F., Fawcett, J. and Runciman, P.J. (2006). *Nursing Practice – Hospitals and Home*, 3rd edn. Edinburgh: Churchill Livingstone.

Blows, W.T. (2005). *The Biological Basis of Nursing: Cancer*. London: Routledge.

Bullock, B.A. and Henze, R.L. (2000). *Focus on Pathophysiology*. Philadelphia: Lippincott.

Hogan, M.A. and Hill, K. (2004). *Pathophysiology: Reviews and Rationale*. New Jersey: Prentice Hall.

Jamieson, E.M., McCall, J.M. and Whyte, C.A. (2002). *Clinical Nursing Practice*, 4th edn. Edinburgh: Churchill Livingstone.

Kozier, B., Erb, G., Berman, A. and Snyder, S.J. (2004). *Fundamentals of Nursing*, 7th edn. New Jersey: Pearson Prentice Hall.

Mader, S.S. (2005). *Understanding Human Anatomy and Physiology*, 5th edn. Boston: McGraw Hill.

Marieb, E.N. and Hoehn, K. (2007). *Human Anatomy and Physiology*, 7th edn. San Francisco: Pearson Benjamin Cummings.

Mehta, A. and Hoffbrand, V. (2000). *Haematology at a Glance*. Oxford: Blackwell.

Nursing and Midwifery Council (2005). *Guidelines for Record and Record Keeping*. London: NMC.

Porth, C.M. (2005). *Pathophysiology: Concepts of Altered Health States*, 7th edn. Philadelphia: Lippincott Williams & Wilkins.

Seeley, R.R., Stephens, T.D. and Tate, P. (2006). *Anatomy and Physiology*, 7th edn. Boston: McGraw Hill.

Waugh, A. and Grant, A. (2006). *Ross and Wilson: Anatomy and Physiology in Health and Illness*, 10th edn. Edinburgh: Churchill Livingstone.

Wynsberghe, D.V., Noback, C.R. and Carola, R. (1995). *Human Anatomy and Physiology*, 3rd edn. New York: McGraw Hill.

Chapter 8

The renal system and associated disorders

Muralitharan Nair

KEY WORDS

- Kidneys
- Hilus
- Renal artery
- Nephron
- Ureter
- Renal medulla
- Renal vein
- Glomerulus
- Urethra
- Renal cortex
- Renal pelvis
- Filtration

Test your prior knowledge

- Name four functions of the kidneys?
- Which substances are reabsorbed and which are excreted by the kidneys?
- List the composition of urine.
- What is the colour of urine? Think about the destruction of the red blood cells.

Introduction

The **kidneys** play an important role in maintaining homeostasis. They remove waste products through the production and **excretion** of urine and regulate fluid balance in the body. As part of their function, the kidneys filter essential substances such as sodium and potassium from the blood and selectively reabsorb substances essential to maintain homeostasis. Any substances not essential are excreted in the urine. The formation of urine is achieved through the processes of **filtration**, selective reabsorption and excretion. The kidney has also an endocrine function, secreting hormones such as **renin** and **erythropoietin**. This chapter discusses the structure and functions of the renal system. It also includes some common disorders and their related nursing management and treatment.

Renal system

The renal system, also known as the urinary system consists of:

■ kidneys
■ ureters
■ urinary bladder
■ urethra

See Figure 8.1 for the organs of the renal system.

The organs of the renal system ensure that a stable internal environment is maintained for the survival of cells and tissues in the body – homeostasis.

Kidneys
External structures
There are two kidneys, one on each side of the spinal column. They are approximately 11 cm long, 5–6 cm wide and 3–4 cm thick (Marieb and Hoehn, 2007). They are said to be bean-shaped organs where the outer border is convex; the inner border is known as the hilum (also known as **hilus**), and it is from here that the renal arteries, renal veins, nerves and the ureters enter and leave the kidneys. The

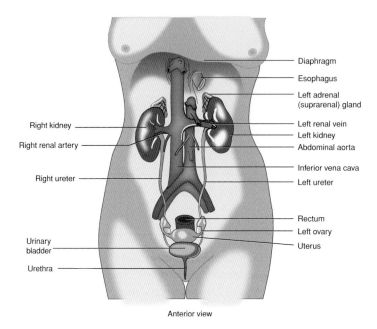

Diaphragm

Esophagus

Left adrenal
(suprarenal) gland

Right kidney

Left renal vein

Right renal artery

Left kidney

Abdominal aorta

Inferior vena cava

Right ureter

Left ureter

Rectum

Left ovary

Urinary
bladder

Uterus

Urethra

Anterior view

Figure 8.1 Renal system.

right kidney is in contact with the liver's large right lobe and hence the right kidney is approximately 2–4 cm lower than the left kidney.

Covering and supporting the kidneys consist of three layers and they are:

- renal fascia – outer layer
- adipose tissue – middle layer
- renal capsule – inner layer

See Figure 8.2 for the external layers.

Internal structures

There are three distinct regions inside a kidney and they are:

- renal cortex
- renal medulla
- renal pelvis

The renal cortex is the outermost part of the kidney. It is reddish brown and has a granular appearance, which is due to the capillaries and the structures of the nephron. The medulla is lighter in colour and has an abundance of blood vessels and tubules of the nephron (see Figure 8.3). The medulla consists of approximately 8–12 **renal pyramids** (see Figure 8.3) (Wynsberghe *et al.*, 1995). The renal pelvis is formed from the expanded upper portion of the ureter and is funnel shaped. It collects urine from the **calyces** (see Figure 8.2) and transports it to the urinary bladder.

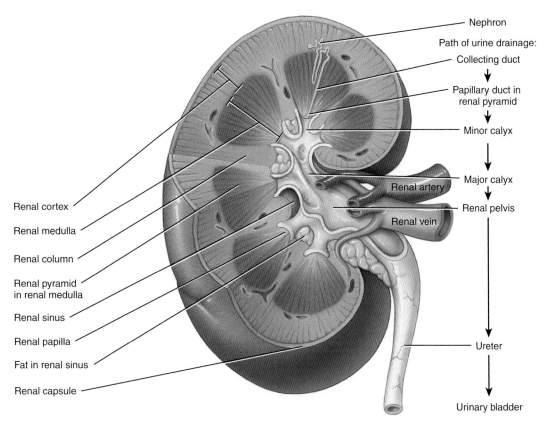

Figure 8.2 External layers of the kidney.

Nephrons

These are small structures found in the kidney. There are approximately over one million nephrons per kidney and it is in these structures where urine is formed (see Figure 8.4). The nephrons:

- filter blood
- perform selective reabsorption
- excrete unwanted waste products from the filtered blood

The nephron is divided into several sections and each section performs a different function; these are discussed in the following sections.

Bowman's capsule

Also known as glomerular capsule (see Figure 8.5) is the first portion of the nephron. It is in this section that the network of capillaries called **glomerulus** (Marieb and Hoehn 2007) are found. Filtration of blood takes place in this portion of the **nephron**.

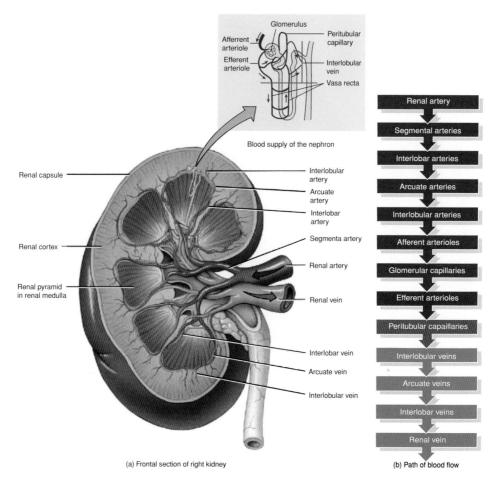

Figure 8.3 Internal structures showing blood vessels.

Proximal convoluted tubule

From the Bowman's capsule, the filtrate drains into the proximal convoluted tubule (see Figure 8.4). The cells lining this portion of the tubule actively reabsorb water, nutrients and ions into the peritubular fluid (the interstitial fluid surrounding the renal tubule).

Loop of Henle

The proximal convoluted tubule then bends into a loop called the loop of Henle (see Figure 8.4). The loop of Henle is divided into the descending and ascending loop. The ascending loop of Henle is much thicker than the descending portion.

Distal convoluted tubule

The thick ascending portion of the loop of Henle leads into the distal convoluted tubule (see Figure 8.4). The distal convoluted tubule is an important site for:

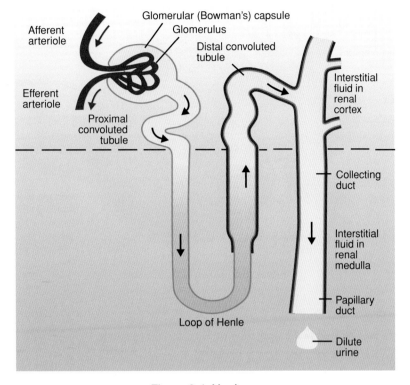

Figure 8.4 Nephron.

- active secretion of ions and acids
- selective reabsorption of sodium and calcium ions
- selective reabsorption of water

Collecting ducts

The distal convoluted tubule then drains into the collecting ducts (see Figure 8.4). Several collecting ducts converge and drain into a larger system called the papillary ducts, which in turn empties into the minor calyx (plural – calices). From here the filtrate, now called urine, drains into the renal pelvis.

Functions of the kidney

The kidneys maintain fluid balance, electrolyte balance and acid–base balance of the blood. For the summary of the functions of the kidney, see Box 8.1.

Blood supply

Approximately, 1200 mL of blood flows through the kidney each minute. Each kidney receives its blood supply directly from the aorta via the renal artery (see Figure 8.2) which is divided into anterior and posterior renal arteries. Two large veins emerge from the hilus and empty into the inferior vena cava.

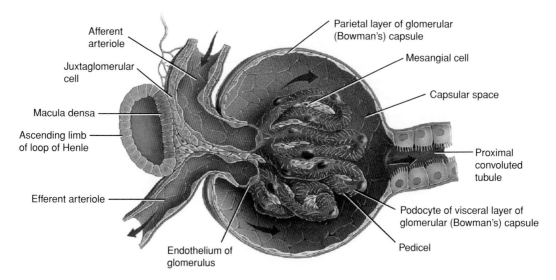

Afferent arteriole

Juxtaglomerular cell

Macula densa

Ascending limb of loop of Henle

Efferent arteriole

Endothelium of glomerulus

Parietal layer of glomerular (Bowman's) capsule

Mesangial cell

Capsular space

Proximal convoluted tubule

Podocyte of visceral layer of glomerular (Bowman's) capsule

Pedicel

Figure 8.5 Bowman's capsule.

Urine formation

Three processes are involved in the formation of urine and they include:

- filtration
- selective reabsorption
- secretion

Filtration

Filtration takes place in the glomerulus which lies in the Bowman's capsule. The blood for filtration is supplied by the **renal artery**. In the kidney, the renal artery divides into smaller arterioles. The arteriole entering the Bowman's capsule is called the afferent arteriole, which further subdivides into a cluster of capillaries called the glomerulus. The fluid from the filtered blood is protein free but contains electrolytes

---

Box 8.1 Summary of the functions of the kidney

- Filtration
- Regulate blood volume
- Regulate **osmolarity**
- Secrete renin and erythropoietin
- Maintain acid–base balance
- Synthesis of vitamin D
- Detoxify free radicals and drugs
- Gluconeogenesis

such as sodium chloride, potassium and waste products of cellular metabolism, for example urea, uric acid and creatinine (McCance and Huether, 2006). The filtered blood then returns into circulation via the efferent arteriole and finally into the **renal vein**.

Selective reabsorption

Selective reabsorption processes ensure that any substances in the filtrate that are essential for body function are reabsorbed into the plasma. Substances such as sodium, calcium, potassium and chloride are reabsorbed to maintain fluid and electrolyte balance and the pH of blood. However, if these substances are in excess to body requirements, they are excreted in the urine.

Secretion

Any substances not removed through filtration are secreted into the renal tubules from the peritubular capillaries (see Figure 8.6) of the nephron (Waugh and Grant, 2006); these include drugs and hydrogen ions.

Composition of urine

Urine is a sterile and clear fluid containing nitrogenous wastes and salts. It is transparent with an amber or light yellow colour. It is slightly acidic and the pH may range from 4.5 to 8. The pH is affected by an individual's dietary intake. Diet that is high in animal protein tends to make the urine more acidic while a vegetarian diet may make the urine more alkaline.

Urine is 96% water and approximately 4% solutes. The solutes include organic and inorganic waste products. For a summary of solutes, see Box 8.2.

Ureters

The **ureters** are approximately 25–30 cm in length and 5 mm in diameter (Mader, 2005) and they extend from the kidney to the bladder. The ureters terminate at the bladder and enter obliquely through the muscle wall of the bladder. They pass over the pelvic brim at the **bifurcation** of the common iliac arteries (see Figure 8.7).

The ureters have three layers and they are:

- transitional epithelial mucosa (inner layer)
- smooth muscle layer (middle layer)
- fibrous connective tissue (outer layer)

Urine is propelled from the kidney to the bladder by peristaltic contraction of the ureters.

Urinary bladder

The urinary bladder is located in the pelvic cavity **posterior** to the symphysis pubis. In the male, the bladder lies anterior to the rectum and in the female, it lies **anterior** to the vagina and inferior to the uterus (Mader, 2005); it is a smooth muscular sac which stores urine. As urine accumulates, the bladder

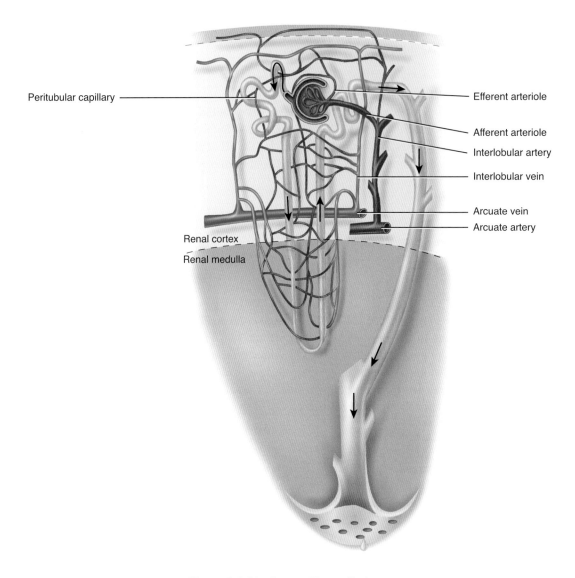

Peritubular capillary

Efferent arteriole

Afferent arteriole

Interlobular artery

Interlobular vein

Arcuate vein

Arcuate artery

Renal cortex

Renal medulla

Figure 8.6 Nephron with capillaries.

expands without a significant rise in the internal pressure of the bladder. The bladder normally distends and holds approximately 350 mL of urine.

The urinary bladder has three layers:

- transitional epithelial mucosa
- a thick muscular layer
- a fibrous outer layer

See Figure 8.8 for the layers of the urinary bladder.

Box 8.2 Summary of the solutes of the kidney

Inorganic solutes: *Organic solutes*:
Sodium   Urea
Potassium   Creatinine
Calcium   Uric acid
Magnesium
Iron
Chloride
Sulphate
Phosphate
Bicarbonate
Ammonia

Adapted from Mader (2005).

Urethra

The **urethra** is a muscular tube that drains urine from the bladder and conveys it out of the body. The urethra varies in length in both males and females. Sphincters keep the urethra closed when urine is not being passed. The internal urethral **sphincter** is under **involuntary** control and lies at the bladder–urethra junction. The external urethral sphincter is under **voluntary** control.

The male urethra passes through three different regions:

■ prostatic region – passes through the prostate gland
■ membranous portion – passes through the pelvis diaphragm
■ penile region – extends the length of the penis

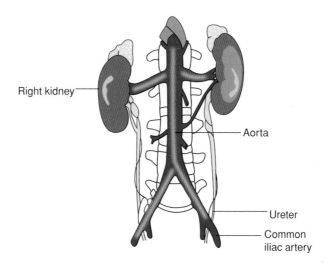

Figure 8.7 Common iliac vessels and ureter.

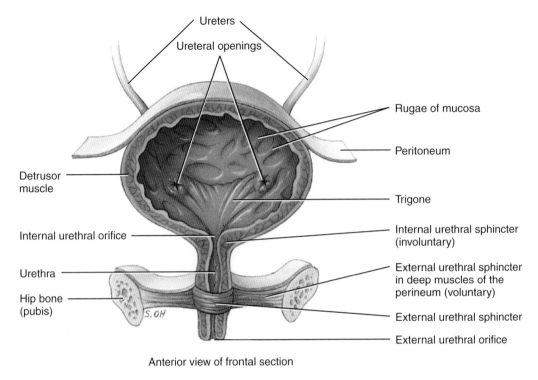

Anterior view of frontal section

Figure 8.8 Layers of the urinary bladder.

The female urethra is bound to the anterior vaginal wall. The external opening of the urethra is anterior to the vagina and posterior to the clitoris (see Figure 8.9).

Disorders of the renal system

Learning outcomes

On completion of this section, the reader will be able to:

- List some of the common diseases of the renal system and identify risk factors associated with the diseases.
- Describe the pathophysiological processes related to specific renal disorders.
- Outline the nursing management and interventions related to the disorders described.

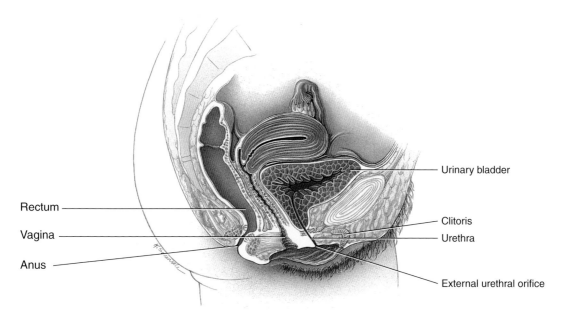

Figure 8.9 Location of the female urethra.

Pyelonephritis

Pyelonephritis is the inflammation of the renal pelvis and the functional units of the kidney (nephrons). It involves the cortex and the medulla which is called the **parenchyma** of the kidney. The incidence is higher in women than in men. There are two main types: acute and chronic pyelonephritis.

Acute pyelonephritis

In acute pyelonephritis, there is sudden or severe infection of the kidney by Gram-negative bacteria such as *Escherichia coli* and *Proteus mirabilis*. Gram-negative bacteria are those that do not retain crystal violet dye after an alcohol wash. They may have a red or pink colouration when another dye such as safranin is added to the slide. Gram-positive bacteria will retain the dye and have a purple colouration, the organism usually ascends from the lower urinary tract (urethra and the urinary bladder). In men, prostatitis and prostatic hypertrophy causing urethral obstruction predispose to bacterial infection. Acute pyelonephritis can occur by blood infection such as septicaemia.

Signs and symptoms of acute pyelonephritis

Patients with acute pyelonephritis may present with the following signs and symptoms:

- sudden onset of fever
- chills
- nausea
- vomiting
- groin pain

- haematuria
- dysuria
- rigor

Investigations to confirm diagnosis

The following may be carried out to confirm diagnosis:

- midstream specimen or catheter specimen of urine to identify causative organism
- full blood count – raised white blood cells may indicate urine infection
- intravenous pyelogram to identify any obstruction in the urinary tract
- full nursing and medical history to identify any previous urinary tract infection and kidney stones

Nursing management of acute pyelonephritis

Patients with acute pyelonephritis should be encouraged to be on bed rest until symptoms of **pyrexia** and the severe groin pain subsides. It is important to observe and report for signs of pain such as restlessness, tachycardia and sweating in order to take prompt action.

Intravenous fluid therapy may be commenced in the early stages if the patient is unable to take oral fluids due to nausea and vomiting. When able to take oral fluids, encourage patient to take 2.5–3 L (Thomas, 2002) of fluid per day to increase urine production and lessen the irritation of urethral mucosa on **micturition**.

Lemone and Burke (2004) report that the female patient should be instructed for proper cleansing of the perineal region. Instruct them to wipe front to back after voiding urine or defecating. Advise them to void urine before and after sexual intercourse in an attempt to flush out bacteria that may have been introduced into the urethra and the bladder.

Vital signs such as temperature, heart rate and respiratory rate should be monitored hourly for the first 24–48 hours to check the effect of treatment.

Patients will need psychological support and reassurance during the course of the illness and should have the opportunity to ask questions and voice their anxiety (Alexander *et al.*, 2006). Patients will need information on how to recognise the signs and symptoms of urinary tract infection and to take preventative measures.

Pharmacological interventions for acute pyelonephritis

The following medications may be prescribed to treat acute pyelonephritis:

- analgesics for pain management
- antibiotics to treat the infection
- antiemetics for nausea and vomiting
- antipyretics to treat the pyrexia

Chronic pyelonephritis

Chronic pyelonephritis progresses from acute pyelonephritis. The calices and the pelvis of the kidney are affected. Chronic pyelonephritis can begin in childhood. Repeated urinary tract infections can lead to scaring and **fibrosis** of the kidney destroys the parenchyma. Over a period of time, the kidneys become small and irregular in shape resulting in renal failure.

Signs and symptoms of chronic pyelonephritis

This condition may be asymptomatic in the early stages until the patient presents with renal failure. The patient may present with:

- fever
- abdominal and groin pain
- hypertension
- dysuria
- uraemia
- proteinuria

Investigations to confirm diagnosis

The investigations are the same as acute pyelonephritis.

Nursing management for chronic pyelonephritis

The nursing management of the patient with chronic pyelonephritis would be same as for acute pyelonephritis. However, patients who have recurrence of urinary tract infection may require long-term antibiotic therapy. In the event of renal failure as a result of kidney damage, the patient may need kidney dialysis. The nurse should prepare and educate the patient in lifestyle changes resulting from kidney dialysis such as diet and fluid intake.

Cystitis

Cystitis is the inflammation of the urinary bladder and the inflamed bladder may haemorrhage. Cystitis is the most common form of urinary tract infection and affects women more than men. The bacteria responsible for the infection are *E. coli*, which is found in the lower gastrointestinal tract and *P. mirabilis*. In women, the bacteria gain entry into the urinary bladder through the short female urethra. Cystitis could also result from non-bacterial infection such as clothing that is made from synthetic fibres, hygiene sprays and talcum powder.

Aetiology of cystitis

There are several causes and they include:

- bacterial infection
- sexual intercourse
- pregnancy
- rectal intercourse
- urinary tract obstruction as a result of enlarged prostate gland
- chemicals in washing powder
- nylon underwear
- talcum powder
- stress

Investigations to confirm diagnosis

Midstream specimen urine for culture to identify the organism.

Signs and symptoms

The patient may present with the following signs and symptoms.

- dysuria
- urgency
- pyuria
- haematuria
- abdominal discomfort
- nocturia
- urinary incontinence

Nursing management for cystitis

The main objective is to identify the cause of cystitis in order to offer the correct treatment as cystitis may not be the result of bacterial contamination. The patient will need reassurance, psychological support and health education. With recurrent urinary tract infection the patient may need long-term antibiotic therapy. The patient should be advised on the importance of taking the prescribed medication. Information on side effects of antibiotics such as diarrhoea, vomiting and allergic reactions should be provided by the nurses.

Unless contraindicated, the patient should be advised to take 2.5–3 L of fluid per day (Thomas, 2002). This would help in the production of urine and help to flush out any bacteria in the renal tract. Measurements of vital signs, for example temperature and pulse, should be recorded every 4 hours until symptoms of cystitis subside or as the patient's condition dictates. Health education would be the same as for the patient with acute pyelonephritis. Unless contraindicated, advise the patient to drink two glasses of cranberry or blueberry juice per day to maintain acidic urine (Lemone and Burke, 2004). These fruit juices contain benzoic acid, which coats the lining of the bladder wall and prevents bacteria from infiltrating into the bladder wall. Advise the patient to avoid materials or chemicals that may cause bladder irritation, such as briefs made from synthetic material, the use of hygiene sprays or bubble bath.

Renal failure

Renal failure is a condition when the kidneys are unable to remove waste products of metabolism by filtration of the blood and urine production is less than 30 mL/hour. The condition can be subdivided into acute and chronic renal failure. In acute renal failure (ARF) the condition may be sudden while in chronic renal failure (CRF) onset is gradual.

Acute renal failure

ARF is an acute decline in renal function leading to azotemia (accumulation of nitrogenous waste in the blood), fluid and electrolyte imbalance. The condition is often reversible; however, if left untreated it leads to permanent renal damage.

Pathophysiology of ARF

The causes of ARF can be categorised into prerenal, intrarenal and postrenal.

Prerenal

Prerenal causes include insufficient blood flow to the kidneys, resulting in reduced cardiac output as a result of heart failure, hypovolaemia resulting from haemorrhage and shock. The kidneys receive 20–25% of cardiac output to maintain glomerular filtration (Lemone and Burke, 2004). With a reduction of renal blood flow, this affects glomerular filtration and causes ischaemic changes to renal tissues.

Intrarenal

Intrarenal failure results from conditions that impair renal function. The renal parenchyma and nephrons are damaged leading to renal failure. Glomerulonephritis, hypertension, chemicals such as ethyl glycol and drugs, for example antibiotics, can all affect renal function.

The nephrons of the kidneys are susceptible to trauma from poor renal blood flow, hypertension and shock. The cell membranes of the nephrons are damaged as a result of the trauma. The renal tubules become blocked with debris, thus increasing tubular pressure resulting in poor elimination of sodium, water and metabolic waste.

Nephrotoxic drugs such as aminoglycoside antibiotics, non-steroidal anti-inflammatory drugs and toxins from bacteria destroy tubular cells. The damaged tubular cells become permeable to water, sodium and metabolic waste.

Postrenal

Postrenal failure results from obstruction along the ureters, urinary bladder and urethra. Obstruction resulting from stones in the ureters, prostatic hyperplasia and urethral stricture could restrict urine flow leading to postrenal failure. See Table 8.1 for summary of aetiology of ARF.

Prerenal	Intrarenal	Postrenal
Haemorrhage	Glomerulonephritis	Ureteric calculi
Low cardiac output	Hypertension	Neoplasm
Myocardial disease	Nephrotoxic drugs	Prostatic hyperplasia
Shock	Bacterial toxins	Phimosis
Heart failure	Chemicals	Urethral stricture
Liver failure		
Severe dehydration		
Adapted from Bullock and Henze (2000).		

Table 8.1 Summary of aetiology of ARF

Investigations to confirm diagnosis

The following investigations may be carried out:

- full blood count may indicate reduced red blood cell count, anaemia
- urea and electrolyte studies may indicate an increase in urea level and electrolyte imbalance such as **hyperkalemia** and **hyponatremia**
- urinalysis may indicate **proteinuria**, **haematuria** and increased cell casts
- intravenous pyelogram is carried out to evaluate renal function
- abdominal X-ray may be performed in order to identify obstructions
- renal biopsy may be necessary to differentiate between acute and chronic renal failure
- ultrasound may be carried out to identify causes of renal failure
- arterial blood gases may indicate metabolic acidosis

Signs and symptoms of ARF

- sudden onset
- **oliguria** to **anuria**
- nausea
- vomiting
- hyperkalaemia

Stages of ARF

ARF goes through three phases, namely anuric, oliguric and diuretic.

The anuric phase could last hours to days. During this period, kidney function is suppressed. The patient is oliguric or anuric during this phase. Haemorrhage may be a problem if there is tubular damage.

During the oliguric phase, urine output is minimal and could last 1–2 weeks (Alexander *et al.*, 2006). Fluid and electrolyte imbalance occurs during this phase and the **specific gravity** of urine is the same as plasma. Serum creatinine and blood urea and nitrogen (BUN) levels are elevated.

The final stage is the diuretic phase. During this phase, kidney function returns and urine production increases (**diuresis**). Diuresis could last for 24 hours and the patient may pass approximately 4–6 L of urine per day. Although there is a large volume of urine produced, full renal function is still impaired. Dehydration is a problem as a result of increased fluid loss and the inability of the kidneys to perform selective reabsorption.

Nursing management of the patient with ARF

A full nursing assessment of vital signs, weight, fluid intake and output, nursing history and assessment of the patient's knowledge of the disease process should all be carried out in order to provide high-quality care.

It is important to alleviate patient's and relative's worries and anxieties. Nurses should give time to the patient to ask questions and respond appropriately. Psychological care is important in the nursing management of the patient with ARF.

An accurate fluid intake and output should be maintained to prevent fluid overload in the early stages of the disease and to prevent dehydration in the diuretic phase.

Strict nutritional status should be maintained. Protein intake should be limited to minimise the increase of nitrogenous compounds. Carbohydrate should be increased to provide energy (Lemone and Burke, 2004).

Patient's vital signs should be monitored hourly to 2 hourly in the initial stages of the disease. Any changes should be reported immediately in order to take prompt action.

The nurse should provide education for patient to monitor weight, vital signs and fluid intake.

Pharmacological interventions for ARF

The patient may be prescribed the following medications. It is the nurse's duty to educate the patient to recognise side effects of the prescribed medications.

- furosemide may be prescribed to induce diuresis
- antihypertensives such angiotensin converting enzyme (ACE) inhibitors may be prescribed for the patient's hypertension
- antacids to prevent gastric ulcers
- analgesia may be prescribed for pain

Chronic renal failure

CRF is defined as the progressive reduction in renal function over months to years. The condition is irreversible and eventually affects all the organs of the body. The parenchyma and the nephrons are destroyed and the renal function progressively diminishes.

Aetiology of CRF

There are many causes for CRF; see Box 8.3 for the causes.

Investigations to confirm diagnosis

- urinalysis to detect abnormalities and specific gravity
- blood urea nitrogen and electrolyte levels are carried out to determine renal function
- urine culture to identify urinary tract infection

Box 8.3 Aetiology of CRF

Renal disease such as polycystic kidney
Arteriosclerosis
Chronic glomerularnephritis
Chronic pyelonephritis
Tuberculosis of the kidneys
Diabetes nephropathy
Hypertension
Renal calculi
Prostatic hypertrophy

Adapted from Alexander et al. (2006).

- renal biopsy to detect kidney diseases
- full blood count to identify the extent of anaemia
- renal ultrasound to determine the size of the kidney

Signs and symptoms of CRF

In the early stages of the disease the patient may be asymptomatic. As the disease progresses the patient may present with the following symptoms:

- lethargy
- headache
- breathlessness
- proteinuria
- haematuria
- oliguria, anuria
- symptoms of anaemia
- hypertension
- pallor

Pathophysiology of CRF

The pathophysiology of CRF involves the gradual loss of nephrons and the renal mass progressively gets smaller. There are three phases to CRF: early phase, second phase and third phase. In the early phase, the BUN levels are 20–50 mg/dL (Hogan and Hill, 2004). The glomerular filtration rate is greatly reduced and the BUN levels are elevated. During this phase, the unaffected nephrons compensate until they are damaged. The patient may be asymptomatic.

In the second phase, the BUN levels are above 100 mg/dL and creatinine is above 4 mg/dL (Hogan and Hill, 2004). The glomerular filtration rate is greatly reduced. The patient may present with symptoms such as nocturia and anaemia.

In the third phase, the BUN levels are above 200 mg/dL and the creatinine is above 5 mg/dL (Hogan and Hill, 2004). The glomerular filtration rate is greatly reduced and most of the nephrons are damaged. The patient may present with symptoms of CRF (see above for signs and symptoms).

Nursing management of the patient with CRF

The patient and his/her relatives will require support to come to terms with the disease. The disease is not curable and could lead to death. The nurse should encourage the patient to express their feelings or concerns and assist the patient in coping strategies. If necessary, refer the patient to specialist nurses such as the palliative care team.

A full nursing assessment of the patient is important in order to plan and implement high-quality care. The assessment should include the general condition of the patient, vital signs, and patient's knowledge of the disease and support systems.

Monitor and record vital signs every 2–4 hours and report any changes immediately in order to take prompt action.

Provide assistance in maintaining personal hygiene such oral hygiene, washing and dressing.

Monitor fluid intake and output to prevent fluid depletion or fluid overload.

Recommend dietary restrictions that are low in sodium, protein and high in carbohydrate.

The patient with CRF may need dialysis and it is the nurse's duty to ensure that safety is maintained at all times. Strict asepsis should be adhered to when the patient is receiving dialysis. Whether the patient has arteriovenous fistula or peritoneal dialysis, the nurse should observe the wound site for any signs of infection such as pyrexia, tachycardia and inflammation. This should be reported immediately for prompt action. All care given should be documented in accordance with Nursing and Midwifery Council guidelines on record keeping (Nursing and Midwifery Council, 2005). Administer and document effects and side effects of prescribed medications (Nursing and Midwifery Council, 2004).

Pharmacological interventions for CRF

The following medications may be prescribed for CRF:

- diuretics such furosemide to decrease fluid load
- antihypertensive, for example ACE inhibitors
- iron and folic acid for the treatment of anaemia
- analgesia if the patient is in pain

Renal calculi

Renal **calculi** are stones in the urinary tract and are the most common cause of upper urinary tract obstruction (see Figure 8.10) (Porth, 2005). Men are more at risk than women. Stones may develop and obstruct any part of the urinary tract.

Aetiology of renal calculi

Some of the causes include:

- dehydration
- immobility
- carcinoma of the bone
- urinary tract infection

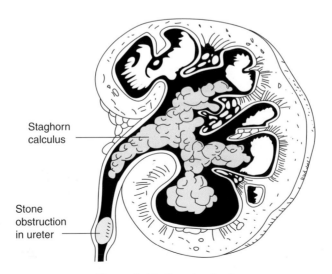

Staghorn calculus

Stone obstruction in ureter

Figure 8.10 Renal calculi.

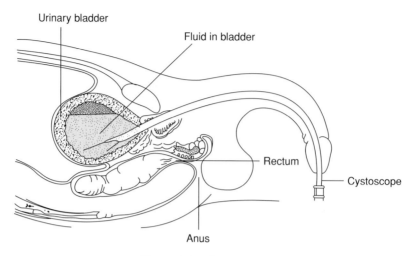

Figure 8.11 Cystoscopy.

- excessive dietary intake of calcium
- excessive dietary intake of vitamin D
- excessive dietary intake of protein
- gout
- hyperparathyroidism
- family history of kidney stones increases the risk of developing kidney stones

Investigations to confirm diagnosis
- urinalysis to detect urinary tract infection and haematuria
- abdominal X-ray to identify urinary obstruction
- ultrasound to determine urinary obstruction
- intravenous pyelogram carried out to show position of stone
- full blood count
- urea and electrolyte to detect electrolyte imbalance
- cystoscopy (see Figure 8.11)

Signs and symptoms of renal calculi
In the early stages, the condition may be asymptomatic. The presenting symptoms depend on the location of the renal stone. Stones formed in the kidney may go undetected for years until identified by routine abdominal X-ray. The patient with stones obstructing the ureters may present with colicky pain, haematuria, nausea and vomiting. Stones in the urinary bladder may not have any symptoms except dull pain in the suprapubic region after voiding urine.

Nursing management for renal calculi
Full nursing assessment should be carried out to establish the cause of renal calculi. The nursing management and treatment will depend on the identified risk factors.

Dietary modification should be encouraged if the renal calculi are as the result of excessive intake of calcium, protein, oxalate or vitamin D. Food rich in oxalate includes chocolate, rhubarb and nuts.

The patient should be encouraged to drink 2–3 L of fluid per day to flush the kidneys of any bacteria that may cause urinary tract infection and to prevent dehydration. The patient should be taught how to recognise the signs and symptoms of urinary tract infection and preventative measures.

Encourage the patient to undertake exercise such as walking, swimming or running to prevent urinary stasis. Exercise improves heart rate and circulation. It also improves blood flow to the kidneys resulting in good urine output.

Instruct the patient to take the medications as prescribed and educate the patient in the benefit of taking medications as prescribed. The patient should be taught to recognise any side effects of the prescribed medications.

Teach the patient to test and strain their urine for stones, saving any passed stone for analysis. The patient should be advised to pass all urine into a urinal as small stones can be passed in the urine unobserved by the patient. Kumar and Clark (2002) report that stones less than 0.5 cm diameter may be passed in the urine without any intervention.

Some patients will require surgery to remove the stones. Approximately, one in five stones will not pass spontaneously and may require surgical intervention. If the stone is small, shock wave lithotripsy may be used to break the stone into smaller pieces, larger stones may be removed using ureteroscopy (Parmar, 2004).

The nurse should provide psychological support to reduce anxiety by actively listening to the patient and relatives and offer information about the prevention of renal calculi.

Pharmacological interventions for renal calculi

The following medications may be prescribed for patients with renal calculi:

- analgesia for persistent pain
- antibiotics, if the patient presents with urinary tract infection

Conclusion

The renal system consists of kidneys, ureters, urinary bladder and the urethra. This chapter has provided the reader with an overview of the renal system and has discussed some of the disease processes related to the system. It is not the remit of this chapter to discuss all the diseases of the renal system. Nurses play a vital role in caring for the patient with renal disorders. In order to deliver high-quality care, nurses need a sound understanding of anatomy and physiology of the renal system. Apart from the physical aspects nurses need to consider the psychosocial aspects of care.

Patients and their relatives will need advice and support to come to terms with the disease, for example CRF where the disease is not curable and could lead to death. Often nurses are good at providing physical aspects of care for the patient but fail to include the relatives when planning the patient's care. Chronic renal conditions could lead to lifestyle changes for the patient and their relatives, and the nurse is in the forefront to offer support and guidance to the patient and their relatives.

Multiple choice questions

1. Which of the following parts of the nephron is in the renal medulla?
(a) loop of Henle
(b) glomerulus
(c) distal convoluted tubule
(d) proximal convoluted tubule

2. Urine passes through the:
(a) afferent artery → to the bladder → to the urethra
(b) efferent artery → to the bladder → to the urethra
(c) pelvis of the kidney → to the ureter → to the bladder → to the urethra
(d) pelvis of the kidney → to the urethra → to the bladder → to the ureter

3. The functional units of the kidney are:
(a) the nephron
(b) glomerulus
(c) collecting duct
(d) loop of Henle

4. Which of the following statement is true of urine?
(a) urine is slightly alkaline
(b) haemoglobin colours the urine yellow
(c) urine contains nitrogenous waste
(d) urine has white blood cells

5. Haematuria:
(a) indicates that the urine has white blood cells
(b) indicates that the urine is acidic
(c) indicates that the urine is alkaline
(d) indicates the presence of blood in the urine

6. Cystitis is:
(a) inflammation of the gallbladder
(b) inflammation of the urinary bladder
(c) inflammation of joints
(d) inflammation of the stomach

7. Glucose:
(a) is in the filtrate and not in the urine
(b) is in the filtrate and in the urine
(c) undergoes tubular excretion and is in the urine
(d) undergoes tubular excretion and is not in the urine

8. Urine is:
(a) 90% water and 10% solutes
(b) 96% water and 4% solutes
(c) 99% water and 1% solutes
(d) 80% water and 20% solutes

9. In the early stages of acute renal failure patients should:
(a) drink 4 L of fluid
(b) not have any fluid
(c) restrict fluid intake
(d) drink any amount of fluid

10. Renal calculi are:
(a) stones in the gallbladder
(b) stones in the cystic duct
(c) stones in the stomach
(d) stones in the urinary system

Answers: 1.a, 2.c, 3.a, 4.c, 5.d, 6.b, 7.a, 8.b, 9.c, 10.d.

Test your knowledge

❓ What happens to the urine output in a patient who is hypovolaemic?

❓ What happens to urine output if you eat large quantities of salty potato crisps?

❓ List the functions of the kidney.

❓ Explain the effect of alcohol on urine production?

❓ Are males or females more prone to cystitis? Explain.

Glossary of terms

Anterior: Front.

Anuria: Absence of urine.

Bifurcation: Dividing into two branches.

Calculi: Stones.

Calyces: Small funnel-shaped cavities formed from the renal pelvis.

Diuresis: Excess urine production.

Dysuria: Painful urination.

Erythropoietin: Hormone produced by the kidneys that regulates red blood cell production.

Excretion: The elimination of waste products of metabolism.

Fibrosis: Growth of fibrous connective tissue.

Filtration: A passive transport system.

Glomerulus: A network of capillaries found in the Bowman's capsule.

Haematuria: Blood in the urine.

Hilus: A small indented part of the kidney.

Hyperkalemia: High potassium level in the blood.

Hyponatremia: Low sodium level in the blood.

Involuntary: Cannot be controlled.

Kidneys: Organs situated in the posterior wall of the abdominal cavity.

Micturition: The act of voiding urine.

Nephron: Functional unit of the kidney.

Nocturia: Excessive urination at night.

Oliguria: Diminished urine output.

Osmolarity: The osmotic pressure of a fluid.

Parenchyma: Soft tissue of the kidney involving the cortex and the medulla.

Posterior: Behind.

Proteinuria: Protein in the urine.

Pyrexia: Fever.

Pyuria: Presence of white blood cells in the urine.

Renal artery: Blood vessel that takes blood to the kidney.

Renal cortex: The outermost part of the kidney.

Renal medulla: The middle layer of the kidney.

Renal pelvis: The funnel-shaped section of the kidney.

Renal pyramids: Cone-shaped structures of the medulla.

Renal vein: Blood vessel that returns filtered blood into circulation.

Renin: A renal hormone that alters systemic blood pressure.

Specific gravity: Density.

Sphincter: A ring-like muscle fibre that can constrict.

Ureters: Membranous tube that drains urine from the kidneys to the bladder.

Urethra: Muscular tube that drains urine from the bladder.

Urgency: Feeling of the need to void urine immediately.

Voluntary: Can be controlled.

References

Alexander, M.F., Fawcett, J. and Runciman, P.J. (2006). *Nursing Practice – Hospitals and Home*. Edinburgh: Churchill Livingstone.

Bullock, B.A. and Henze, R.L. (2000). *Focus on Pathophysiology*. Philadelphia: Lippincott.

Hogan, M.A. and Hill, K. (2004). *Pathophysiology: Reviews and Rationale*. New Jersey: Prentice Hall.

Kumar, P. and Clark, M. (2002). *Clinical Medicine*, 5th edn. Edinburgh: W.B. Saunders.

Lemone, P. and Burke, K. (2004). *Medical – Surgical Nursing: Critical Thinking in Client Care*. New Jersey: Pearson Education.

Mader, S.S. (2005). *Understanding Human Anatomy and Physiology*, 5th edn. Boston: McGraw Hill.

Marieb, E.N. and Hoehn, K. (2007). *Human Anatomy and Physiology*, 7th edn. San Francisco: Pearson Benjamin Cummings.

McCance, K.L. and Huether, S.E. (2006). *Pathophysiology: The Biological Basis for Disease in Adults and Children*, 5th edn. St. Lewis: Mosby.

Nursing and Midwifery Council (2004). *Guidelines for Administration of Medicines*. London: NMC.

Nursing and Midwifery Council (2005). *Guideline for Record and Record Keeping*. London: NMC.

Parmar, M.S. (2004). Kidney stones. *BMJ*, *328*(7453), 1420–1424.

Porth, C.M. (2005). *Pathophysiology: Concepts of Altered Health States*, 7th edn. Philadelphia: Lippincott Williams & Wilkins.

Thomas, N. (ed) (2002). *Renal Nursing*, 2nd edn. London: Bailliere Tindall.

Waugh, A. and Grant, A. (2006). *Ross and Wilson: Anatomy and Physiology in Health and Illness*, 10th edn. Edinburgh: Churchill Livingstone.

Wynsberghe, D.V., Noback, C.R. and Carola, R. (1995). *Human Anatomy and Physiology*, 3rd edn. New York: McGraw Hill.

Chapter 9

The respiratory system and associated disorders

Anthony Wheeldon

KEY WORDS

- Carbon dioxide (CO_2)
- External respiration
- Hypoxaemia
- Oxygen (O_2)
- Dyspnoea
- Haemoglobin (Hb)
- Hypercapnia
- Respiration
- Expiration
- Hypoxia
- Inspiration
- Respiratory failure

Test your prior knowledge

- Name five major anatomical structures of the lower respiratory tract.
- What is the main function of the respiratory system?
- What nursing observations would you use to assess a patient's respiratory status?

Learning outcomes

On completion of this section, the reader will be able to:

- List the main anatomical structures of both the upper and the lower respiratory tracts.
- Describe the process of pulmonary ventilation.
- Discuss the principles of external respiration.
- Explain how the body is able to control the rate and depth of breathing.

Introduction

All human cells require a continuous supply of oxygen; indeed, cells will only survive for a few minutes without it. Fortunately, around 21% of the air within our atmosphere is oxygen, providing a plentiful supply. As cells use oxygen, the waste gas (carbon dioxide) is produced. If allowed to build up, carbon dioxide can affect cellular activity and disrupt homeostasis. Therefore, the principal function of the respiratory system is to ensure that the body extracts enough oxygen from the atmosphere whilst disposing excess carbon dioxide. The collection of oxygen and removal of carbon dioxide is referred to as respiration. Respiration involves the following four distinct processes, **pulmonary ventilation**, **external respiration**, **transport of gases** and **internal respiration**. Although all four are examined in this chapter, only pulmonary ventilation and external respiration are the sole responsibility of the respiratory system. As oxygen and carbon dioxide are transported around the body in blood, effective respiration is also reliant upon a fully functioning cardiovascular system.

The respiratory system is divided into upper and lower respiratory tracts. It is within the lower respiratory tract that external respiration takes place and the structures involved are microscopic, very fragile and easily damaged by infection. For this reason, both the upper and the lower respiratory tracts are equipped to fight off any invading airborne bacterial or viral pathogens. However, the air we breathe is also contaminated by a wide variety of pollutants (e.g. exhaust fumes, industrial gases, cigarette smoke) and as a result respiratory diseases are highly prevalent throughout the world.

Respiratory disease accounts for 20% of all deaths in the United Kingdom (UK), more than coronary heart disease. The most common respiratory diseases include lung cancer, asthma, chronic obstructive pulmonary disease (COPD), pneumonia and tuberculosis (TB). Together they place a heavy burden on the National Health Service (NHS), costing an estimated £3 billion pounds a year. Every year in the UK, one in every five men and one in every four women consult their GP regarding a respiratory complaint, resulting in around 62 million prescriptions (British Thoracic Society, 2006).

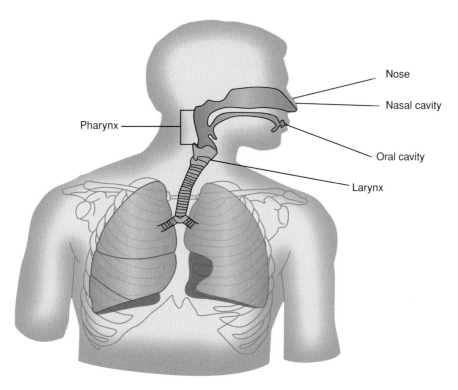

Figure 9.1 The main structures of the upper respiratory tract.

Anatomy and physiology

The upper respiratory tract

The upper respiratory tract consists of the oral cavity (mouth), the nasal cavity (the nose), the pharynx and the larynx (see Figure 9.1). As well as providing also smell and speech the upper respiratory tract ensures that the air entering the lower respiratory tract is warm, damp and clean. First and foremost, the spaces just inside the nostrils are lined with course hairs that filter incoming air, ensuring that large dust particles do not enter the airways. The nasal cavity is also lined with a mucus membrane made from **pseudostratified ciliated columnar epithelium**, which contains a network of capillaries and a plentiful supply of mucus-secreting **goblet cells**. The blood flowing through the capillaries warms the passing air while the mucus moistens it and traps any passing dust particles. The mucus-covered dust particles are then propelled by the **cilia** towards the pharynx where they can be swallowed or **expectorated**. To add further protection the upper respiratory tract is lined with irritant receptors, which when stimulated by invading particles (dust or pollen for example) force a sneeze ensuring the offending material is ejected through the nose or mouth.

Unlike the nasal cavity and larynx, the pharynx acts as a passage for food as well as air. The pharynx also contains five tonsils. The two tonsils visible when the mouth is open are the palatine tonsils, behind the tongue lie the lingual tonsils and the pharyngeal tonsil or adenoid sits on the upper back wall of the pharynx. Tonsils are **lymph nodules** and part of the body's defence system. The epithelial lining

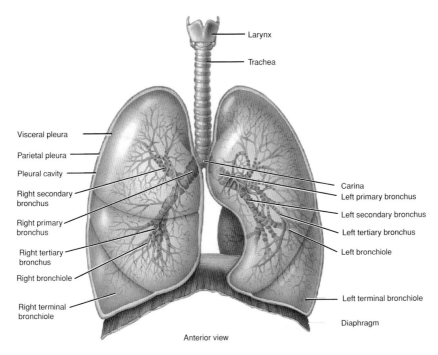

Figure 9.2 Gross anatomy of the lower respiratory tract.

of their surface has deep folds, called crypts. Inhaled bacteria or particles become entangled within the crypts and are then engulfed and destroyed.

The larynx (voice box) also provides a degree of protection, this time from food. The larynx occupies the space between the pharynx and the trachea – the first section of the lower respiratory tract. Also nearby is the oesophagus, which propels food towards the stomach. Attached to the top of the larynx is a leaf-shaped piece of epithelial-covered **elastic cartilage**, called the epiglottis. On swallowing the epiglottis blocks entry to the larynx and food and liquid is diverted towards the oesophagus. Inhalation of solid or liquid substances can block the lower respiratory tract and cut off the body's supply of oxygen – this medical emergency is referred to as aspiration and necessitates the swift removal of the offending substance.

The lower respiratory tract

The lower respiratory tract includes the trachea, the right and left primary bronchi and all the constituents of both lungs (see Figure 9.2). The trachea (or windpipe) is a tubular vessel that carries air from the larynx down towards the lungs. The trachea is also lined with pseudostratified ciliated columnar epithelium so that any inhaled debris are trapped and propelled upwards towards the oesophagus and pharynx to be swallowed or expectorated. The trachea and the bronchi also contain irritant receptors, which stimulate a cough forcing larger invading particles upwards. The outermost layer of the trachea contains connective tissue that is reinforced by a series of 16–20 C-shaped **cartilage** rings. The rings prevent the trachea from collapsing despite the pressure changes that occur during an active breathing cycle. If any obstruction occurs above the larynx, be it a foreign object, inflammation or trauma, a hole or stoma may

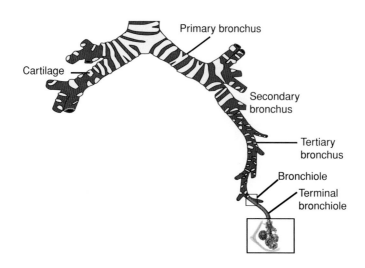

Figure 9.3 The bronchial tree.

be created in the trachea and a small tube inserted. This procedure is called a **tracheostomy** and can ensure that the blocked portion of the upper airway is bypassed, enabling the patient to breathe (Russell and Metta, 2004).

The lungs are two cone-shaped organs that almost fill the **thorax**. They are protected by a framework of bones, the thoracic cage, which consists of the ribs, sternum (breast bone) and vertebrae (spine). The tip of each lung, the apex, extends just above the clavicle (collar bone) and their wider bases sit just above a concave muscle called the diaphragm. The lungs are divided into distinct regions called lobes. There are three lobes in the right lung and two in the left. The heart along with its major blood vessels sits in a space between the two lungs called the cardiac notch. Each lung is surrounded by a two thin protective membranes called the parietal and visceral pleura (see Figure 9.2). The parietal pleura lines the walls of the thorax whereas the visceral pleura lines the lungs themselves. The space between the two pleura, the pleural space, is minute and contains a thin film of lubricating fluid. This reduces friction between the two pleura, allowing both layers to slide over one another during breathing. The fluid also helps the visceral and parietal pleura to adhere to one another, in the same way two pieces of glass stick together when wet.

The airways of the lower respiratory tract divide into branches; for this reason they are often called the bronchial tree. Within the lungs, the primary bronchi divide into the secondary bronchi, each serving a lobe (three secondary bronchi on the right and two on the left). The secondary bronchi split into tertiary bronchi (see Figures 9.2 and 9.3) of which there are ten in each lung. Tertiary bronchi continue to divide into a network of bronchioles which eventually lead to a terminal bronchiole. The section of the lung supplied by a terminal bronchiole is referred to as a lobule and each lobule has its own arterial blood supply and **lymph vessels**. The bronchial tree continues to subdivide with the terminal bronchiole leading to a series of respiratory bronchioles which in turn generate several alveolar ducts. The airways terminate with numerous sphere-like structures called alveoli which are clustered together to form alveolar sacs (see Figure 9.4). There are approximately 490 million alveoli in your lungs (Ochs *et al.*, 2004).

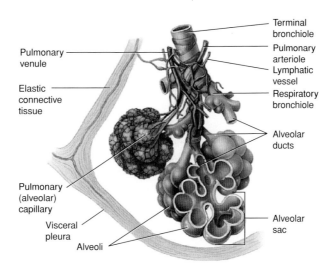

Figure 9.4 Microscopic anatomy of a lobule.

Pulmonary ventilation

Pulmonary ventilation describes the process more commonly known as breathing. In order to understand breathing some knowledge of the behaviour of gases is needed. For instance air always flows from an area of high pressure to low pressure. All the gases in the atmosphere collectively exert a pressure called atmospheric pressure. The gases in the lungs also exert a pressure known as alveolar pressure (McGowan et al., 2003). During inspiration, the thorax expands and alveolar pressure, falls below atmospheric pressure. Because alveolar pressure is now less than atmospheric pressure, air will naturally move into our airways until the pressure difference no longer exists. This phenomenon is explained by Boyle's law, which states that, at a constant temperature, the pressure of gas in the lungs is inversely proportional to their size. In other words, as the size of the thorax increases the pressure inside falls as the gas molecules have more room to circulate (Hlastala and Berger, 2001).

A range of respiratory muscles are used to achieve thoracic expansion during inspiration (see Figure 9.5). The rib cage is pulled outwards and upwards by the **external intercostal muscles**, whilst the diaphragm contracts downward pulling the lungs with it. Expiration is a more passive process. The external intercostal muscles and the diaphragm relax allowing the natural elastic recoil of the lung tissue to spring back into shape, forcing air back into the atmosphere (see Figure 9.6). Other respiratory muscles can also be utilised. The abdominal wall muscles and **internal intercostal muscles**, for instance, are utilised to force air out beyond a normal breath, when playing a musical instrument or blowing out candles on a birthday cake, for example. The sternocleidomastoids, the scalenes and the pectoralis can also be used to produce a deep forceful inspiration. These muscles are referred to as accessory muscles, so called because they are rarely used in normal quiet breathing (Simpson, 2006).

External respiration

External respiration only occurs beyond the respiratory bronchioles. For this reason, the end portion of the bronchial tree is called the respiratory zone. The remainder of the bronchial tree from the trachea down to the terminal bronchioles is the conducting zone. Because the air present in the conducting zone

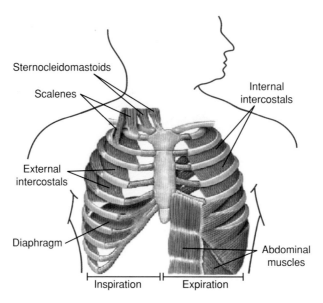

Figure 9.5 Muscles involved in pulmonary ventilation.

plays no part in supplying the body with oxygen, it is also referred to as anatomical dead space. External respiration is the **diffusion** of oxygen from the alveoli into pulmonary circulation (blood flow through the lungs) and the diffusion of carbon dioxide in the opposite direction. Diffusion occurs because gas molecules always move from areas of high concentration to low concentration. Each lobule of the lung has its own arterial blood supply; this blood supply originates from the pulmonary artery, which stems from the right ventricle of the heart. The blood present in the pulmonary artery has been collected

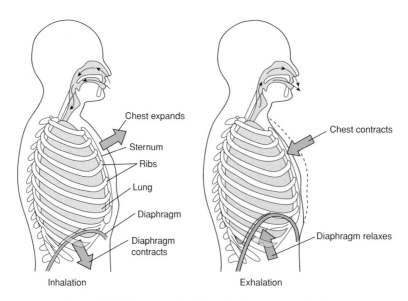

Figure 9.6 Movements of inspiration and expiration.

from **systemic circulation** and is therefore low in oxygen and relatively high in carbon dioxide. The amount (and therefore concentration) of oxygen in the alveoli is far greater than in the passing arterial blood supply. Oxygen therefore moves passively out of the alveoli and into pulmonary circulation and on towards the left-hand side of the heart. Because there is less carbon dioxide in the alveoli than in pulmonary circulation, carbon dioxide transfers into the alveoli ready to be exhaled (see Figure 9.7).

Transport of gases and internal respiration

Blood transports oxygen and carbon dioxide between the lungs and all the tissue cells of the body. Cells utilise oxygen when manufacturing the cells' prime energy source, adenosine triphosphate (ATP). In addition to ATP, the cells also produce water and carbon dioxide. Internal respiration describes the exchange of oxygen and carbon dioxide between blood and tissue cells, a phenomenon governed by the same principles of external respiration. Because cells are continually using oxygen, its concentration within tissue is always lower than within blood. Likewise, the continual use of oxygen ensures that the level of carbon dioxide within tissue is always higher than within blood. As blood flows through the capillaries, oxygen and carbon dioxide follow their concentration gradients and continually diffuse between blood and tissue (see Figure 9.7).

Control of breathing

Respiratory centres within the **medulla oblongata** and **pons** are responsible for controlling the rate and depth of breathing (see Figure 9.8). Within the medulla oblongata there are **chemoreceptors**, which continually analyse carbon dioxide levels within **cerebrospinal fluid**. As levels of carbon dioxide rise, messages are sent via the **phrenic** and **intercostal nerves** to the diaphragm and intercostal muscles instructing them to contract. Another set of chemoreceptors found in the **aorta** and **carotid arteries** analyse levels of oxygen as well as carbon dioxide. If oxygen falls or carbon dioxide rises, messages are sent to the respiratory centres via the glossopharyngeal nerve and vagus nerve, stimulating further contraction (see Figure 9.9). Throughout the day, whether at work, rest or play our respiration rate changes in order to meet our body's oxygen demands.

Although breathing is essentially a subconscious activity, the rate and depth of breathing can be controlled voluntarily or even stopped altogether when swimming under water, for example. However, this voluntary control is limited as your respiratory centres have a strong urge to take over. Breathing can also be influenced by state of mind. The inspiratory area of the respiratory centres (see Figure 9.8) can be stimulated by both the limbic system and hypothalamus, two areas of the brain responsible for processing our emotions. Fear, anxiety or even the anticipation of stressful activities can cause an involuntary increase in the rate and depth of breathing. Other factors that can affect breathing include **pyrexia** and pain. Because breathing is largely beyond an individual's control, any changes in respiration rate are clinically significant (see Table 9.1).

Pathophysiology

On completion of this section, the reader will be able to:

- Explain the principles of respiratory failure.
- Describe the pathophysiology of TB and pneumonia.

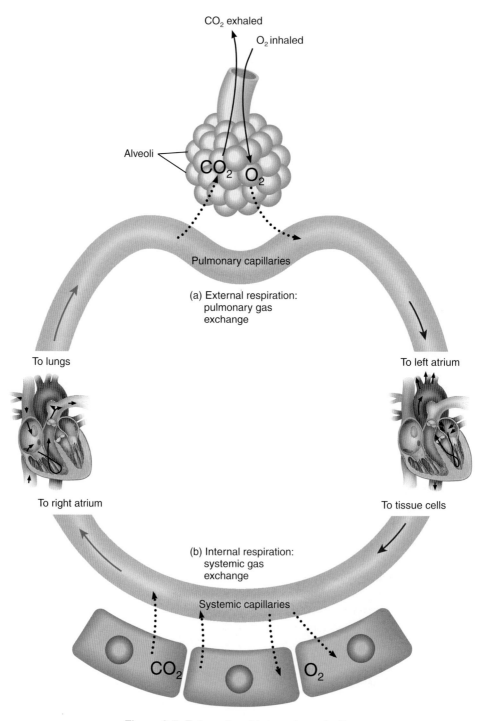

Figure 9.7 External and internal respiration.

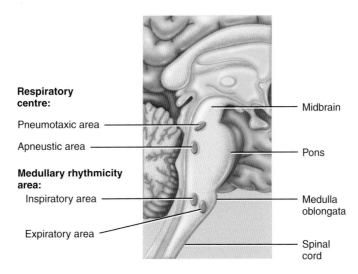

Figure 9.8 The respiratory centres of the brainstem.

- Discuss the pathophysiology of obstructive and restrictive disorders.
- Describe the physiological changes that occur due to pleural disorders.
- Outline the nursing management of pneumonia, asthma, COPD and pleural disorders.

Respiratory failure

Respiratory failure occurs when respiration is unable to sustain the metabolic needs of the body (Schwartzstein and Parker, 2006). In other words, the lungs are not extracting enough oxygen from the atmosphere. The majority of oxygen (around 98%) is attached to **haemoglobin (Hb)** which is

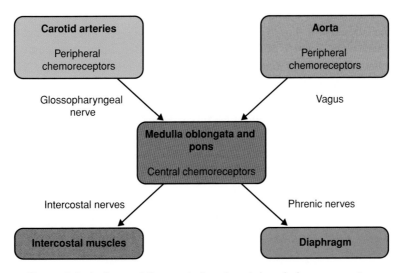

Figure 9.9 Actions of the central and peripheral chemoreceptors.

Term	Definition
Eupnoea	Easy or normal breathing, with a respiration between 12 and 16 breaths per minute
Tachypnoea	Rapid and usually shallow respiration rate, more than 20 breaths per minute
Bradypnoea	Slow respiration rate less than 10 breaths per minute
Hyperventilation	Increased respiration rate associated with increased ventilation – increased amounts of air entering the alveoli
Hypoventilation	Decreased ventilation – lack of air entering the alveoli
Apnoea	The absence of breathing for more than 15 seconds
Hypopnoea	Shallow breathing with inadequate ventilation
Dyspnoea	Difficult or laboured breathing
Orthopnoea	Difficulty in breathing while lying flat
Cheyne–Stokes breathing	Irregular breathing cycles associated with drugs overdose, neurological disturbances and the dying patient

Table 9.1 Important terminology of breathing

found in abundance in **erythrocytes** (red blood cells). A **pulse oximiter** can gauge what percentage of haemoglobin is carrying oxygen. This reading is called 'oxygen saturation' (SpO_2). In health, SpO_2 should be between 95 and 99%; however, tremors, **anaemia**, **polycythaemia**, cold extremities and nail varnish can all reduce the accuracy of the reading. For this reason, SpO_2 should only be used in conjunction with other nursing observations (Clark *et al.*, 2006). A reduced amount of oxygen in arterial blood is called **hypoxaemia**. One major symptom of severe hypoxaemia is **central cyanosis**, a visible bluish hue or tinge visible in the lips and mouth. Hypoxaemia naturally leads to the development of **hypoxia**, a lack of oxygen in tissue cells. However, hypoxaemia is not the only cause of hypoxia; if you recall, effective transport of oxygen also requires a fully functioning cardiovascular system. Heart failure or haemorrhage, for example, could also result in hypoxia. When a patient is hypoxaemic they are said to be in *respiratory failure type 1*. Ultimately the underlying cause should be treated but oxygen may be prescribed to increase SpO_2.

Around 10% of all carbon dioxide is dissolved in plasma and the rest diffuses into the erythrocytes. Once inside the erythrocyte, 20% of the carbon dioxide binds to haemoglobin and the remainder combines with water to form carbonic acid. The carbonic acid then quickly dissociates into bicarbonate ions and hydrogen ions (see equation below).

$$\underset{\text{Carbon dioxide}}{CO_2} + \underset{\text{Water}}{H_2O} \rightleftarrows \underset{\text{Carbonic acid}}{H_2CO_3} \rightleftarrows \underset{\text{Hydrogen ions}}{H^+} + \underset{\text{Bicarbonate ions}}{HCO_3^-}$$

Naturally, the carbon dioxide dissolved in plasma will also generate carbonic acid. However, the reaction which occurs within the erythrocyte is much faster due to the presence of the **enzyme** carbonic anhydrase. The production of hydrogen and bicarbonate helps to regulate arterial blood pH. A normal arterial blood pH should rest between a very narrow range (7.35–7.45). As levels of hydrogen ion rise and pH starts to fall below 7.35, more hydrogen ions are combined with bicarbonate to form carbonic acid. As hydrogen ion levels fall and pH starts to rise, more carbonic acid dissociates. Respiration therefore can regulate hydrogen ion concentration (West, 2005).

Respiratory disease often leads to respiratory muscle fatigue which in turn may lead to a more shallow and weaker rate and depth of breathing. Any reduction in ventilation will lead to an accumulation of carbon dioxide, a phenomenon known as **hypercapnia**. Any patient that is hypoxaemic and hypercapnic is said to be in *respiratory failure type 2*. Because high carbon dioxide levels lead to a reduction in arterial blood pH, respiratory failure type 2 is often referred to as **respiratory acidosis**. Respiratory failure type 2 is a medical emergency and the only way to reduce carbon dioxide is to 'breathe' it away by improving ventilation. Ventilation can be improved by placing the patient onto a mechanical ventilator which can increase the patient's depth of breathing. One common example of mechanical ventilation used in both hospital and community settings is **non-invasive positive pressure ventilation (NIPPV)**. NIPPV is delivered by a special portable machine that delivers breaths via a flexible hose and special facial mask (British Thoracic Society, 2002). Patients with respiratory diseases may have chronic respiratory failure. In such cases, the body develops compensatory mechanisms to cope with the diminished oxygen supply and possible elevated carbon dioxide levels (Margereson, 2001).

Lower respiratory tract infections

Tuberculosis

TB is a lung infection mainly caused by *Mycobacterium tuberculosis*, an airborne slow-growing **bacillus**. The signs and symptoms of TB include **haemoptysis**, weight loss, pyrexia, fatigue and night sweats. When the individual is first infected, usually in the upper lobes, **lymphocytes** and **nuetrophils** congregate at the infection site. The bacilli are then trapped and walled off by **fibrous** tissue. This phase of TB is referred to as the primary infection and the infected individual is often asymptomatic and unaware. At some point thereafter re-exposure to TB or another form of bacteria causes a secondary infection. The bacilli are then reactivated and start to multiply after which the patient soon becomes symptomatic and infectious. Bacilli are very arduous and can survive trapped in fibrous tissue for long periods. Individuals can remain unaware that they have TB for many years.

Incidence of TB is growing worldwide and its rise is attributed to increased international travel, immigration and poverty. TB, however, can be successfully treated on an outpatient basis with a 6-month course of a combination of antibiotics. Because of the recent increases in drug resistant strains of TB the major aspects of nursing care are health promotion and the maintenance of compliance (National Collaboration Centre for Chronic Conditions, 2006).

Pneumonia

Pneumonia is an infection of the alveoli and small airways. Inflammation and **oedema** cause the alveoli to fill with debris and **exudate**. The exudate quickly fills with neutrophils, erythrocytes and **fibrin** and a solid mass called consolidation is formed. Consolidation can be patchy and spread throughout both lungs or concentrated in one mass affecting one or more lobes. Consolidation in the alveoli disturbs external

Box 9.1 Signs and symptoms of pneumonia

- ■ Hypoxaemia
- ■ Tachypnoea and dyspnoea
- ■ Tachycardia
- ■ Pyrexia – in response to bacterial infection
- ■ Dehydration – pyrexia causes fluid loss, also body loses humidified air on expiration
- ■ Reduced lung expansion – consolidation makes it hard to expand the lungs and breathing becomes difficult
- ■ Pain – inflammation could spread to the pleura, causing pleuritic pain (pleurisy)
- ■ Productive cough – the exudate present in the alveoli often produces rusty coloured sputum
- ■ Lethargy

respiration and less oxygen diffuses from the alveoli into pulmonary circulation; as a result the patient becomes hypoxaemic and breathless (see Box 9.1). Pneumonia can develop secondary to aspiration or other airway infections (i.e. influenza); however, in the majority of cases people catch pneumonia from inhaled pathogens. Up to 12% of all GP prescriptions for lower respiratory tract infections are for pneumonia (British Thoracic Society, 2004). Table 9.2 summarises the investigations used to establish a diagnosis of pneumonia.

Pneumonia can either be community or hospital-acquired. In one third of cases of community-acquired pneumonia the cause remains unknown; however, key known pathogens include *Streptococcus pnuemoniae*, *Chlamidya pnuemoniae* and *Legionella* (Legionnaire's disease). Alcoholism, smoking, drug abuse and chronic heart and lung disease all increase the risk of contracting pneumonia. The

Investigation	Rationale
Full blood count	A white blood cell count above 11×10^9 per litre indicates inflammation, infection or an immune system response
Urea and electrolytes	Raised urea (>7 mmol/L) is an indicator of severe infection
Blood and sputum cultures	To identify the causative agent and appropriate antibiotic treatment
Liver function test	Acute pneumonia can effect liver function
X-ray	To establish the extent of infected lung tissue
Hoare and Lim (2006).	

Table 9.2 The main investigations of pneumonia

immunosuppressed are also vulnerable; however, the invading bacteria in such cases are usually either candida (fungus) or *Pneumocystic carinii* (PCP).

As its name suggests hospital-acquired pneumonia is contracted during a hospital admission. Inpatients are exposed to a wide variety of risks whilst in hospital. Unconscious patients, for example, require **intubation** and postoperative patients may have a suppressed cough, increasing the risk of aspiration. Furthermore, long-term patients are often immunosuppressed and repeatedly exposed to a multitude of pathogens. Hospital-acquired pneumonia is often caused by bacteria such as *Escherichia*, *Klebsiella* and *Psuedomonas* and, regrettably, occurs in 1–5% of all admissions (McGowan *et al.*, 2003).

Nursing management of pneumonia

Pneumonia can develop into a severe infection. However, up to 42% of cases will require inpatient care and between 5 and 10% of patients will require an admission to intensive care (British Thoracic Society, 2004). The nurse can play an important role in the early detection of deterioration. The main nursing goals include:

- Safe administration of prescribed antibiotics.
- Safe administration of prescribed oxygen – to correct hypoxaemia and maintain oxygen saturations above 90%.
- Patient positioning – placing the patient in an upright position will promote diaphragm and intercostal muscle activity and enhance ventilation.
- Establishing and minimising pain levels – to make the patient more comfortable and enhance breathing. Utilise an appropriate pain assessment tool (see Chapter 15).
- Temperature management – safe administration of **antipyretic agents**, such as aspirin, paracetamol or ibuprofen, electric fans, reducing bed clothes.
- Close monitoring of vital signs – respiration rate greater than 30 respirations per minute, new **hypotension** (systolic less than 90 mm Hg or diastolic less than 60 mm Hg) and new mental confusion could indicate life-threatening pneumonia (British Thoracic Society, 2004). Vital signs should therefore be recorded hourly until patient's condition stabilises.
- Fluid balance – as patient is dehydrated. A minimum of 2.5 L every 24 hours is required. Fluids may be administered intravenously if required (Dunn, 2005).
- Communication – to reduce anxiety and promote comfort.

Obstructive disorders

Obstructive lung disorders involve a degree of obstruction to airflow. In conditions such as asthma and COPD the obstruction to airflow is associated with narrow airways and increased airflow resistance. If the lumen of an airway is halved, then resistance to airflow will increase 16 times. As resistance increases and more and more gas molecules collide a noise is generated, accounting for the characteristic wheeze often heard in respiratory patients (Middleton and Middleton, 2002). In many patients, airway resistance can be overcome by increasing the respiratory muscle work. However, normal passive expiration may not be enough to promote adequate alveoli emptying. Forced expiration generates high intrathoracic pressures that force smaller airways to close, trapping air in the chest.

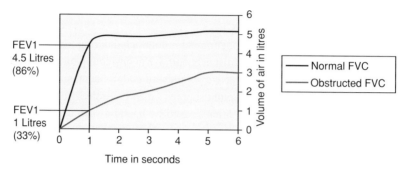

Figure 9.10 Spirometry – a normal forced vital capacity compared to an obstructed forced vital capacity.

Investigations for obstructive airways disorders

The extent of air trapping can be measured by using **spirometry**, which measures the force and volume of a maximum expiration after a full inspiration. The volume of air one is able to force out is referred to as forced vital capacity (FVC) and the volume one can exhale in the first second of expiration is their forced expiratory volume (FEV_1) (see Figure 9.10). By comparing FEV_1 with FVC, the FEV_1:FVC ratio and the severity of airway obstruction can be ascertained. An individual with an FEV_1:FVC ratio of less than 80% has obstructed airways (Sheldon, 2005). Another important measure of airway resistance is **peak expiratory flow rate (PEFR)** or 'peak flow'. PEFR measures the force of expiration in litres per minute. It measures the patient's maximum expiratory flow rate via their mouth. An inability to meet a predicted value based on age, sex and height could indicate airway obstruction. Peak expiratory flow rates provide a quick and simple assessment of the airways; however, regular peak flow measurements are more revealing than single arbitrary readings and nurses should be mindful that peak expiratory flow rates are effort dependent (Talley and O'Connor, 2001).

Asthma

Asthma is a chronic inflammatory disorder of the lungs. It causes the bronchi and bronchioles to become inflamed and constricted. As a result, airflow becomes obstructed, often resulting in a characteristic wheeze. In the UK, 11% of men and 12% of women have doctor-diagnosed asthma (British Thoracic Society, 2006).

Asthmatics periodically react to triggers. Triggers are substances or situations that would not normally trouble an asthma-free person. Asthma is said to be either **extrinsic** or **intrinsic**. In extrinsic asthma, airway inflammation is a consequence of hypersensitive reactions associated with allergy, i.e. pollen, dust mites or foodstuffs. Whereas intrinsic asthma is linked to hyperresponsive reactions to other forms of stimuli, infection, sudden exposure to cold, exercise, stress or cigarette smoke, for example. Extrinsic asthma is more common in childhood, with many sufferers 'growing out' of it in adolescence, intrinsic asthma on the other hand usually develops in adulthood. Many patients, however, have a combination of both types and irrespective of causative agents the physiological changes, symptoms and treatments are the same.

The pathophysiology of asthma is complicated and intricate. The bronchi and bronchioles contain smooth muscle and are lined with mucus-secreting glands and ciliated cells (see Figure 9.11). Close to

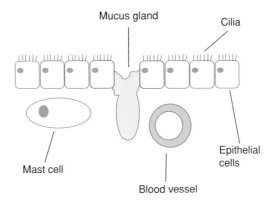

Figure 9.11 Cellular structure of airway the airways.

the airways' blood supply, there are large quantities of **mast cells**. Once stimulated mast cells release a number of cytokines (chemical messengers), which cause physiological changes to the lining of the bronchi and bronchioles. Three such cytokines are histamine, kinins and prostaglandins, which cause smooth muscle contraction, increased mucus production and capillary permeability. The airways soon narrow and become flooded with mucus and fluid leaking from blood vessels (see Figure 9.12). As the airways become obstructed, the patient finds it increasingly hard to breathe and to cough up the mucus. If unresolved fatigue can occur and the patient's respiratory effort becomes weak and inadequate, causing hypoxaemia and in severe cases hypercapnia (Sims, 2006).

Nursing management of asthma

In the UK, around 1500 people a year dic from asthma (British Thoracic Society, 2006); therefore, health professionals must be aware of the signs of severe and life-threatening asthma (see Box 9.2). Asthma is reversible and nursing management should focus on close monitoring and health promotion. The main nursing goals are:

- Continuous monitoring of vital signs until patient is stabilised.
- Safe administration of prescribed oxygen to maintain oxygen saturation above 92%.

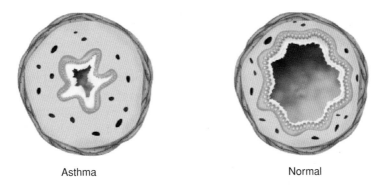

Figure 9.12 Airway pathophysiology, normal compared to status asthmaticus.

Box 9.2 Features of acute/severe and life-threatening asthma

Main symptoms of asthma

- Cough, which may become productive with thick sticky mucus
- Dyspnoea and chest tightness
- Wheeze
- Peak flow less than predicted or best

Features of acute-severe asthma

- Peak flow of less than 50% predicted or best
- Dyspnoea – unable to complete a sentence in one breath
- Tachypnoea – respiration rate greater than 25 breaths per minute
- Tachycardia – Pulse greater than 110 beats per minute

Features of life-threatening asthma

- Peak flow less than 33% of predicted or best
- Oxygen saturation (SpO_2) less than 92%
- Silent chest
- Weak and feeble respiratory effort
- Cyanosis
- Bradycardia or hypotension
- Confusion, exhaustion or coma

Adapted British Thoracic Society and Scottish Intercollegiate Guidelines Network (2005).

- Safe administration of prescribed bronchodilators and steroids – to alleviate dyspnoea (see Tables 9.3 and 9.4).
- Communication – as speaking requires a constant flow of air, patients experiencing acute breathlessness are only able to talk for very short periods before the need to breathe interrupts them. The patient's inability to complete a sentence, therefore, provides a sensitive measure of the extent of a patient's respiratory distress.
- Regular PEFR measurement – singular or infrequent peak flows will not accurately reflect the patient's status. PEFR should be measured every 15–30 minutes after commencement of treatment until conditions stabilise. PEFR can also be used to measure the effectiveness of bronchodilator therapy; therefore, PEFR should be measured pre- and post-inhaled or nebulised beta-2 agonists at least 4 times a day throughout their stay in hospital.
- Comfort and re-assurance – dyspnoea can be a traumatic experience and fear and anxiety also promote hyperventilation. Listen to the patient's anxieties and provide continuous explanations for the multidisciplinary team's actions.
- Sputum collection – yellow or green sputum can indicate infection.
- Health promotion – avoidance of triggers, compliance with prescribed pharmacological therapies, smoking cessation and weight reduction in obese patients may reduce the frequency of asthma attacks.

Type	Actions	Examples	Routes	Nursing considerations
Beta-2 agonists	Mimics the actions of adrenaline. Beta-2 agonists stimulate beta-2 receptor sites in the airways promoting rapid bronchodilation within 15 minutes, with a duration of 4–8 hours – depending on dose	Salbutamol Terbutaline Fenoterol Salmeterol	Inhaler Nebuliser Oral Subcutaneous	Patient will need to be advised of the potential for tachycardia and hand tremor
Anticholergenics	Blocks the action of acetylcholine, a neurotransmitter released by the parasympathetic nervous system. Acetylcholine promotes bronchoconstriction and bronchial secretion. Peak bronchodilator effects occur within 1 hour, with a duration similar to beta-2 agonists	Ipratropium bromide	Inhaler Nebuliser	Patient may need frequent mouthwashes may cause dry mouth and a bitter taste
Methylxanthines	Increases concentration of intracellular cyclic adenosine monophosphate (cAMP). Increased cAMP causes bronchodilation	Theophylline	Oral Intravenous (as aminophylline)	Optimal effects occur when plasma theophylline levels are between 10 and 20 mg/L. Regular blood tests are required

Adapted Murphy (2001).

Table 9.3 Summary of bronchodilator therapies given in asthma and chronic obstructive pulmonary disease

Indication	Corticosteroids[a]	Route	Nursing considerations
Prophylaxis and reduction of frequency of exacerbations	Beclametasone Budesonide Fluticasone	Inhaler	Inhaled corticosteroids can cause hoarseness, loss of voice and candidiasis. Advised to rinse out their mouths after taking these inhalers
Exacerbation	Prednisolone Hydrocortisone	Oral Intravenous	Patients taking prednisolone and hydrocortisone will need careful monitoring can cause the following side effects: ■ osteoporosis ■ diabetes ■ weight gain ■ increased body hair ■ altered mood

[a]Corticosteroids are potent anti-inflammatory agents. They are used to reduce bronchial hyperactivity in patients with asthma, chronic obstructive pulmonary disease and other respiratory diseases where reversibility is present. The table shows the main corticosteroids currently utilised.

Adapted Murphy (2001).

Table 9.4 Summary of corticosteroids used in the treatment of respiratory disease

Chronic obstructive pulmonary disease

Approximately 600 000 people in UK have COPD and it accounts for 5.4% of all male deaths and 4.2% of all female deaths. COPD has been defined as airflow obstruction that is progressive, not fully reversible and does not change markedly over several months. The main symptoms of COPD are summarised in Box 9.3. It has one major cause – smoking. COPD is a term now used to describe the patients traditionally diagnosed with chronic bronchitis or emphysema. Chronic asthma sufferers are also at risk of developing fixed airway obstruction as airways become re-modelled over time. Their symptoms may be

---

Box 9.3 The main symptoms of COPD

■ Reduced FEV_1 less than predicted
■ Dyspnoea – due to airway obstruction and air trapping
■ Productive cough
■ Reduced exercise tolerance
■ Respiratory failure types 1 and 2
■ **Cor pulmonale** – chronic hypoxia causes **hypertension** within pulmonary circulation. Eventually, the right ventricle becomes enlarged and fails, ultimately leading to peripheral oedema

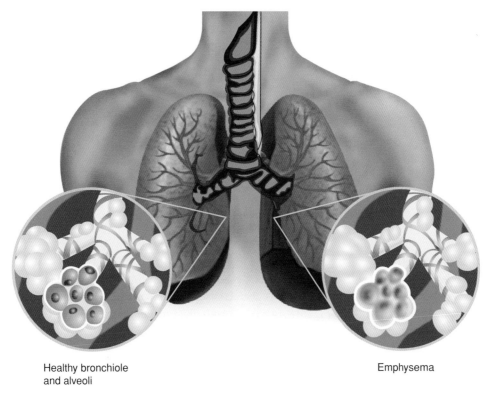

Healthy bronchiole
and alveoli

Emphysema

Figure 9.13 Comparison of a normal bronchiole and alveoli to that of an emphysema sufferer.

indistinguishable from COPD and many COPD patients may also have asthma. Accurate diagnosis therefore is often problematic (Devereux, 2006; National Institute for Health and Clinical Excellence, 2004).

Emphysema

Emphysema is defined as the permanent enlargement of airspaces beyond the terminal bronchiole and the destruction of the alveolar wall. The mechanisms behind this degeneration of tissue are thought to relate to the actions of proteases, which are destructive enzymes released from nuetrophils and **macrophages** in response to infection. In health, lung tissue produces a substance called alpha antitrypsin, which counteracts the destructive action of protease. Smoking, however, is thought to reduce the effect of alpha antitrypsin and increase protease activity, allowing alveolar destruction to continue unabated (Hogg and Senior, 2002). For example, proteases destroy the elastic fibres essential for elastic recoil much needed during exhalation. As a result, the alveoli become overinflated as air becomes trapped within the lung (see Figure 9.13). The increased volume of air within the thorax pushes the diaphragm downwards, disturbing its natural concave shape and making breathing difficult. Frequent infections can also develop as it becomes increasingly difficult to cough up secretions. The destruction of the alveolar wall and adjacent capillaries will mean that there is less lung tissue available for external respiration and the patient will be at risk of developing hypoxaemia and hypoxia (Gould, 2006).

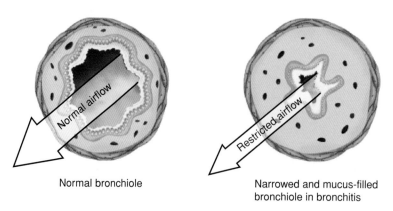

Normal bronchiole

Narrowed and mucus-filled
bronchiole in bronchitis

Figure 9.14 Comparison of a normal bronchiole to that of a chronic bronchitis sufferer.

Chronic bronchitis

Chronic bronchitis is defined as the presence of a productive cough lasting for 3 months in each of 2 consecutive years (Enright *et al.*, 1994). It is characterised by an increase in mucus production and damaged cilia in the bronchi (see Figure 9.14). As a result, the bronchi become clogged with mucus, which continues to stimulate the airway's irritant receptors, producing a cough. This chronic irritation causes inflammation and the bronchial wall thickens causing airway obstruction. Mucus clearance is difficult because of the damaged cilia and it collects and blocks the smaller airways. Secondary infection of these retained secretions then occurs, causing yet more irritation and inflammation. As more and more airways become blocked, external respiration is reduced and less oxygen is transferred into the bloodstream. The pathophysiological processes behind increased mucus production and cilia dysfunction are thought to involve an inflammatory response to the constant bombardment of cigarette smoke (MacNee, 2006).

Management of COPD

The severity of COPD is determined by FEV_1 (see Table 9.5). However, wherever possible the patient should be managed by the multidisciplinary team in their own home. In certain circumstances, however, acute exacerbation may necessitate a hospital admission (see Box 9.4). COPD is a diverse and varied

FEV_1	Severity of airway obstruction
50–80% predicted	Mild
30–49% predicted	Moderate
Less than 30%	Severe
NICE (2004).	

Table 9.5 FEV_1 as an assessment of airway obstruction

Box 9.4 Factors that may lead to hospital admission for patients with COPD

Inability to cope at home
Poor social circumstances
Cyanosis
Rapid onset
Impaired level of consciousness
On long-term oxygen therapy
Confusion or disorientation
SpO_2 less than 90%
Respiratory failure type 2
Chest X-ray changes
Significant co-morbidity – i.e. diabetes, heart disease

NICE (2004).

condition and its management requires a holistic approach centred upon self-management and symptom control. The main management goals are:

- education on prescribed oxygen and bronchodilator therapies – to maximise relief of breathlessness
- smoking cessation advice
- immunisation – to minimise frequency of exacerbations
- dietary advice – severe weight loss is a feature of both emphysema and chronic bronchitis
- pulmonary rehabilitation
- promotion of self-management techniques – COPD is associated with high levels of anxiety and depression

Bronchiectasis

Bronchiectasis describes an irreversible lung condition caused by recurrent infection and inflammation. The condition is associated with abnormal dilation of the bronchi together with a loss of functioning cilia. Destruction of alveolar walls and **fibrosis** also occurs. It is characterised by a chronic productive cough, in which the patient produces large amounts of purulent sputum. Other symptoms include dyspnoea, pleuritic pain and wheeze. Treatments include chest physiotherapy and antibiotics.

Bronchiectasis is a chronic lung disorder that usually develops secondary to a problem during childhood. Inflammation as a result of severe pneumonia, measles or whooping cough during childhood damages and weakens the bronchial walls. Diseases that cause bronchial obstruction, such as tumours and TB, can also lead to bronchiectasis when infections occur beyond the obstruction. Less common are congenital causes such as cystic fibrosis, in which the overproduction of viscous mucus causes recurrent lung infections, and immunoglobulin deficiencies which cause recurrent infections (Barker, 2002).

Restrictive disorders

Patients with restrictive disorders have difficulties expanding their thorax. Spirometry would show a reduced FVC and FEV_1 but unlike obstructive disorders the FEV_1:FVC ratio would be normal. This is because the airways are not obstructed, but rather chest expansion is restricted. There are two main reasons why chest expansion could be impeded. The patient may have a condition that directly affects the chest wall, such as **kyphosis** or **scoliosis** or they may have a disease that affects lung compliance. **Poliomyelitis, amyotrophic lateral sclerosis**, and **botulism**, for example, can cause respiratory muscle paralysis, whereas **muscular dystrophy** causes muscle weakness.

Disorders that restrict lung tissue are in the main chronic conditions caused by the inhalation of industrial or commercial pollutants. The upper respiratory tract is often unable to handle the vast quantities of airborne particles generated by various work practices, coal dust for example. Small particles that become lodged within the lungs cause chronic inflammation. Over time connective tissue within the lungs is eroded and the lungs become less compliant, making chest expansion difficult. This group of respiratory diseases are called pneumoconioses and are often named after the job or pastime that generated them, for example coal worker's lung (Bourke and Brewis, 1998). Chest expansion can also be restricted by acute problems such as adult respiratory distress syndrome, which occurs after lung trauma or pulmonary oedema.

Lung cancer

Lung cancer has the highest mortality rate of all known cancers in the Western world. In the UK alone, it accounts for around 36 000 deaths a year (British Thoracic Society, 2006). The most significant risk factor is smoking. Ex-smokers remain at risk although the likelihood reduces over time. Also susceptible are those exposed to passive smoking, albeit at a much lower probability. Smoking or other irritants (i.e. occupational pollutants) damage the pseudostratified epithelium of lung tissue rendering more susceptible to inflammation. Certain chemicals present within cigarette smoke are **carcinogenic**, and promote the development of tumours within the lung tissue. The vast majority of lung cancers (95%) are bronchial carcinomas of which there are two major types: *non-small cell* and *small cell*. Non-small cell carcinomas account for 70% of all lung cancers and can be subdivided again into *squamous cell carcinomas*, which tend to develop within the larger bronchi, and *adencarcinomas* and *large cell carcinomas*, which are found in the smaller airways making them much harder to detect. Small cell carcinomas tend to grow near a large bronchi and are the most aggressive bronchial carcinomas. There are no specific signs of lung cancer but a diagnosis is usually made in smokers who present with the following symptoms, cough, haemoptysis, dyspnoea, chest pain, wheezing and in some cases **finger clubbing** (Olson and Jett, 2000).

Pleural disorders

Only a minute amount of fluid occupies the pleural space (the space between the parietal and visceral pleura). Any condition that causes air or fluid to collect in the pleural space can cause the lung to partially or fully collapse (see Figure 9.15). The collapse of a lung results in areas that are underventilated, a phenomenon known as **atelectasis**. The surface area for external respiration is dramatically reduced and the patient may develop hypoxaemia (West, 2003). The main investigation for pleural disorders is a chest X-ray; the critically ill patient, however, may require a **computed tomographic (CT) scan**.

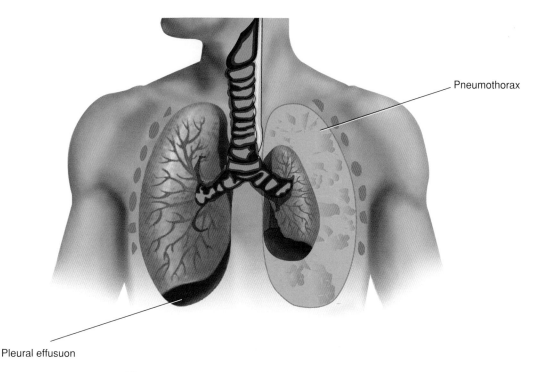

Pneumothorax

Pleural effusuon

Figure 9.15 Pleural effusion and a pneumothorax.

One fluid that can leak in the pleural space is blood. Trauma, cancer and surgery can all cause bleeding into the pleural space, a phenomenon referred to as haemothorax. Exudate and transudate pleural effusions can cause other kinds of fluid to collect in the pleural space. Exudate pleural effusions occur when there is a problem within lung tissue. The fluid that collects in the pleural space is rich in protein and white blood cells because it is generated as a result of inflammation secondary to a tumour or an infection, such as pneumonia or TB. Inflammation increases capillary permeability, allowing fluid to leak out of blood vessels and into the pleural space. Transudate pleural effusions occur as a result of a problem outside of the lungs. A prime example is left ventricular failure, which causes an increase in capillary **hydrostatic pressure** forcing fluid out of the blood stream and into the pleural space. A decrease in blood **osmotic pressure** will also force fluid from blood vessels into the pleural space; causes of reduced blood osmotic pressure include **hypoproteinaemia**. Some patients may develop an empyema, the formation of pus in the pleural effusion (Bono, 2004). Table 9.6 summarises the signs and symptoms of pleural effusions.

The presence of air in the pleural cavity is called a pneumothorax. A pneumothorax can occur as a result of chest trauma such as a stabbing or a broken rib, for example. Patients with chronic respiratory disease are also at risk of developing a pneumothorax. Some individuals have a congenital defect or bleb within the alveolar wall which can rupture spontaneously. Tall young men are at particular risk of this kind of pneumothorax (Ryan, 2005). In certain circumstances, a flap of tissue creates a one-way valve effect and airflow into the pleural space is promoted with each inspiration. As the pneumothorax

Signs and symptoms of a pleural effusion	Signs and symptoms of a pneumothorax
■ Dyspnoea ■ Pleuritic pain ■ Dry cough ■ Cyanosis ■ Tachycardia	■ Tachypnoea ■ Use of accessory muscles ■ Asymmetrical chest expansion ■ Cyanosis ■ Tachycardia ■ Hypertension or hypotension ■ **Pulsus paradoxus** ■ Sweating ■ Dry cough ■ Restlessness or confusion

Table 9.6 Signs and symptoms of pleural disorders

grows, pressure is exerted on the inferior vena cava impeding the blood flowing back to the heart (venous return). As a result, the patient becomes hypoxic and breathless. This medical emergency is called a tension pneumothorax (see Table 9.6).

Nursing management of pleural disorders

Chest drains are often used to assist the re-inflation of the affected lung. The monitoring of both the patient and the drain is the responsibility of the nurse and attention should be paid to the following (Allibone, 2003):

■ Patient positioning – nursing the patient in an upright position will encourage drainage and aid expansion of the thorax.
■ Position of the chest drain – the drainage bottle must be kept below the patient's chest level to prevent fluid re-entering the pleural space. Coiled and looped tubing should also be avoided as it can impede drainage flow and lead to a tension pneumothorax or **surgical emphysema**.
■ Continuous monitoring of vital signs until patient's condition stabilises.
■ Close monitoring of the chest drain.
  □ Swinging – the level of the fluid in the underwater seal of the drain should fluctuate between 5 and 10 cm when the patient breathes. Absence of swinging could indicate a kink or blockage in the tubing.
  □ Bubbling – bubbles often occur in the water seal bottle without suction when the patient exhales or coughs. Continuous bubbling indicates a problem with the drain or insertion site.
■ Administration of prescribed analgesics for pleuritic pain.
■ Accurate recording of drainage – the nurse should note the quantity, colour and consistency of the fluid being drained.
■ Infection control – the insertion site should be checked daily for signs of infection, i.e. redness, swelling, heat, pain and discharge.

Conclusion

This chapter has examined how respiratory disorders can interfere with respiration. Respiration involves four distinct physiological processes: pulmonary ventilation, external respiration, transport of gases and internal respiration. Respiration ensures that the body receives enough oxygen whilst disposing of excess carbon dioxide. In doing so, respiration plays a vital role in the maintenance of homeostasis. Any disease that interferes with pulmonary ventilation or external respiration will disturb homeostasis by reducing oxygen levels and possibly increasing carbon dioxide. The respiratory system has a complex anatomical structure and therefore there are a multitude of respiratory diseases. TB and pneumonia, for example, affect the alveoli and neighbouring tissue, whereas COPD and asthma obstruct the airways. Whatever the primary cause of the respiratory disorder, pulmonary ventilation and external respiration will almost always be affected and hypoxaemia and hypoxia could result. Patients with respiratory disease present with a multitude of symptoms such as dyspnoea, tachypnoea, pleuritic pain, reduced peak expiratory flow rate, low SpO_2, cyanosis and an inability to speak in complete sentences being just a few examples.

Multiple choice questions

1. Which of the following structures is not found in the lower respiratory tract?

(a) the trachea
(b) the pharynx
(c) right primary bronchus
(d) bronchioles

2. Which of the following statements about pulmonary ventilation is correct?

(a) expiration during quiet breathing is an active process that utilises muscle contraction
(b) inspiration results from passive recoil of the chest wall and lungs
(c) air flow during breathing is due to a pressure gradient between the lungs and atmospheric air
(d) the internal intercostal muscles are important muscles of inspiration

3. Which of the following muscles would be referred to as accessory muscles?

(a) internal intercostal muscles
(b) sternocleidomastoids
(c) external intercostal muscles
(d) abdominal muscles

4. Which of the following occurs during gaseous exchange?

(a) oxygen travels from the alveoli to the red blood cells in the capillary
(b) carbon dioxide travels from the alveoli to the red blood cells in the capillary
(c) carbon dioxide remains in blood plasma
(d) oxygen travels from the red blood cell in the capillary to the alveoli

5. Which of the following statements are correct?

(a) central chemoreceptors respond to elevated levels of carbon dioxide
(b) fear and anxiety can increase an individual's rate of breathing
(c) the peripheral chemoreceptors are found in the aorta and carotid arteries.
(d) all of the above

6. What is the correct definition of dyspnoea?

(a) a respiration rate of 10 respirations per minute or less
(b) difficulty in breathing
(c) difficulty in breathing while lying flat
(d) the absence of breathing for more than 15 seconds

7. Which of the following would indicate that your patient was in respiratory failure type 2?

(a) hypoxaemia

(b) hypocapnia

(c) hypoxaemia and hypercapnia

(d) low SpO_2

8. What colour sputum would most likely indicate pneumonia?

(a) clear

(b) pink and frothy

(c) rusty

(d) white

9. Which of the following treatments for asthma is a beta-2 agonist?

(a) ipratropium bromide

(b) hydrocortisone

(c) theophylline

(d) salbutamol

10. Which of the following statements regarding chronic obstructive pulmonary disease (COPD) is false?

(a) COPD is an umbrella term for emphysema and chronic bronchitis

(b) the main causative agent for COPD is smoking

(c) a patient with COPD will have a FEV_1 of 80% or higher

(d) wherever possible COPD patients should be cared for at home

11. Which of the following is a restrictive lung disorder?

(a) asthma

(b) muscular dystrophy

(c) chronic obstructive pulmonary disease

(d) bronchiectasis

12. The presence of air in the pleural space is called:

(a) pneumothorax

(b) haemothorax

(c) empyema

(d) pleural effusion

Answers: 1.b, 2.c, 3.b, 4.a, 5.d, 6.b, 7.c, 8.c, 9.d, 10.c, 11.b, 12.a.

Test your knowledge

- Explain what happens in the alveoli during normal breathing.
- Why would someone in respiratory failure type 2 have an arterial blood pH < 7.35?
- Explain why someone with asthma might produce a peak expiratory flow rate (PEFR) less than predicted for their age, height and sex.
- Why might someone with a pleural disorder become hypoxaemic?

Glossary of terms

Amyotrophic lateral sclerosis: Serious neurological disease in which motor neurones gradually deteriorate.

Anaemia: A reduced number or function of erythrocytes (red blood cells) or haemoglobin.

Antipyretic agents: Drugs that can reduce high temperatures – i.e. paracetamol, aspirin, ibuprofen.

Aorta: First major blood vessel of arterial circulation. Emerges from the left ventricle of the heart.

Atelectasis: Partial or complete collapse of lung tissue due to a blocked airway.

Bacillus: A form of bacteria. Bacilli are rod-shaped, Gram-positive and usually have motility.

Botulism: A rare but serious bacterial infection which causes muscle weakness and paralysis.

Carcinogenic: Prone to promote the formation of carcinomas (tumours).

Carotid artery: Major artery supplying the brain, stems from the aorta.

Cartilage: Type of connective tissue which contains collagen and elastic fibres. Cartilage can stand up to both tension and compression.

Cerebrospinal fluid (CSF): Fluid found within the brain and spinal cord.

Chemoreceptors: Sensory cells sensitive to a specific chemical.

Central cyanosis: A bluish hue or tingle visible in lips and mouth that occurs when arterial oxygen levels are abnormally low.

Cilia: Hair-like extensions to the plasma membrane.

Cor pulmonale: Right-sided heart failure caused by hypoxia.

Diffusion: The passive movement of molecules or ions from a region of high concentration to low concentration until a state of equilibrium is achieved.

Elastic cartilage: Cartilage that contains more elastin fibres, providing strength and stretchability.

Enzyme: A protein that speeds up chemical reactions.

Erythrocytes: Red blood cells.

Expectorate: To cough up and spit out mucus or sputum.

External intercostal muscles: Muscles that span the spaces between the ribs. As opposed to the internal intercostal muscles the external intercostal muscles sit closer to the outside of the thorax.

External respiration: The transfer of oxygen from the alveoli in the lungs to the blood stream and the transfer of carbon dioxide from the blood stream into alveoli in the lungs.

Extrinsic asthma: Asthma caused by hypersensitive reactions to an allergy.

Exudate: Escaping fluid that spills from a space, contains cellular debris and pus.

Fibrin: A protein essential for clotting.

Fibrosis: The development of scar tissue.

Fibrous: Containing regenerated or scar tissue.

Finger clubbing: Alteration in the angle of finger and toe bases caused by chronic tissue hypoxia.

Goblet cells: Mucus-secreting cells found in epithelial tissue.

Haemoglobin (Hb): Protein consisting of globin and four haeme groups that is found within erythrocytes (red blood cells). Responsible for the transport of oxygen.

Haemoptysis: Coughing up of blood.

Hydrostatic pressure: Pressure exerted by a fluid.

Hypercapnia: Elevated levels of arterial carbon dioxide.

Hypertension: Abnormally high blood pressure.

Hypoproteinaemia: A reduced level of plasma proteins.

Hypotension: Abnormally low blood pressure.

Hypoxaemia: A reduced amount of oxygen within arterial blood.

Hypoxia: A reduced amount of oxygen within the tissues.

Intercostal nerves: Nerves which link the respiratory centres in the brainstem with the intercostal muscles.

Internal intercostal muscles: Muscles that span the spaces between the ribs. As opposed to the external intercostal muscles the internal intercostal muscles sit closer to the inside of the thorax.

Internal respiration: The transfer of oxygen from the blood stream into body cells and the transfer of carbon dioxide from body cells to the blood stream.

Intrinsic asthma: Asthma caused by hyperresponsive reactions to non-allergic stimuli.

Intubation: The insertion of a special tube into the pharynx and down into the trachea, in order to maintain a patent airway in an unconscious patient.

Kyphosis: Curvature of the thoracic spine.

Lymph nodules: Egg-shaped masses of lymph tissues that provide an immune response.

Lymphocytes: Specialist white blood cell involved in immune responses.

Lymph vessel: A vessel that carries lymphatic fluid. Part of the lymphatic system which forms part of the immune system.

Macrophages: A cell which ingests and destroys microbes, cell debris and foreign matter.

Mast cells: A cell found in connective tissue that releases histamine during inflammation.

Medulla oblongata: Lowest region of the brainstem.

Muscular dystrophy: A group of diseases characterised by the progressive loss of muscle fibres. Almost all these diseases are hereditary.

Neutrophils: A type of white blood cell.

Non-invasive positive pressure ventilation (NIPPV): Respiratory support technique that enhances the patient's rate and depth of breathing.

Oedema: An abnormal collection of fluid.

Osmotic pressure: Pressure exerted by fluid flowing through a semipermeable membrane that separates two fluids with different levels of dissolved substances.

Peak expiratory flow rate: The velocity at which a patient can expire their total lung volume.

Phrenic nerve: Nerve which links the diaphragm to the respiratory centre in the brainstem.

Poliomyelitis: An acute viral disease which affects the central nervous system.

Polycythaemia: A condition in which there is an abnormally high number of erythrocytes (red blood cells).

Pons: Upper region of the brainstem. Connects the midbrain to the medulla oblongata.

Pseudostratified ciliated columnar epithelium: Covering or lining of internal body surface that contains cilia and mucus-secreting goblet cells.

Pulmonary ventilation: Breathing. The inspiration and expiration of air into and out of the lungs.

Pulse oximeter: Device that provides an instant pulse and oxygen saturation (SpO_2).

Pulsus paradoxus: A phenomenon in which the pulse is weaker during inspiration than that of expiration.

Pyrexia: Elevated temperature associated with fever.

Respiratory acidosis: A blood pH of less than 7.35 caused by a rise in arterial carbon dioxide.

Scoliosis: A sideways curvature of the thoracic spine.

Spirometry: Diagnostic tool which measures a patient's forced vital capacity (FVC) and forced expiratory volume within the first second of expiration (FEV_1).

Surgical emphysema: Air trapped in the tissues, usually as a result of a surgical or invasive procedure.

Systemic circulation: Arterial and venous blood flow through the body, except the lungs (pulmonary circulation) and the coronary arteries.

Tachycardia: Pulse rate greater than 100 beats per minute.

Thorax: The body trunk above the diaphragm and below the neck.

Tracheostomy: A procedure in which an incision is made in the trachea to facilitate breathing.

Transport of gases: The movement of oxygen and carbon dioxide between the lungs and body cells.

References

Allibone, L. (2003). Nursing management of chest drains. *Nursing Standard, 17*(22), 45–54.

Barker, A.F. (2002). Medical progress: Bronchiectasis. *New England Journal of Medicine, 346*(18), 1383–1393.

Bono, M.J. (2004). Recognising and managing thoracic empyema. *Emergency Medicine, 36*(12), 37–40.

Bourke, S. and Brewis, R. (1998). *Lecture Notes on Respiratory Medicine*, 5th edn. Oxford: Blackwell Science.

British Thoracic Society (2002). BTS guideline non-invasive ventilation in acute respiratory failure. *Thorax, 57*, 192–211.

British Thoracic Society (2004). *Pneumonia Guidelines 2004 Update*. London: BTS.

British Thoracic Society (2006). *The Burden of Lung Disease*. London: BTS.

British Thoracic Society and Scottish Intercollegiate Guidelines Network (2005). *British Guideline on the Management of Asthma: A National Clinical Guideline*. London: BTS.

Clark, A.P., Giuliano, K. and Chen, H. (2006). Pulse oximetry revisited 'but his O_2 sat was normal!'. *Clinical Nurse Specialist, 20*(6), 268–272.

Devereux, G. (2006). ABC of chronic obstructive disease definition, epidemiology and risk factors. *BMJ, 332*, 1142–1144.

Dunn, L. (2005). Pneumonia: Classification, diagnosis and nursing management. *Nursing Standard, 19*, 50–54.

Enright, P.L., Kronmal, R.A., Higgins, M.W., Schenker, M.B. and Haponik, E.F. (1994). Prevalence and correlates of respiratory symptoms and disease in the elderly. *Chest, 108*, 827–834.

Gould, B.E. (2006). *Pathophysiology for the Health Professions*, 3rd edn. Philadelphia: Elsevier.

Hlastala, M.P. and Berger, A.J. (2001). *Physiology of Respiration*, 2nd edn. Oxford: Oxford University Press.

Hoare, Z. and Lim, W.S. (2006). Pneumonia: Update on diagnosis and management. *BMJ, 332*, 1077–1079.

Hogg, J.C. and Senior, R.M. (2002). Chronic obstructive pulmonary disease 2: Pathology and biochemistry of emphysema. *Thorax, 57*, 830–834.

MacNee, W. (2006). ABC of chronic obstructive pulmonary disease pathology, pathogenesis and pathophysiology. *BMJ, 332*, 1202–1204.

Margereson, C. (2001). Anatomy and physiology. In: Esmond, G. (ed) *Respiratory Nursing*. Edinburgh: Bailliere Tindall.

McGowan, P., Jeffries, A. and Turley, A. (2003). *Crash Course Respiratory System*, 2nd edn. London: Mosby.

Middleton, S. and Middleton, P.G. (2002). Assessment and investigation of patients' problems. In: Pryor, J.A. and Ammani Prasad, S. (eds) *Physiotherapy for Respiratory and Cardiac Problems*, 3rd edn. Edinburgh: Churchill Livingstone.

Murphy, S. (2001). Respiratory medication. In: Esmond, G. (ed) *Respiratory Nursing*. Edinburgh: Bailliere Tindall.

National Collaboration Centre for Chronic Conditions (2006). *Tuberculosis: Clinical Diagnosis and Management of Tuberculosis, and Measures for Its Management and Its Control*. London: The Royal College of Physicians.

National Institute for Health and Clinical Excellence (2004). *Clinical Guideline 12. Chronic Obstructive Pulmonary Disease. Management of Chronic Obstructive Pulmonary Disease in Primary and Secondary Care*. London: NICE.

Ochs, M., Nyengaard, A.J., Knudsen, L., Voigt, M., Wahlers, T., Richter, J. and Gundersen, H.J.G. (2004). The number of alveoli in the human lung. *American Journal of Respiratory and Critical Care Medicine*, *169*, 120–124.

Olson, E.J. and Jett, J.R. (2000). Clinical diagnosis and basic evaluation. In: Hansen, H.H. (ed) *Textbook of Lung Cancer*. London: Martin Duntiz.

Russell, C. and Metta, B. (2004). *Tracheostomy: A Multiprofessional Handbook*. Cambridge: Cambridge University Press.

Ryan, B. (2005). Pneumothorax assessment and diagnostic testing. *Journal of Cardiovascular Nursing*, *20*(4), 251–253.

Schwartzstein, R.M. and Parker, M.J. (2006). *Respiratory Physiology: A Clinical Approach*. Philadelphia: Lippincott Williams & Wilkins.

Sheldon, R.L. (2005). Pulmonary function testing. In: Wilkins, R.L., Sheldon, R.L. and Krider, S.J. (eds) *Clinical Assessment in Respiratory Care*, 5th edn. St. Louis: Elsevier Mosby.

Simpson, H. (2006). Respiratory assessment. *British Journal of Nursing*, *15*(9), 484–488.

Sims, J.M. (2006). An overview of asthma. *Dimensions of Critical Care Nursing*, *25*(6), 264–268.

Talley, N.J. and O'Connor, S. (2001). *Clinical Examination: A Systematic Guide to Physical Diagnosis*, 4th edn. Oxford: Blackwell Science.

West, J.B. (2003). *Pulmonary Pathophysiology: The Essentials*, 6th edn. Philadelphia: Lippincott Williams & Wilkins.

West, J.B. (2005). *Respiratory Physiology: The Essentials*, 7th edn. Philadelphia: Lippincott Williams & Wilkins.

Chapter 10

The nervous system and associated disorders

Janet G. Migliozzi

KEY WORDS

- Autonomic nervous system
- Brainstem
- Central nervous system
- Cerebral vascular accident
- Epilepsy
- Glasgow Coma Scale
- Limbic system
- Meninges
- Multiple sclerosis
- Parkinson's disease
- Peripheral nervous system
- Spinal cord

Test your prior knowledge

- List the structures of the central nervous system (CNS) and peripheral nervous system (PNS).
- What are the functions of the four areas of the brain?
- What are the major functions of the spinal cord?

> ## Learning outcomes
>
> On completion of this section, the reader will be able to:
>
> - Outline the structure and function of the central and peripheral nervous systems.
> - Describe the function of the autonomic nervous system and understand the function of its divisions.
> - Understand the nursing care of the patient with a common disorder of the nervous system.

Introduction

The nervous system is the body's 'computer' as it is responsible and controls all aspects of voluntary and involuntary action and plays a major role in the coordination of the body's organ system to maintain homeostasis.

This chapter discusses the structure and function of the central and peripheral nervous systems and common disorders of the nervous system such as multiple sclerosis, stroke, Parkinson's disease, Alzheimer's disease, epilepsy, traumatic head injury are also explored and the nursing management outlined.

Structure of the nervous system

The nervous system is divided into two major sections: the **central nervous system** (CNS) and the **peripheral nervous system** (PNS). The CNS consists of the brain and spinal cord. The PNS lies outside of the CNS and consists of the nerves that carry impulses to and from the spinal cord and includes the cranial nerves from the brain and the spinal nerves from the spinal cord. The PNS can also be divided into the **somatic** and **autonomic nervous system** which is divided further into the **parasympathetic** and **sympathetic** divisions (see Figure 10.1).

The central nervous system
Brain
The brain or **encephalon** which is encased in the **cranium** (or skull) is the body's control system and can be divided into four main parts: the cerebrum, the cerebellum, the diencephalon and the brainstem (see Figure 10.2).

The cerebrum
The cerebrum (or cerebral cortex) makes up the largest part of the brain and lies uppermost in the skull. The cerebrum consists of two frontal lobes, two parietal lobes, two temporal lobes and two occipital lobes and is divided into the right and left cerebral hemispheres by fissures or **sulci**. The cerebral hemispheres are connected at their lower midpoint by the **corpus callosum**. The hemispheres' surface

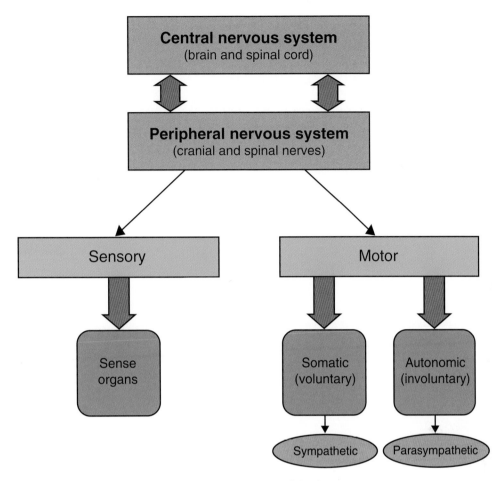

Figure 10.1 Diagram showing divisions of the human nervous system.

appears wrinkled due to the numerous convolutions or **gyri** which are raised areas that fold in on each other to increase the brain's surface area. The surface of the cerebrum is known as the **cerebral cortex** and is composed of a thin layer of grey matter. The inner layer of the cerebrum consists of mainly white matter but does contain some grey matter in the form of **basal ganglia** which play an important role in producing automatic movements and the body's posture.

The cerebrum is divided into four lobes, each of which has a specific function.

The cerebellum

The cerebellum, which is separated from the brainstem by the fourth **ventricle**, lies under the occipital lobe of the cerebrum and is the second largest part of the human brain. It consists of an inner layer of white matter and an outer layer of grey matter and plays a major role in balance, posture and fine movement and coordination.

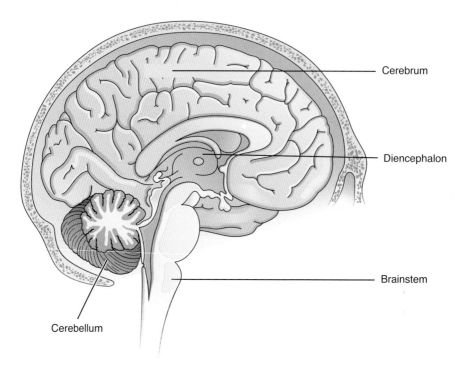

Figure 10.2 The four main parts of the human brain.

Diencephalon

The diencephalon or interbrain lies between the brainstem and the cerebrum where it encircles the third ventricle and consists of the **thalamus** and **hypothalamus**. The **pineal gland** which is responsible for the secretion of the hormone melatonin is also located in the diencephalon.

The **thalamus** consists of grey matter and is a dumb-bell-shaped structure which encloses the third ventricle of the brain and acts as a relay centre which receives information from the body via the spinal

Lobe	Function
Frontal lobe	Conscious thought, abstract thinking, affective reactions, memory, judgement and initiation of motor activity
Parietal lobe	Sensory functioning and sensory perception association
Temporal lobe	Processing of auditory information and auditory association (Wernicke's area)
Occipital lobe	Visual processing and association

Table 10.1 The lobes of the cerebral hemispheres

cord and forwards this on to the appropriate areas of the brain. The thalamus plays a crucial role in the conscious awareness of pain, the **limbic system** of the brain which controls instinctual and emotional drives, e.g. hunger, fear, sexual drive and short-term memory.

The **hypothalamus** is located just below the thalamus (as its name suggests) and is the major link between the body's endocrine and nervous system where it has many roles to play in the regulation of homeostasis (Germann and Standfield, 2002). The hypothalamus also forms part of the limbic system of the brain.

Brainstem

The brainstem connects the spinal cord to the remainder of the brain and is responsible for many essential functions including the entry to and exit from the brain of 10 of the 12 cranial nerves (see Table 10.2).

Nerve	Brain location	Transmits nerve impulses to and from
I Olfactory	Olfactory bulb	Olfactory receptors for sense of smell
II Optic	Thalamus	Retina (sight)
III Oculomotor	Midbrain	Eye muscles (including eyelids and lens, pupil
IV Trochlear	Midbrain	Eye muscles
V Trigeminal	Pons	Teeth, eyes, skin, tongue
VI Abducens	Pons	Jaw muscles (chewing)
		Eye muscles
VII Facial	Pons	Taste buds
		Facial muscles, tear and salivary glands
VIII Vestibulocochlear	Pons	Inner ear (hearing and balance)
IX Glossopharyngeal	Medulla oblongata	Pharyngeal muscles (swallowing)
X Vagus	Medulla oblongata	Internal organs
XI Spinal accessory	Medulla oblongata	Neck and back muscles
XII Hypoglossal	Medulla oblongata	Tongue muscles

Table 10.2 Cranial nerves

The brainstem contains the **midbrain**, the **pons**, the **medulla oblongata** and the **reticular formation.**

The **midbrain** or mesencephalon is a short section of the brainstem between the diencephalon and the pons and is the centre for auditory and visual reflexes (Shier *et al.*, 2004). The midbrain consists of bundles of nerve fibres that join the lower parts of the brainstem and the spinal cord with the higher parts of the brain and also plays a part in the control of the wakefulness of the brain.

The **pons** is latin for 'bridge' and connects the midbrain to the medulla and cerebrum. The pons plays an important role in the control of the rate and length of respiration.

The **medulla oblongata**, which consists of grey and white matter, is approximately 3 cm long and, arguably, an extension of the spinal cord as it lies just inside the cranial cavity above the large hole in the occipital bone called the **foramen magnum**. Within it are contained a number of reflex centres for control of blood vessel diameter, the regulation of heart rate, breathing, coughing, swallowing, vomiting and sneezing. On either side of the medulla oblongata is a round oval protrusion called an **olive** which plays a part in controlling balance, coordination and the intonation of sound impulses from the middle ear.

The **reticular formation** (RF) is a dense network of neurones that evolves from the medulla and midbrain and extends through the brainstem and is important in the control of consciousness, arousal and the sleep–wake cycle (Germann and Standfield, 2002).

The blood supply to the brain

The brain receives approximately 15% of the body's total circulating volume of blood which is equivalent to 750 mL of blood per minute (Hickey, 2003) and is supplied by the vertebral and internal carotid arteries. These two sets of arteries interconnect at the base of the brain to form the cerebral arterial circle or **circle of Willis** (see Figure 10.3) which provides a collateral supply of blood to the whole of the brain in the event that one of the carotid arteries becomes compromised.

The blood–brain barrier

The brain (unlike other organs) is unable to withstand changes in levels of circulating nutrients, hormones and ions. Therefore, maintenance of a constant environment is crucial to the brain's ability to function and the blood–brain barrier which is an impermeable network of brain capillaries acts as a 'filter' between the brain tissue and blood-borne substances to provide the brain with some protection against harmful toxins and metabolites. However, the blood–brain barrier provides little protection against fat-soluble molecules and respiratory gases (Marieb, 2006); consequently some substances, e.g. nicotine, anaesthetic gases and alcohol, can cross the barrier and affect the brain.

The ventricles of the brain

The brain contains four interconnecting ventricles or cavities which produce, circulate and absorb **cerebrospinal fluid** (CSF) and also provide a protective barrier between the CSF and the brain. CSF which protects and nourishes the brain consists of water, glucose, protein and electrolytes is continually secreted by specialised epithelial cells called the **choroid plexus**.

The meninges

The dura mater, arachnoid mater and pia mater or **meninges** are the three layers of connective tissue that protect and cover the brain and spinal cord.

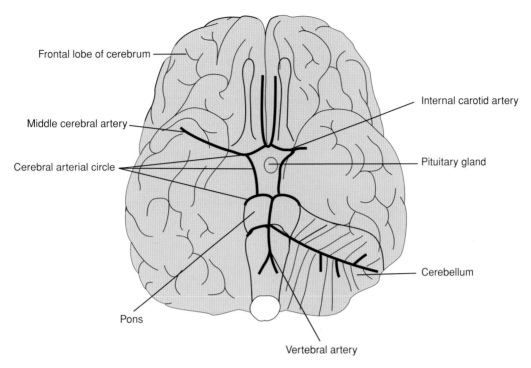

Figure 10.3 The circle of Willis.

The spinal cord

The spinal cord is located in the vertebral column and provides the communication route between the brain and parts of the body not supplied by cranial nerves through 31 pairs of spinal nerves which are grouped as either the cervical, thoracic or lumber spinal nerves according to their location along the vertebral column (see Figure 10.4).

Peripheral nervous system

The peripheral nervous system consists of the nerves connecting the brain and spinal cord to other parts of the body and includes the cranial and spinal nerves (see above) that connect the brain and spinal cord to the peripheral structures, e.g. the skin and skeletal muscles. The PNS is divided into the somatic and autonomic nervous systems of which the autonomic nervous system has two divisions – the parasympathetic and sympathetic divisions.

Somatic nervous system

The somatic nervous system consists of motor neurons that connect the CNS to the skin and skeletal muscles and plays a major role in the regulation of skeletal muscle contractions and conscious activities.

Autonomic nervous system

The autonomic nervous system (ANS) plays a major role in the maintenance of homeostasis by regulating the body's automatic, involuntary functions and in common with the rest of the nervous system, consists of **neurones**, **neuroglia** and other connective tissue. However, its structure is quite unique in that it is divided into two, namely the **sympathetic division** and the **parasympathetic division**.

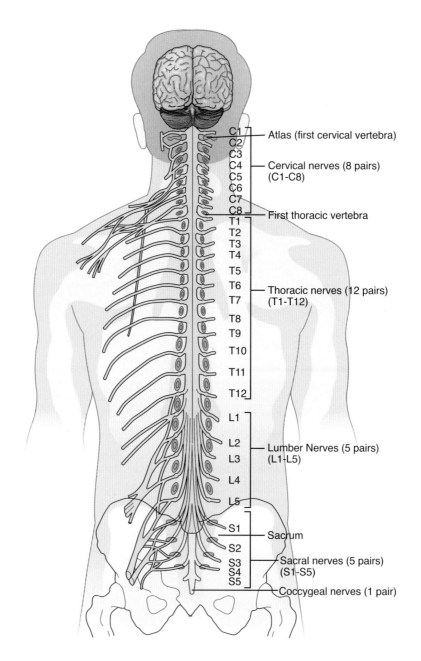

Figure 10.4 The spinal cord and the location of the 31 pairs of spinal nerves.

Organ/system	Sympathetic effects	Parasympathetic effects
Cell metabolism	Increases metabolic rate, stimulates fat breakdown and increases blood sugar levels	No effect
Blood vessels	Constricts blood vessels in viscera and skin Dilates blood vessels in the heart and skeletal muscle	No effect
Eye	Dilates pupils	Constricts pupils
Heart	Increases rate and force of contraction	Decreases rate
Lungs	Dilates bronchioles	Constricts bronchioles
Kidneys	Decreases urine output	No effect
Liver	Causes the release of glucose	No effect
Digestive system	Decreases peristalsis and constricts digestive system sphincters	Increases peristalsis and dilates digestive system sphincters
Adrenal medulla	Stimulates cells to secrete epinephrine and norepinephrine	No effect
Lacrimal glands	Inhibits the production of tears	Increases the production of tears
Salivary glands	Inhibits the production of saliva	Increases the production of saliva
Sweat glands	Stimulates to produce perspiration	No effect

Table 10.3 Physiological effects of the sympathetic and parasympathetic nervous systems

The **sympathetic division** takes control of many internal organs when a stressful situation occurs. This can take the form of physical stress, e.g. if undertaking strenuous exercise, or emotional stress, e.g. at times of anger or anxiety. In emergency situations, the sympathetic nervous system releases **norepinephrine** which assists in the 'fight or flight' response.

The **parasympathetic division** utilises **acetylcholine** to control all the internal responses associated with a state of relaxation and therefore has the opposite effect on the body to the sympathetic nervous system. Table 10.3 provides a summary of the physiological effects of the sympathetic and parasympathetic divisions of the nervous system.

Disorders of the nervous system

Learning outcomes

On completion of this section, the reader will be able to:

- List some of the common diseases associated with disorders of the central nervous system.
- Describe the pathophysiological processes related to some specific central nervous system disorders.
- Outline the nursing management and interventions related to the disorders described.

Raised intracranial pressure

Intracranial pressure (ICP) is the recordable pressure within the skull caused by three intracranial components: brain tissue, cerebrospinal fluid (CSF) and blood. As the skull is a rigid structure, any increase in volume in any of the three components will lead to an increase in ICP. Several conditions can lead to an increase in ICP including bleeding in the brain due to a head injury, a space-occupying lesion, e.g. a brain tumour, or infection, e.g. a brain abscess. Left untreated, raised ICP can lead to poor perfusion of the brain as the cerebral arteries and veins become compressed and the brain herniates or shifts as it becomes compressed within the skull. Common signs and symptoms of increased ICP are summarised in Box 10.1.

Box 10.1 Common symptoms of raised ICP

In the early stages the individual may experience

- Decreasing levels of consciousness
- Headache
- Sluggish pupil reaction
- Visual disturbances
- Abnormal breathing patterns
- Impaired motor responses

In the later stages the individual may experience

- Further deterioration in level of consciousness
- A rise in systolic blood pressure
- A fall in diastolic blood pressure
- Irregular shallow, slow breathing
- Slow pulse
- A high temperature

Nursing management of the patient at risk of increased intracranial pressure

Patients at risk of neurological deterioration require frequent, accurate neurological assessment in order to detect problems early. Therefore, nurses need to not only be able to perform a basic neurological assessment but must also understand the significance of the findings (Waterhouse, 2005).

A neurological assessment should include the following:

■ conscious level
■ pupil size and reactivity
■ vital signs, e.g. temperature, heart rate, respiratory rate, blood pressure and blood oxygen saturation
■ limb movements (National Institute for Health and Clinical Excellence (NICE, 2003))

Glasgow Coma Scale

The NICE advocates the use of the Glasgow Coma Scale (GCS) (Teasdale and Jennett, 1974) for assessment and classification of all head-injured patients (NICE, 2003).

The GSC was specifically designed as a tool for detecting and monitoring changes in the patient's neurological status by evaluating three categories of behaviour: eye opening, verbal response and motor response (see Table 10.4). Within each category, each level of response is allocated a numerical value

Feature	Response	Score
Best eye response	Open spontaneously	4
	Open to verbal command	3
	Open to pain	2
	No eye opening	1
Best verbal response	Orientated	5
	Confused	4
	Inappropriate words	3
	Incomprehensible sounds	2
	No verbal response	1
Best motor response	Obeys commands	6
	Localising pain	5
	Withdrawal from pain	4
	Flexion to pain	3
	Extension to pain	2
	No motor response	1

Adapter NICE (2003).

Table 10.4 The Glasgow Coma Scale (GCS)

(Waterhouse, 2005) and the lower the patient scores on the scale, the more serious the neurological condition, e.g. a score of 15 would indicate a fully conscious, alert, responsive patient whereas a score of 3 would mean that the patient was deeply unconscious.

Vital signs recording

NICE (2003) recommends that head-injured patients with a GCS of less than 15 should have their vital signs monitored half-hourly until a GCS of 15 has been achieved. After the initial assessment (usually in the emergency department) the frequency of observations of patients with GCS equal to 15 should be:

- half-hourly for 2 hours
- then 1-hourly for 4 hours
- then 2-hourly thereafter

If the patient with a GCS equal to 15 deteriorates at any time after the initial 2-hour period, observations should revert back to half-hourly and follow the schedule as outlined above. Additionally, the patient should undergo an urgent reappraisal by medical staff if they experience any of the following (NICE, 2007a):

- development of agitation or abnormal behaviour
- development of severe or increasing headache or persistent vomiting
- a sustained (at least 30 minutes) drop of one point in GCS (a drop of one point in motor response score requires more urgent attention)
- a drop of three or more points in the eye-opening or verbal response scores of the GCS or two or more points in the motor response score
- new or evolving neurological signs or symptoms, e.g. pupil inequality or loss of movement/strength to one side of the body or face

Stroke (cerebrovascular accident)

A cerebrovascular accident (CVA) or 'stroke' occurs as a direct result of impaired blood flow to the brain either as a result of vessel occlusion or haemorrhaging due to a ruptured vessel. The nature and extent of neurological impairment that the patient may suffer is dependent on the amount and location of oxygen starvation that the brain tissue has experienced and/or the severity of cerebral bleeding that has occurred.

Stroke is the third largest cause of death (approximately, 66 000 deaths each year) and a leading cause of adult disability in the United Kingdom (Turner and Jowett, 2006). Whilst stroke is primarily a disease experienced by older people and is more likely to be experienced by men (although women who experience a stroke are more likely to die), other factors exist that make certain groups more at risk of having a stroke (see Box 10.2).

Pathophysiology of stroke

The brain is unable to store nutrients or glucose for use and is therefore dependent on a steady supply of these from the circulation of blood via the internal carotid and vertebral arteries. Any interruption of blood supply to the brain tissue will result in **ischaemia** and, if prolonged, result in the death of brain cells. There are two main types of stroke: **ischaemic** stroke and **haemorrhagic** stroke.

Box 10.2 Risk factors for stroke

■ Smoking
■ Obesity
■ History of heart disease or high blood pressure (**hypertension**)
■ High cholesterol (**hyperlipidaemia**)
■ Diabetes
■ Afro-Caribbean or South Asian descent
■ A family history of stroke at a young age (less than 50 years of age)

The Stroke Association (2004).

Ischaemic stroke, which accounts for 85% of all strokes (Hickey, 2003), occurs when a blood clot blocks an artery to the brain causing an interruption of blood flow to the brain cells. A high cholesterol level causing a 'furring' of the arteries is a common cause of this type of stroke.

Haemorrhagic stroke occurs when a blood vessel in or around the brain bursts causing bleeding and increased pressure in the skull, resulting in compression and eventual ischaemia to brain tissue. Untreated high blood pressure (hypertension) is a common cause of this type of stroke.

Following a stroke, it is possible to determine the area of the brain that has been damaged by observing the signs and symptoms the patient may experience and these are summarised in Table 10.5.

Damage to left side of brain	Damage to right side of brain
Loss of motor function to the right side of the body	Loss of motor function to the left side of the body
Language impairment – either an inability to express self – **expressive aphasia** or difficulty in understanding or using speech appropriately although able to speak fluently – **receptive aphasia**	Language centres not affected
Right visual field deficit	Left visual field deficit
Frustration and depression over loss of independence	Apparent unconcern over loss of independence
Intellectual impairment	Poor judgement and impulsive behaviour

Table 10.5 Signs and symptoms of stroke according to side of brain affected

Transient ischaemic attack

A transient ischaemic attack (TIA) or 'mini' stroke is a temporary interruption in blood flow to the brain which can result in numbness, temporary paralysis and impaired speech. Whilst the symptoms experienced are not permanent and by definition resolve within 24 hours (Monahan *et al.*, 2007), a TIA is often a warning of an impending, more serious CVA.

Pharmacological management of stroke

The pharmacological treatment of stroke aims to prevent the reoccurrence of stroke or TIA whilst also taking into consideration the cause of the stroke.

- In the first 3 hours of an ischaemic stroke occurring the use of thrombolytic therapy, e.g. alteplase is advocated (NICE, 2007b).
- Aspirin or dipyridamole (Persantin) may be prescribed to reduce platelet aggregation in the case of TIA or ischaemic stroke.
- Antihypertensives may be prescribed for patients who have high blood pressure.
- Cholesterol-reducing drugs such as simvastatin should be prescribed to prevent recurrent ischaemic stroke or TIA (Turner and Jowett, 2006).

Non-pharmacological management of stroke

- Carotid **endarterectomy** (removal of fatty plaques from the wall of the carotid artery) may be performed in patients with **stenosis** (narrowing) of the carotid arteries that supply blood to the brain.
- The patient should be educated as to the importance of a varied diet that is low in fat in order to keep blood cholesterol within safe limits. Patients who are overweight need support to lose weight and should be encouraged to take regular exercise.
- Patients should be offered support to stop smoking and reduce alcohol intake.
- Regular monitoring of blood pressure is important to ensure that it is kept within safe limits and patients should be encouraged to reduce their salt intake.

Nursing management of stroke

Nursing management of a patient who has suffered from a stroke varies according to the area of the brain affected and the neurological and functional deficits that the individual experiences. However, the nursing care of the patient during the acute phase of stroke will differ to the care required once the patient has stabilised and is in the rehabilitative phase.

Key nursing considerations during the acute phase focus on early detection and prevention of neurological deterioration and life-threatening complications and include:

- frequent monitoring of the patient's vital signs and neurological function during the acute phase using an appropriate assessment tool, e.g. the GCS (see above), to detect any deterioration in the patient's level of consciousness
- keeping the patient nil by mouth until an assessment of the swallowing reflex can be carried out
- undertaking a nutritional status assessment within the first 48 hours of admission
- protecting the patient from injury due to possible seizures, motor and visual deficits
- the prevention of pressure sore formation as due to immobility and incontinence, the patient is at increased risk

During the rehabilitative phase of stroke, care is geared towards maximising the patient's independence and key nursing considerations include:

- collaborating with other health care professionals to teach the patient adaptive measures to enable them to carry out their activities of living, e.g. bathing, eating, dressing and toileting, as independently as possible
- minimising the risk of injury and complications associated with impaired mobility
- involvement of a speech therapist to ensure that patients who have impaired communication are able to express themselves effectively
- provision of information and support for the patient and their carers/family
- liaising with other health care professionals and social services prior to the patient's discharge from hospital to ensure that the patient's home environment is suitably adapted to deal with any residual disabilities that the patient may have

Parkinson's disease (paralysis agitans)

Parkinson's disease (PD) is a disease of the brain that mainly affects older people and progresses over time (NICE, 2006b). This is caused by the loss of cells that produce a messenger called **dopamine**, which is involved in controlling muscles.

The causes of PD are unknown; however, the disease is estimated to affect between 100 and 180 people per 100 000 of the UK population and has an incidence of 4–20 per 100 000 (NICE, 2006b). There is an increased risk of PD with age and men are more likely to be affected.

Pathophysiology of PD

The symptoms of PD are directly attributable to the loss of the neurotransmitter **dopamine** from the **basal nuclei** nerve cells in the **substantia nigra** of the **basal ganglia** within the cerebrum.

Levels of dopamine are closely linked with the levels of other chemicals in the brain, including **acetylcholine**, and the low levels of dopamine, together with changes in other chemicals, lead to the symptoms of PD (see Box 10.3). At present, it is not known what causes the loss of the cells that produce dopamine; however, both inherited and sporadic forms of PD have been identified and in both cases degenerative changes have been found within the affected brain tissue (Hickey, 2003).

Box 10.3 Some typical symptoms of PD

- Slow movements (**bradykinesia**)
- Tremors (initially in the hand but also seen in the limbs, head, face and jaw
- Muscle stiffness and rigidity
- A tendency to walk forward on the toes with small, shuffling steps
- Changes in balance
- A stooped posture
- Confusion
- Depression
- Difficulty with fine motor functions, e.g. writing and eating
- 'Mask'-like face
- General weakness and muscle fatigue

Adapted from Monahan *et al.* (2007).

Pharmacological management of PD

Treatment for PD aims to primarily replace dopamine in the brain and minimise the effects of the disease. Drugs commonly used include:

- L-dopa or levodopa, which is the precursor to dopamine, is the mainstay of treatment for PD. However, as the drug does not cross the blood–brain barrier effectively, it has to be combined with either carbidopa (Sinemet) or benserazide (Madopar) to increase its uptake by the brain.
- Selegiline (Eldepryl) is commonly prescribed for patients who are newly diagnosed with PD as it delays the progression of the disease by blocking the metabolism of dopamine and delaying the need for L-dopa (Monahan *et al.*, 2007).
- Amantadine (Symmetrel), an antiviral agent, is also used in the early stages of PD as it acts by allowing more dopamine to accumulate at and enter the nerve synapse, which delays the need for L-dopa.
- Anticholenergic drugs such as trihexyphenidyl (Artane) and benztropine mesylate (Cogentin) are often used in addition to L-dopa (or in patients who cannot tolerate it) to treat tremor and rigidity.

Non-pharmacological management of PD

- Surgery to create lesions to one side of the thalamus (Thalamotomy) or destroy part of the basal ganglia (pallidotomy) to control rigidity and tremor, which was the treatment for PD prior to L-dopa becoming available, has become popular once again due to the complication associated with the long-term use of, or intolerance to, L-dopa (Hickey, 2003).
- More recent therapy has involved the use of deep-brain stimulation to send impulses deep into the brain and block the signals that cause Parkinsonian movements (Mader, 2005).
- The use of stem cells either from the umbilical cords of newborns or by the creation of the patient's genetically identical cells using donor eggs are experimental treatments currently being explored (Hickey, 2003).

Nursing management of PD

Whilst the majority of patients with PD are managed in the community, as the disease progresses to the later stages, the patient may require residential/nursing home care. Key nursing considerations include:

- Reducing the threat of injury from falls as due to the physical immobility, weakness, rigidity and slow movement the patient with PD is at greater risk. This may also require undertaking a risk assessment of the patient's home environment to ensure that any potential hazards are removed.
- Ensuring that the patient is able to express themselves effectively, as due to vocal changes and difficulty with writing the patient's ability to communicate may be affected. Therefore, it might be necessary to gain the involvement of a speech therapist and other support measures to ensure that the patient will be able to communicate effectively.
- Monitoring of the patient's body weight and the provision of adequate nutrition that the patient is able to tolerate, as due to possible difficulties with swallowing (**dysphagia**) there is a risk of malnutrition and weight loss.
- Assisting the patient with meeting their hygiene needs as necessary.

Stage of disease	Common signs and symptoms
1 (2–4 years)	Loss of interest in people, environment and present affairs Hesitant in using own initiative, becomes uncertain about making decisions/actions and is forgetful
2 (2–12 years)	Memory loss becomes more apparent, has difficulty in undertaking simple tasks or carrying out simple instructions. Loses documents, forgets to pay bills or undertake household chores Unable to meet own needs, loses inhibitions, has periods of irritability, paranoia and anxiety Prone to wandering particularly at night, becomes lost in familiar surroundings and may forget way home
3 (Final stage)	Loses the ability to communicate verbally or in writing Becomes bedridden and incontinent of urine and faeces Does not recognise loved ones Becomes emaciated due to lack of eating

Table 10.6 Stages of Alzheimer's disease

Alzheimer's disease

Alzheimer's disease (AD) is the most common form of **dementia** and affects around 450 000 people in the UK (Alzheimer's Society, 2007).

Pathophysiology of AD

Although the cause of AD remains unclear, the disease does cause structural changes in the brain predominately the presence of plaques and tangles. Additionally, the disease has also been associated with a shortage of acetylcholine, loss of nerve cells and structural changes in the memory and cognition areas of the brain. Therefore, the sufferer exhibits memory loss, poor judgement, disorientation, confusion, changes in personality which can lead to mood swings, and sometimes violent outbursts. Inability to maintain self-care, wandering and hallucinations are common in the later stages. Table 10.6 outlines the stages of the disease.

Pharmacological management of AD

Whilst there is no cure for AD, there are a number of drug treatments available that can alleviate or slow down the symptoms of the disease. These include:

■ Aricept, Exelon and Reminyl which work by maintaining existing levels of acetylcholine in patients with mild to moderate dementia.
■ Ebixa which can be used in patients with middle- to late-stage dementia and prevents excess entry of calcium ions into brain cells. Excess calcium is known to damage brain cells and prevent them from receiving messages from other brain cells (Alzheimer's Society, 2007).

In addition, drug therapy can be used to manage behavioural changes associated with the disease. These include:

- antidepressant medication to treat depressive symptoms
- neuroleptic drugs to treat psychosis and delusional behaviour
- sedatives to treat agitation

Non-pharmacological management of AD
- Patients with mild to moderate disease should be offered the opportunity to participate in a structured group cognitive stimulation programme (NICE, 2006a).

Nursing management of AD
The progressive nature of AD which results in the patient's loss of independence, personality and cognitive function presents the nurse and the patient's family with many challenges. Key nursing considerations include:

- maintenance of a safe environment, as due to loss of judgement, cognitive decline and poor memory the patient is at increased risk of injury
- maintenance of hygiene and nutritional needs, as due to loss of independence and inability to make decisions the patient is unable to meet or plan for own needs
- promotion of restful sleep as the patient is likely to be awake at night and prone to wandering
- provision of information and support for caregivers/family

Multiple sclerosis
Multiple sclerosis or MS is a chronic, degenerative disease in which **demyelination** of the brain and spinal cord leads to damage to the nerve pathways and loss of function to the affected area. The disease is progressive; however, the patient may experience periods of remission before relapsing again.

Whilst the cause of MS is unclear it is thought to be linked to an impaired immune system following a viral infection that initiates an **autoimmune response**.

Pathophysiology of MS
MS affects primarily the white matter of the brain and spinal cord by causing areas of demyelination and a breakdown of the myelin sheath that surrounds the nerve fibres and axons (see Figure 10.5) preventing conduction of normal nerve impulses.

The signs and symptoms of MS vary greatly from patient to patient and may vary over time in the same patient (Hickey, 2003). Common signs and symptoms are summarised in Box 10.4.

Pharmacological management of MS
Whilst MS is an incurable, extremely debilitating disease it is rarely fatal (Monahan *et al.*, 2007) and drug therapy can help with the management of the condition. Drug therapy falls into two broad categories: treatment to slow or stop the disease process and treatment to manage the symptoms of MS:

- Treatment to arrest the disease process includes the use of interferon and steroids, e.g. prednisolone which may be used to treat acute relapses and aid recovery.
- Treatment to manage the symptoms of MS include:

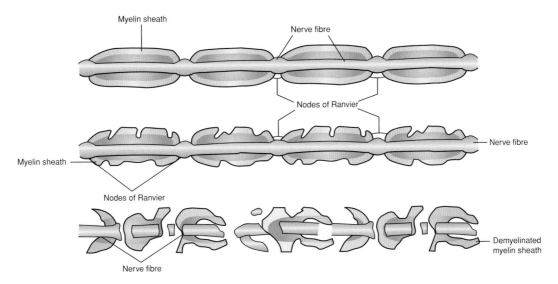

Figure 10.5 The process of demyelination.

☐ baclofen to treat muscle spasticity
☐ stool softeners and laxatives to manage constipation
☐ oxybutynen (Ditropan) to manage bladder function
☐ fluoxetine (Prozac), amitriptyline (Elavil) or imipramine (Tofranil) to treat depression

Nursing management of MS

Because of the unpredictable nature of its progression, MS presents the nurse, the patient and their family with many challenges. Therefore, the care of the patient with MS will require a multidisciplinary approach to ensure that all aspects of the patient's care are met. The nurse plays a key role in this process and key nursing considerations include:

■ minimising risk of injury due to weakness, impaired coordination and sensory deficits
■ prevention of complications related to immobility and physical weakness
■ ensuring that the patient's activities of living are met

Box 10.4 Typical signs and symptoms of MS

■ Muscular weakness/feeling of heaviness to the legs
■ Numbness to face or extremities
■ Loss of short-term memory
■ Visual field defects
■ Bladder and bowel dysfunction
■ Sexual dysfunction
■ Fatigue
■ Depression

- providing the patient with education and psychological support to understand and adapt to the unpredictable nature of their illness
- educating the patient as to how to avoid relapses where possible, e.g. keeping stress to a minimum, reducing the risk of infection

Epilepsy

Epilepsy is a term often used to describe a chronic disorder characterised by recurring seizures of unknown cause (Walsh, 2002). Within the UK, 1 in every 131 people have epilepsy (National Society for Epilepsy, 2007) and the disease affects all age groups.

Pathophysiology of epilepsy

A seizure or 'fit' is caused by an abnormal electrical discharge in the brain in either the sensory system, motor system or autonomic nervous system and in the majority of cases the cause is unknown (Martini, 2001). However, seizures of all kinds are accompanied by a marked change in the pattern of electrical activity in the brain. The change starts in one part of the brain and may spread to nearby areas or continue across the whole of the cerebral cortex. Consequently, a seizure may take many different forms depending on the area and amount of the brain involved and the International League against Epilepsy (2006) has developed a widely used system of classifying seizures as outlined in Table 10.7.

Status epilepticus

Status epilepticus is an episode of seizure activity lasting at least 30 minutes or repeated seizures without a full recovery period in between (Monahan *et al.*, 2007). Prolonged seizures can be life-threatening as they lead to cellular destruction and death if not stopped and should be treated as a medical emergency.

Nursing management of seizures

Nurses need to act quickly when a patient has a seizure. Key nursing considerations include:

- easing the patient to the floor if seated when the seizure occurs
- protecting the patient from injury by moving nearby furniture or objects out of the way and putting a pillow under the head
- not restraining the patient or forcing anything into the patient's mouth
- when the seizure has stopped, ensuring that the airway is clear and administering oxygen if necessary
- documenting the duration and type of seizure as well as how long it takes for the patient to become fully responsive to their surrounding (postictal phase)
- staying with the patient throughout the seizure and orientating/informing the patient about the event once they are awake

Nursing management of status epilepticus

Status epilepticus is a medical emergency; therefore, key nursing considerations include:

- maintenance of the patient's airway to ensure adequate ventilation – this may include suction of the airway to prevent obstruction

Type of seizure	Effect on consciousness	Signs and symptoms

Partial or focal onset
 A. Local
   1. Neocortical
   2. Hippocampal or
      parahippocampal
	Not impaired	Twitching or tingling and numbness of a body area
		 Loss of speech
		 Sensory disturbance or 'aura', e.g. seeing lights, strange smells, feeling of deja vu
		 Feeling of fear or doom

B. With ipsilateral propagation C. With contralateral spread	Impaired	Begins as a partial seizure but progresses to a tonic–clonic (see below). Automatic behaviour or automatism experienced, e.g. chewing, lip smacking or picking at clothes
D. Secondarily generalised		
1. Tonic–clonic (formerly grand mal)	Impaired	Tonic phase involving rigidity of all muscles followed by clonic phase involving rhythmic jerking of muscles and possible tongue biting and urinary/faecal incontinence
2. ?Absence	Impaired for only a few seconds	Brief loss of muscle tone which may cause patient to fall or drop something – referred to as drop attacks
3. ?Epileptic spasm	Impaired for only a few seconds or not at all	Brief jerking of a muscle group which may cause a patient to fall

Adapted from International League against Epilepsy (2006).

Table 10.7 Classification of seizures

- providing oxygen therapy via nasal cannulae as prescribed
- protecting the patient from injury
- administering prescribed medication usually diazepam or lorazepam until the seizures stop

Pharmacological management of epilepsy

- Up to 70% of people with epilepsy have the condition controlled with antiepileptic (also known as anticonvulsant) drugs and many people become seizure-free on the first drug that is used (Bingham, 2004). Common drugs used include carbamazepine (Tegretol), sodium valporate (Epilim) and phenytoin (Dilantin).

Non-pharmacological management of epilepsy

- Surgical intervention such as removal of the temporal lobe (temporal lobectomy) and vagal nerve stimulation may be performed for patients who do not respond to medication or who are not considered suitable for certain forms of surgery.
- As treatment for epilepsy is usually long-term or lifelong, the patient needs to be educated as to the importance of compliance with drug therapy.
- The patient needs to be educated as to lifestyle changes that may be required as a result of having epilepsy, e.g. occupation and driving.

Conclusion

Because of the complex nature of the nervous system impairment to any part of it will mean that the symptoms that the patient experiences are dependent on the areas of the nervous system affected and the extent of damage incurred. Therefore, caring for the patient with a neurological disorder presents nurses with many challenges and the overall aim of this chapter was to provide the reader with insight into some of the more common, related problems of the nervous system and their nursing management.

Multiple choice questions

1. The structures which connect the brain to the spinal cord are collectively known as the:
(a) basal ganglia
(b) corpus callosum
(c) brainstem
(d) cerebellum

2. The brain requires how much of the body's circulating blood volume per minute?
(a) 2%
(b) 15%
(c) 20%
(d) 40%

3. Cerebrospinal fluid is produced in the:
(a) choroid plexus
(b) limbic system
(c) ventricles
(d) meninges

4. The reticular formation plays an important role in:
(a) the maintenance of body posture
(b) the control of body temperature
(c) the sleep–wake cycle
(d) the intonation of sound

5. Which of the following is not a layer of the meninges?
(a) arachnoid mater
(b) dura mater
(c) erathnoid mater
(d) pia mater

6. Parkinson's disease is caused by:
(a) a loss of myelin sheath to the nerve cell
(b) fatty plaques in the brain
(c) an interruption in blood flow to the brain
(d) a loss of dopamine

7. A bleed to the left side of the brain will result in:
(a) loss of movement to the left side of the body
(b) difficulty with speech
(c) visual impairment to the left eye
(d) all of the above

8. The parasympathetic division of the autonomic nervous system:
(a) utilises norephinephrine to initiate internal responses
(b) increases the heart rate
(c) dilates the pupils
(d) constricts the bronchioles in the lungs

9. The diencephalon:
(a) is also known as the midbrain
(b) contains the hypothalamus
(c) plays a major role in fine movement and coordination
(d) is divided into four lobes

10. The presence of Schwann cells (myelin sheath) is important in:
(a) the release of a neurotransmitter
(b) protection of the brain from injury
(c) the rapid transmission of a nerve impulse
(d) the control of specific muscle groups

Answers: 1.c, 2.b, 3.a, 4.c, 5.c, 6.d, 7.b, 8.d, 9.b, 10.c.

Test your knowledge

❷ Compare and contrast the differing function of the parasympathetic and sympathetic divisions of the autonomic nervous system.

❷ Describe the structure and function of the four areas of the brain.

❷ Devise a nursing care plan for a patient who has sustained a traumatic head injury.

Glossary of terms

Acetylcholine: A neurotransmitter found widely in the central and peripheral nervous system.

Choroid plexus: Tissues in the ventricles of the brain which produce cerebrospinal fluid.

Dementia: A loss of mental ability.

Demyelination: The loss of the myelin sheath from around the axon of the nerve cell.

Dopamine: A neurotransmitter found in the central nervous system.

Foramen magnum: A large hole in the occipital bone through which the vertebral column and spinal cord pass.

Norephinepherine: A neurotransmitter in the central and peripheral nervous system.

Schwann cells: Cells that form myelin around the axon of a nerve cell.

Substantia nigra: A part of the midbrain which connects to the basal ganglia.

Ventricle: A cavity filled with cerebrospinal fluid.

References

Alzheimer's Society (2007). www.alzheimer's.org.uk.

Bingham, E. (2004). Diagnosis and support for people with epilepsy. *Practice Nursing, 15*(2), 64–70.

Germann, W.J. and Standfield, C.L. (2002). *Principles of Human Physiology*. London: Benjamin Cummings.

Hickey, J. (2003). *The Clinical Practice of Neurological and Neurosurgical Nursing*, 5th edn. Philadelphia: Lippincott Williams & Wilkins.

International league against epilepsy (ILEA) (2006). www.ilea.org.

Mader, S. (2005). *Understanding Human Anatomy and Physiology*. London: McGraw Hill.

Marieb, E.N. (2006). *Essentials of Human Anatomy and Physiology*, 8th edn. London: Pearson Benjamin Cummings.

Martini, F.H. (2001). *Fundamentals of Anatomy and Physiology*, 5th edn. New Jersey: Prentice Hall.

Monahan, F.D., Neighbors, M., Sands, J.K. and Marek, J.F. (2007). *Phipps' Medical and Surgical Nursing – Health and Illness Perspectives*, 8th edn. St. Louis: Mosby.

National Institute for Clinical Excellence (2003). *Head Injury: Triage, Assessment, Investigation and Early Management of Head Injury in Infants, Children and Adults*. Clinical Guideline 4. London: NICE.

National Institute for Clinical Excellence (2006a). *Dementia: Supporting People with Dementia and Their Carers in Health and Social Care*. Clinical Guideline 42. London: NICE.

National Institute for Clinical Excellence (2006b). *Parkinson's Disease: Diagnosis and Management in Primary Care*. Clinical Guideline 3. London: NICE.

National Institute for Clinical Excellence (2007a). *Head Injury: Triage, Assessment, Investigation and Early Management of Head Injury in Infants, Children and Adults*. Clinical Guideline 56 (a partial update of clinical guideline 4). London: NICE.

National Institute for Clinical Excellence (2007b). *Alteplase for the Treatment of Acute Ischaemic Stroke*. NICE technology appraisal guidance 122. London: NICE.

National Society for Epilepsy (2007). Available at http//www.epilepsynse.org.uk.

Shier, D., Butler, J. and Lewis, R. (2004). *Human Anatomy and Physiology*. London: McGraw Hill.

Teasdale, G. and Jennett, B. (1974). Assessment of coma and impaired consciousness: A practical scale. *Lancet, 2*(7872), 81–84.

The Stroke Association (2004). Available at http:// www.stroke.org.uk.

Turner, A.M. and Jowett, N.I. (2006). The role of statin therapy in preventing recurrent stroke. *Nursing Times, 102*(38), 25–26.

Walsh, M. (2002): *Watson's Clinical Nursing and Related Sciences*. London: Bailliere Tindall.

Waterhouse, C. (2005): The Glasgow Coma Scale and other neurological observations. *Nursing Standard, 19*(33), 56–64.

Chapter 11

The gastrointestinal system and associated disorders

Muralitharan Nair

KEY WORDS

- Oral cavity
- Duodenum
- Large intestine
- Peristalsis
- Oesophagus
- Jejunum
- Digestion
- Peritoneum
- Stomach
- Small intestine
- Chyme

Test your prior knowledge

- ❓ What are the main functions of saliva?
- ❓ List five functions of the stomach.
- ❓ Differentiate between chemical and mechanical digestion.
- ❓ Name the accessory organs of digestion?

Learning outcomes

On completion of this section, the reader will be able to:

■ Describe the organs of digestion.

■ List the accessory organs of digestion.

■ List the main functions of the gastrointestinal tract.

■ Explain the differences between chemical and mechanical digestion.

Introduction

The gastrointestinal tract is also known as the digestive system or alimentary canal. It involves the mouth, **pharynx**, **oesophagus**, **stomach** and the **intestines** (see Figure 11.1). The main function of the gastrointestinal tract is to provide water, nutrients and electrolytes for bodily function. These are obtained from food eaten and fluids drunk; to carry out this function the gastrointestinal tract performs the role of **digestion, absorption** and the **elimination** of unwanted materials.

The gastrointestinal tract is a continuous tract and is approximately 10 m long from the mouth to the anus. The accessory organs are the salivary glands, liver, pancreas and gallbladder. The accessory organs produce various enzymes that help break down foodstuffs, for example salivary amylase (ptyalin) will act on sugars and starch in the diet whereas pepsin will act on proteins. Other accessory organs include the lips, teeth, tongue and palate. This chapter discusses the structure and functions of the gastrointestinal tract, the accessory organs of digestion and some common disorders and their related nursing management and treatment.

The oral cavity

The mouth, also known as the oral cavity, is the start of the gastrointestinal tract. It receives food and the mechanical breakdown of food particles begins here and food is mixed with saliva (Shier *et al.*, 2004) which eases the passage of food down the oesophagus. Saliva, secreted by the salivary glands, contains a digestive enzyme called salivary amylase. Salivary amylase breaks down carbohydrates into smaller sugar molecules.

The activity of breaking down foodstuff and mixing it with saliva is called **mastication**. The brokendown foodstuff is then swallowed and it enters the stomach via the oesophagus. The mouth is surrounded by and contains the lips, gums, teeth, cheeks, tongue and palate. The space between the tongue and the palate is the cavity of the mouth and the space between the lips, gums and the teeth is called the vestibule (see Figure 11.2).

Lips
The lips form the orifice of the mouth. They are fleshy folds, which contain skeletal muscles and sensory receptors (Shier *et al.*, 2004). These structures help in the assessment of temperature and texture of foods

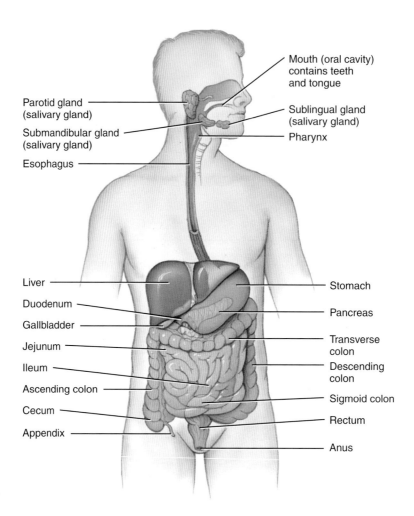

Figure 11.1 Gastrointestinal tract.

eaten. The reddish colour of the lips results from numerous blood vessels. The lips also assist food into the mouth. The junction between the upper and the lower lips forms the angle of the mouth.

Cheeks
Cheeks form the fleshy sides of the face and they run from the corner of the mouth to the side of the nose. Subcutaneous fat, muscles and mucous membranes line the cheeks. The cheeks assist in the chewing of food.

Palate
The **palate** is divided into the hard and the soft palates (see Figure 11.2); both form the roof of the mouth whereas the tongue lies at the bottom of the oral cavity and forms the floor of the mouth. The hard and the soft palates are covered by mucous membranes.

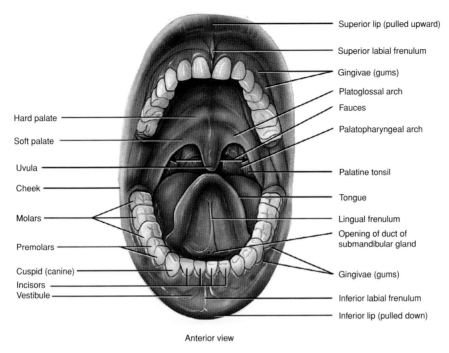

Superior lip (pulled upward)

Superior labial frenulum

Gingivae (gums)

Platoglossal arch

Fauces

Palatopharyngeal arch

Hard palate

Soft palate

Uvula

Cheek

Molars

Premolars

Cuspid (canine)

Incisors

Vestibule

Palatine tonsil

Tongue

Lingual frenulum

Opening of duct of
submandibular gland

Gingivae (gums)

Inferior labial frenulum

Inferior lip (pulled down)

Anterior view

Figure 11.2 The oral cavity.

Tongue

The tongue is a thick muscular organ composed of skeletal muscles and mucous membranes. It contains approximately 10 000 taste buds (Silverthorn, 1998). It tells the person about the taste of food, for example whether the food is sweet or sour. Marieb and Hoehn (2007) state that the tongue detects four basic tastes: sweet, salt, bitter and sour. Silverthorn (1998) identified a fifth taste called umami. This word is derived from the Japanese word meaning 'deliciousness', and the taste is associated with glutamate and some **nucleotides**. Hence, in some Asian countries monosodium glutamate (MSG) is sometimes used to enhance flavour when cooking.

The tongue is an accessory organ, which forms the floor of the mouth; it helps to blend food when chewing and to push food particles to the back of the mouth when swallowing. Tongue movement can alter the volume of the oral cavity and also has an important role in speech, chewing, swallowing and taste.

Teeth

Humans develop two sets of teeth: milk teeth and permanent teeth. There are approximately 20 milk teeth (see Figure 11.3) which begin to develop, usually from the age of 6 months. Often one pair of milk teeth grow per month and they usually fall out between the ages of 6 and 12 years. Once the milk teeth fall out, they are replaced by permanent teeth. Usually, there are 32 permanent teeth (see Figure 11.4), which have the potential to last a lifetime. However, permanent molars do not replace milk teeth. The first permanent molars appear at the age of 6 years, the second at the age of 12 years and the third may develop after the age of 13 years. The functions of the teeth include cutting, tearing and chewing food.

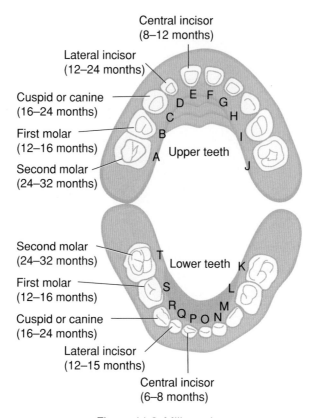

Central incisor
(8–12 months)

Lateral incisor
(12–24 months)

Cuspid or canine
(16–24 months)

First molar
(12–16 months)

Second molar
(24–32 months)

Upper teeth

Second molar
(24–32 months)

First molar
(12–16 months)

Cuspid or canine
(16–24 months)

Lateral incisor
(12–15 months)

Central incisor
(6–8 months)

Lower teeth

Figure 11.3 Milk teeth.

Salivary glands

There are three main pairs of salivary glands and they include these:

- parotid
- submandibular
- sublingual

See Figure 11.5 for the salivary glands.

The salivary glands are covered by a fibrous capsule and contain secretory cells. The saliva from these secretory cells drain into larger ducts leading into the mouth. These salivary glands secrete approximately 1 L of saliva per day (Marieb and Hoehn, 2007).

Composition of saliva

Saliva consists of:

- water
- salts
- salivary amylase

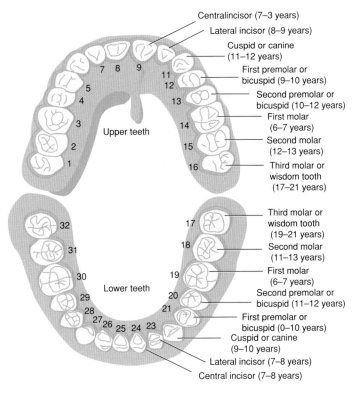

Centralincisor (7–3 years)
Lateral incisor (8–9 years)
Cuspid or canine (11–12 years)
First premolar or bicuspid (9–10 years)
Second premolar or bicuspid (10–12 years)
First molar (6–7 years)
Second molar (12–13 years)
Third molar or wisdom tooth (17–21 years)
Third molar or wisdom tooth (19–21 years)
Second molar (11–13 years)
First molar (6–7 years)
Second premolar or bicuspid (11–12 years)
First premolar or bicuspid (0–10 years)
Cuspid or canine (9–10 years)
Lateral incisor (7–8 years)
Central incisor (7–8 years)

Upper teeth

Lower teeth

Figure 11.4 Permanent teeth.

- mucin (a protein that help form mucous)
- lysozyme (a bacteriolytic enzyme)

Functions of saliva

Insert sevifence. Saliva keeps the oral cavity moist at all times and moisten food to aid swallowing. The secretion of saliva is under autonomic nerve control with no hormonal stimulation. The breakdown of carbohydrate begins in the mouth with the aid of salivary amylase. The pH of saliva ranges from 5.8 to 7.4 (Waugh and Grant, 2006). Saliva helps to clean the mouth and keep it free from infection through the action of lysozyme.

Pharynx

The pharynx lies behind the nose, mouth and larynx. It is approximately 12 cm in length and is divided into three sections: the nasopharynx, oral pharynx and laryngeal pharynx. There are several openings into the pharynx (Mader, 2005): the mouth, larynx, oesophagus, two small nasal cavities and two eustachian tubes. When food is swallowed, the soft palate closes the nasal passages and the epiglottis moves over the glottis to close the larynx and the trachea (see Figure 11.6). This allows the foodstuff to move down the oesophagus rather than into the respiratory tract (see Figure 11.7).

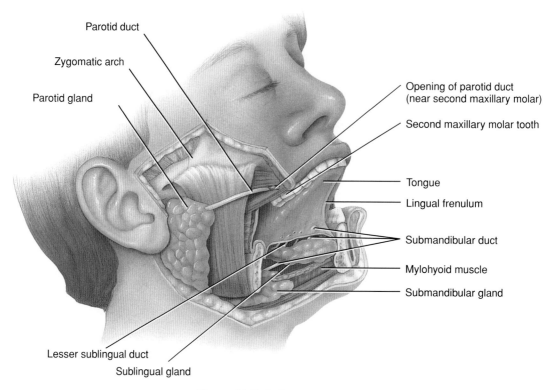

Figure 11.5 Salivary glands.

Oesophagus

This is a muscular tube approximately 25 cm long, running from the pharynx to the stomach. It lies at the back of the trachea and in front of the spinal column (backbone). The oesophagus is sometimes known as the food pipe (gullet) (Mader, 2005). It is a collapsible muscular tube that channels food into the stomach. The movement of food down the oesophagus occurs as a result of peristaltic action. It is not possible for a person to swallow and breathe at the same time; this part of swallowing is a reflex action.

Stomach

The stomach is a 'J'-shaped muscular organ situated below the diaphragm, made up of four regions. The upper portion is called the cardiac region, an elevated part the **fundus**, a middle section the body and a **pyloric region** (see Figure 11.8). The layers of the stomach include an outer layer called the visceral peritoneum also known as serosa, muscularis layer, submucosa layer and mucosa layer (see Figure 11.9).

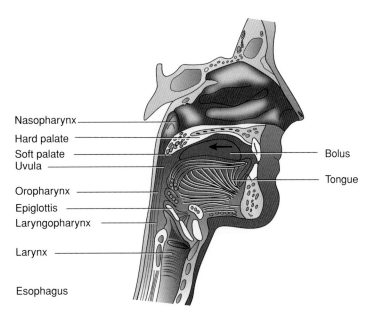

Nasopharynx
Hard palate
Soft palate
Uvula
Oropharynx
Epiglottis
Laryngopharynx
Larynx
Esophagus
Bolus
Tongue

Position of structures before swallowing

Figure 11.6 The pharynx.

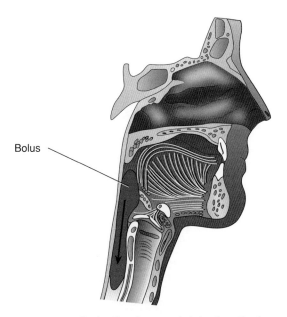

Bolus

During the pharyngeal state of swallowing

Figure 11.7 Swallowing action.

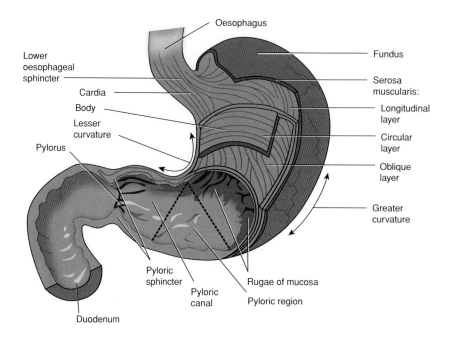

Figure 11.8 The stomach.

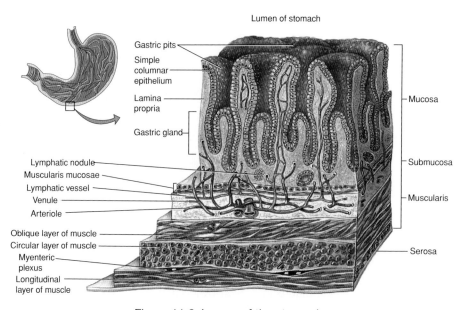

Figure 11.9 Layers of the stomach.

The cells of the mucosa protect the stomach from acid secretions and digestive enzymes of the stomach.

Secretions of the stomach

The stomach secretes numerous enzymes and other substances. These are:

- mucus – protects the lining and provides lubrication for food
- hydrochloric acid – protects the stomach from bacteria
- intrinsic factor – helps in the absorption of vitamin B_{12}
- gastrin – stimulates the secretion of hydrochloric acid
- pepsinogen – helps in the digestion of protein

The secretions and the ingested food are mixed together into a thick, pasty, semisolid and acidic substance called chyme. **Chyme** leaves the stomach by way of the pyloric sphincter (see Figure 11.8) and enters the duodenum.

Functions of the stomach

The stomach performs numerous functions:

- It is a temporary reservoir for food until it is ready to be passed into the duodenum. All nutrients are liquefied, broken down and mixed with hydrochloric acid and forms a semisolid substance called chyme.
- Proteins are converted into peptones by pepsins.
- Milk is curdled and casein is released from the milk.
- Digestion of fats begins in the stomach.
- Production of intrinsic factor essential for the absorption of vitamin B_{12}.

Digestion

Digestion involves two processes: mechanical and chemical digestion. The mechanical process is whereby the stomach churns the food by the muscular action of the muscle layers of the stomach (see Figure 11.8). The brokendown food boli (singular – bolus) are then mixed with the chemical secretions of the stomach gastric juice. The gastric juice renders the semisolid boli into a semiliquid form which is called chyme.

Small intestine

The small intestine extends from the pylorus of the stomach to the ileocaecal valve and is divided into three sections: duodenum, jejunum and the ileum (see Figure 11.10).

The small intestine is approximately 6 m long and 3 cm in diameter and is situated in the abdominal cavity. The small intestine is supported by mesenteries (see Figure 11.11) which convey blood vessels, lymphatic vessels and nerves for its function.

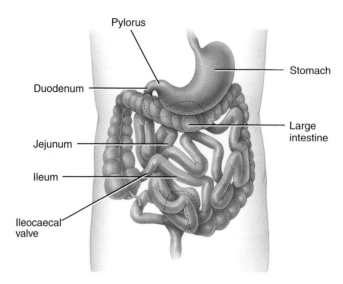

Figure 11.10 Small intestine.

Duodenum

The duodenum is the 'C'-shaped section of the small intestine (see Figure 11.10). This is the shortest section and it is approximately 25 cm in length. The duodenum commences from the pyloric sphincter and ends at the beginning of the jejunum. This section is involved with further digestion of nutrients from the stomach.

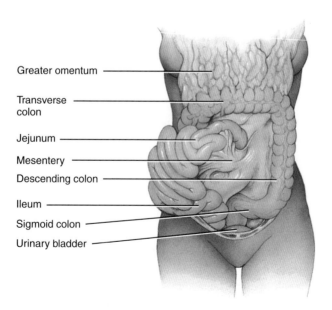

Figure 11.11 Mesentery of the small intestine.

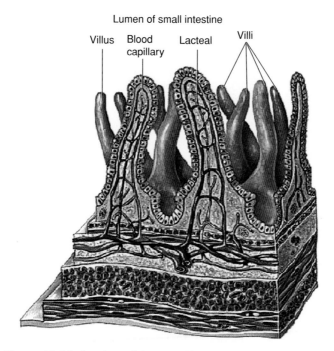

Figure 11.12 Section of the small intestine showing the villi.

Jejunum

The jejunum is approximately 2.5 m in length and it commences from the end of the duodenum and **terminates** at the beginning of the ileum. The main function of the jejunum is to further break down the nutrients coming from the duodenum.

Ileum

The ileum commences from the end of the jejunum and terminates at the ileocaecal valve. It is approximately 3.5 m in length. Absorption mainly takes place in the ileum. The absorption is carried out by small structures called villi (singular – villus) (see Figure 11.12).

Large intestine

The **large intestine**, also known as the colon, commences from the ileocaecal valve and terminates at the rectum. The large intestine is approximately 2 m in length and 6 cm in diameter. The large intestine consists of the caecum, the ascending, transverse, descending and sigmoid colons; the rectum and the anus (see Figure 11.13) (Wynsberghe *et al.*, 1995).

The functions of the large intestine include:

- absorption of water, electrolytes and vitamins
- secretion of mucus for the lubrication of faeces
- storage of indigestible food stuff such as cellulose and vegetable fibres
- production of vitamin K and some B complexes (B_1, B_2 and folic acid)
- defecation

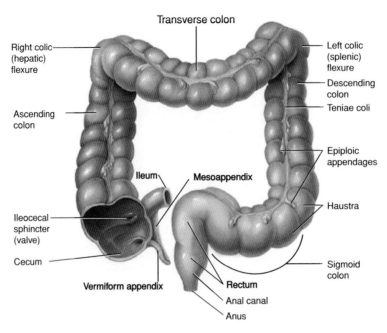

Figure 11.13 Large intestine.

Accessory organs of digestion

Liver

The liver is the largest organ in the body and weighs approximately 1.5 kg. The liver is reddish in colour, wedge-shaped and covered by connective tissue (Wynsberghe *et al.*, 1995) and is divided into the right and left lobes (see Figure 11.14). It is situated in the upper right quadrant of the abdominal cavity beneath the diaphragm. It is partially protected by the ribs. The right and the left lobes are separated by the falciform ligament and the liver is covered by a serous membrane called **peritoneum**.

Vessels of the liver

The main blood vessels of the liver include:

■ the hepatic artery – this is a branch of the celiac artery and it supplies oxygenated blood to the liver
■ the hepatic portal vein drains venous blood from the gastrointestinal tract, which contains nutrients absorbed from the small intestine into the liver
■ the hepatic vein drains venous blood from the liver to the inferior vena cava

Functions of the liver

The liver has numerous functions and they include:

■ aids metabolism through chemical reactions from the absorbed nutrients
■ modifies waste products and toxic substances, i.e. drugs such as paracetamol, aspirin and alcohol
■ produces and stores **glycogen**

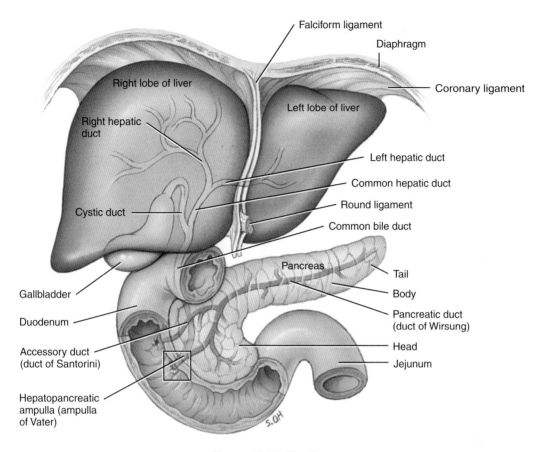

Figure 11.14 The liver.

- maintains blood glucose levels
- produces **bile**, which emulsifies fats in the diet for absorption
- converts ammonia into urea which is a waste product
- forms red blood cells in fetal life
- plays a part in the destruction of red blood cells
- stores iron, fat-soluble vitamins A, D, E and K and water-soluble vitamin B_{12}; and minerals such as iron and copper
- manufactures plasma proteins such as prothrombin
- produces anticoagulants

Gallbladder

The gallbladder is a pear-shaped muscular sac, which lies beneath the right lobe of the liver (see Figure 11.14). It is divided into the fundus, the body and the neck. The gallbladder is approximately 7–9 cm in length and its main function is to store and concentrate bile which is produced in the liver. See Figure 11.15 for the production and storage of bile. Bile is released from the gallbladder in the presence of a hormone called cholecystokinin (CCK). The presence of chyme in the duodenum stimulates the

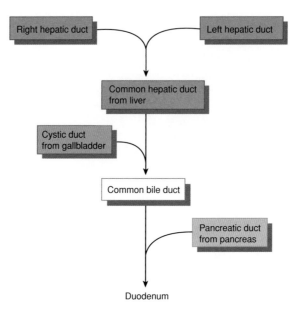

Figure 11.15 Production and storage of bile.

production of CCK by the enteroendocrine cells of the duodenum. This hormone is transported in the blood stream to the gallbladder where it stimulates the smooth muscles of the gallbladder to contract, thus ejecting bile.

Pancreas

The pancreas is a triangular-shaped organ. It is approximately 12–15 cm in length and 2.5 cm thick. It is divided into three sections: head, body and the tail. The head of the pancreas lies in the loop of the duodenum (see Figure 11.14) and the tail touches the spleen. It has two functions: exocrine and endocrine.

Exocrine functions

Exocrine pertains to the process of secreting outwardly through a duct such as the pancreatic **duct** which directs the flow of pancreatic juices to the duodenum (see Figure 11.14). The exocrine cells of the pancreas secrete **enzymes** that break down food particles and these enzymes are:

- pancreatic amylase for the digestion of starch
- trypsin for the digestion of proteins
- lipase for the digestion of fats

Approximately, 1500 mL of pancreatic juices are produced per day.

Endocrine functions

Endocrine pertains to the process of secreting directly into the blood stream without the aid of ducts. The endocrine functions include:

- production of the hormone glucagon by the alpha cells – increases blood glucose levels
- production of the hormone insulin by the beta cells – lowers blood glucose levels
- production of the hormone somatostatin by the delta cells – regulate both glucagons and insulin levels

For more detailed discussion on pancreas, see Chapter 13.

Disorders of the gastrointestinal tract

On completion of this section, the reader will be able to:

- List some of the common disorders of the gastrointestinal tract.
- Describe the pathophysiology of specific gastrointestinal disorders.
- Discuss the nursing management of gastrointestinal disorders.

Gingivitis

Also known as inflammation of the gums, gingivitis may lead to ulceration and necrosis of the gums. It may be caused by plague, which is a sticky substance deposited on the exposed portion of the teeth, consisting of bacteria, food particles and mucous. Other possible causes of gingivitis are vigorous brushing and flossing of the teeth. Some individuals who have diabetes mellitus and certain pregnant women can develop gingivitis which may be the result of hormonal changes (Kozier *et al.*, 2004).

Aetiology of gingivitis

Gingivitis may be caused by poor oral hygiene whereby bacteria infect the gums and the toxins produced by the bacteria cause inflammation of the gums. Long-term plaque deposits may also cause gingivitis. Dental plague is made up of mucin and colloid materials found in saliva. Colloid materials can mineralise into hard deposits called tartar and accumulate at the base of the teeth. Certain drugs, for example phenytoin, some birth control pills and ingestion of heavy metals such as lead and bismuth may cause inflammation of the gums. Badly fitting orthodontic appliances, i.e. dentures, bridges and crowns, can irritate the gums and cause inflammation, leading to gingivitis.

Signs and symptoms

These include:

- swollen and painful gums; tender when touched
- bleeding from the gums and blood may be visible on the toothbrush even with gentle brushing
- excessive salivation
- bad breath (halitosis)
- gums may appear shinny and or bright red

Nursing management of gingivitis

A dentist should be consulted when signs of gingivitis are suspected. The dentist may use dental instruments to remove the plaque and clean the teeth. Meticulous oral hygiene is essential after visiting the dentist. The dentist or the dental hygienist will demonstrate the correct method of brushing and

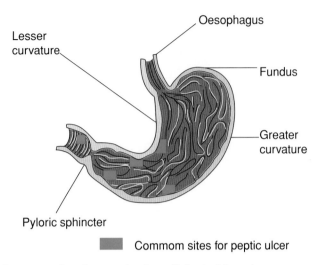

Figure 11.16 Common sites for peptic ulcer. (Adapted from Lemone and Burke, 2004.)

flossing the teeth. The mouth should be rinsed using copious amounts of water after brushing and flossing.

The nurse should encourage patients who are at risk of contracting gingivitis to brush and floss their teeth after each meal. This will help to remove particles that may become lodged between the teeth.

Peptic ulcer

Peptic ulcer is a term used to define the development of an ulcer along the gastrointestinal tract namely in the stomach or the duodenum. Duodenal ulcers are more common than gastric ulcers. The ulcer develops as a result of exposure to acidic gastric secretions of the stomach. The prevalence of the disease is equal in both sexes. Peptic ulcer usually responds well to drug treatment, but if left untreated can cause severe complications such as perforation of the gastrointestinal wall and even stomach cancer. See Figure 11.16 for the common sites for peptic ulcer.

Aetiology of peptic ulcers

The causes of peptic ulcers include:

- infection from *Helicobacter pylori* (Gram-negative bacteria)
- excessive consumption of alcohol and cigarette smoking
- excessive gastric section as a result of stress
- excessive use of non-steroidal anti-inflammatory drugs (NSAIDs) and aspirin derivatives
- excessive consumption of caffeine
- familial history of peptic ulcer

Investigations to confirm diagnosis

The following investigations may be carried out:

- The patient's full nursing and medical history.

- ***Gastroscopy*** and biopsy of stomach lining to detect changes as a result of *H. pylori* infection.
- **Barium swallow** may be performed to detect ulcer formation. This involves swallowing a drink containing barium, which shows up radio opaque. The barium coats the lining of the stomach and the duodenum and if an ulcer is present this is detected on the X-ray.
- Full blood analysis.

Signs and symptoms of peptic ulcer

Some patients with peptic ulcer have no symptoms. However, the following symptoms have been reported in patients with peptic ulcer:

- dyspepsia
- epigastric pain
- heart burn as a result of regurgitation of gastric secretion
- nausea and vomiting
- blood may be present in the vomit, if the ulcer bleeds
- loss of weight
- eructation (belching)

Pathophysiology of peptic ulcer

A peptic ulcer can occur as a result of excess acid secretions which can lead to destruction of the mucous membrane and decreased mucous production can leave mucosal lining unprotected. The mucous acts as a barrier for the mucosal lining of the gastrointestinal tract against acid damage. Erosion of the mucosal lining may result in the formation of a **fistula**. The fistula would allow the acidic gastric contents to leak out into the peritoneum resulting in **peritonitis** (Burkitt *et al.*, 2002). Stress, caffeine, cigarette smoking and alcohol consumption increase acid production. Medications such as NSAID and aspirin inhibit **prostaglandins** which protects mucosal lining (Hogan and Hill, 2004).

H. pylori bacterial infection leads to death of the mucosal epithelial cells of the stomach and duodenum. The bacteria release toxins and enzymes that reduce the efficiency of mucous in protecting the mucosal lining of the gastrointestinal tract. In response to the bacterial infection, the body initiates an inflammatory response which results in further destruction of the mucosal lining.

Nursing management of peptic ulcer

Identify and advise the patient to avoid risk factors associated with peptic ulcer such as stress, heavy alcohol consumption and caffeine as this increases acid production resulting in mucosal damage of the gastrointestinal tract. The patient may be taught relaxation therapy such as listening to music in order to reduce stress level. Encourage the patient to stop smoking as the nicotine in cigarettes could result in mucosal damage.

Dietary advice should be offered to the patient. Small regular meals are encouraged, approximately five small meals per day to prevent hunger pain. Spicy food should be avoided as it may cause irritation on the mucosal membrane of the stomach resulting in inflammation and epigastric pain. If necessary encourage patient to drink milk during mealtime (one glass per meal).

Avoid taking medications such as aspirin and NSAID as these drugs may inhibit the action of prostaglandins and may lead to gastrointestinal bleeding.

Pharmacological interventions for the treatment of peptic ulcer

The patient with peptic ulcer may be prescribed the following medications:

- antibiotics to treat the bacterial infection as a result of *H. pylori*
- H$_2$ antagonists such as zantac or tagamet may be prescribed
- proton pump inhibitor such as omeprazole

Ulcerative colitis

Ulcerative colitis is the chronic inflammation of the mucous membrane of the colon and the rectum. The lining becomes inflamed and ulcerated. Some possible causes of ulcerative colitis include factors such as nutrition, stress, bowel infections, genetic factors and autoimmune dysfunction (Paradiso, 1999).

Investigations to confirm diagnosis

The following investigations may be performed:

- Sigmoidoscopy or colonoscopy may be carried out to examine the mucous membrane of the colon and the rectum. The procedure involves passing a flexible scope via the rectum to examine the lining.
- A barium enema to identify bowel strictures or ulcerations.
- Stool cultures may be performed to rule out any infection.
- Full blood count to exclude anaemia and other complications from ulcerative colitis such raised white blood cell count to indicate infection.
- Plain abdominal X-ray.
- Ultrasound to identify ulcerations.

Signs and symptoms of ulcerative colitis

The following symptoms have been reported:

- severe diarrhoea
- blood, pus or mucous in the diarrhoea
- weight loss
- poor appetite
- abdominal pain
- nausea and vomiting

Pathophysiology of ulcerative colitis

Inflammatory process occurs in the mucosa and the submucosa of the rectum (**proctitis**) and spreads along the colon. The inflammation may involve the entire colon up to the junction of the ileocaecal valve. The inflammation results in swelling, oedema and bleeding and as the disease progresses ulceration develops. The ulceration spreads through the submucosa causing necrosis and sloughing of the mucous membrane (Lemone and Burke, 2004). In later stages of the disease, the walls of the colon thicken and become **fibrous**. Complications such as intestinal obstruction, iron-deficiency anaemia and electrolyte imbalance may develop.

Nursing management of ulcerative colitis

The patient with ulcerative colitis may need psychological support and counselling. Depression may be a result of the debilitating disease and the person may feel isolated. As a result of diarrhoea and bowel habits, the patient may be reluctant to engage in social activity and feel a burden to their family. The patient should be allowed to express their anxieties and worries about the disease (Russell, 1999).

Fluid intake and output must be monitored, ensure that the patient is not dehydrated. Dehydration may be a possibility as a result of the diarrhoea. Electrolyte balance needs to be monitored daily as a result of the loss of electrolytes such as sodium and potassium in the vomit and diarrhoea.

Dietary intake should be monitored. A low-residue diet should be advised to prevent irritation of the mucosal lining of the colon from the bulk formation. During the early stage of the disease, the patient may be unable to eat and therefore may need **parenteral nutrition** (Miller *et al.*, 2006) when diarrhoea is severe. The patient may need vitamin and mineral supplements in the diet. Healthy eating should be advised once the diarrhoea has settled.

Blood transfusion may be necessary if the patient is anaemic as a result of the bleeding. The nurse must ensure the safe administration of blood transfusion and be able to recognise incompatible blood transfusion reactions such as pyrexia, tachycardia and rashes.

Bowel movements should be monitored and findings recorded such as frequency, consistency and volume. The stool should be tested for blood and the findings recorded on a stool chart. Diarrhoea is an indication of the severity of the disease and it can indicate the amount of fluid and electrolytes lost.

Assist the patient in personal cleansing and dressing. Observe signs of inflammation or any bleeding around the perianal area from frequent wiping after the diarrhoea. The patient should lie in a warm bath for a soothing effect and if necessary apply soothing barrier cream to the perianal region.

Pharmacological intervention for ulcerative colitis

The following medications may be prescribed in the treatment of ulcerative colitis:

- analgesia for pain
- anti-inflammatory drugs (steroid therapy)
- anti-diarrhoeal drugs

Peritonitis

Peritonitis is the inflammation of the peritoneum which is the lining that covers the abdominal viscera. It may be caused by bacteria or through contamination of the acidic contents of the stomach as a result of perforation or from the rupture of any of the abdominal organs such as the appendix or urinary bladder. The condition can also occur postoperatively as a result of a leakage from intestinal **anastomosis**.

Signs and symptoms of peritonitis

The following signs and symptoms may be present in a patient with peritonitis:

- abdominal pain with rebound tenderness
- nausea and vomiting
- board-like rigidity of the abdomen

- **paralytic ileus**
- dehydration
- shallow respiration
- tachycardia
- hypotension

Pathophysiology of peritonitis

The peritoneum is a serous membrane that lines the organs of the peritoneum and the peritoneal cavity. When the peritoneum is infected, an inflammatory response is initiated. The surrounding tissues become oedematous with accumulation of fluid in the peritoneal cavity. The patient may become dehydrated as fluid and electrolytes are lost from systemic circulation into the peritoneal cavity.

The patient may experience severe abdominal pain as a result of the infection and inflammation of the peritoneum. The patient may develop **oliguria**, electrolyte imbalance and shock. As the inflammation worsens, septicaemia may develop resulting in multi-organ failure.

Nursing management of the patient with peritonitis

In the early stages of the disease, the patient should be on bed rest due to extreme weakness and shock. Vital signs should be monitored hourly until they are stable; any changes in the vital signs should be reported immediately in order to take prompt action.

The patient may require a nasogastric tube inserted as a result of abdominal distension and paralytic ileus. The contents of the stomach should be aspirated 2-hourly and record the amount of aspirate and the content recorded on a fluid chart.

Intravenous fluid therapy may be commenced for fluid replacement and to correct electrolyte imbalance. The nurse should ensure that the fluid is administered as per regimen and a record of fluid input and output maintained. Urine output is monitored hourly until the patient is stable. Some patients may need parenteral nutrition in the early stages of the disease as the patient may be able to take nutrients orally (Finlay, 1997).

If surgery is needed, it is the nurse's duty in the safe preparation of the patient for theatre taking into account local protocol in preparing patients for theatre. Document all care given pre- and postoperatively in accordance with Nursing and Midwifery Council on guidelines on record and record keeping (Nursing and Midwifery Council, 2005) as well as local policy and procedure.

Provide assistance in maintaining personal hygiene and inform the patient the importance of moving their limbs in bed to prevent deep vein thrombosis and to improve circulation. Observe pressure areas, for example the sacral region, for signs of redness or inflammation as it is the early sign of pressure sore (decubitus ulcer) developing.

Pharmacological interventions for peritonitis

The following medications may be prescribed for the patient with peritonitis:

- analgesia for pain
- antibiotics for bacterial infection

Conclusion

The gastrointestinal tract also referred to as the digestive system provides water, nutrients and electrolytes for bodily functions. Nutrients are extracted from food and transported throughout the body for cellular function. Any undigested food with water, bacteria and dead cells are eliminated from the body in the formed faeces. Digestive enzymes help to break down foodstuff into smaller molecules which are then absorbed along the gastrointestinal tract. This chapter has provided the reader with insight into the normal anatomy and physiology of the gastrointestinal tract and some of the disorders associated with the system. It is not the remit of this chapter to discuss all the related disorders; the reader is advised to read further.

Nurses are in the forefront in a multidisciplinary team in assisting or giving advice to patients with gastrointestinal problems. These problems could affect the patient both physically and psychologically and this may impinge on the patient's ability to perform activities of living.

Multiple choice questions

1. An adult has all of the following except:
(a) four incisors
(b) two canines
(c) two cuspids
(d) six molars

2. Which of the following is not a major region of the stomach?
(a) cardiac
(b) oesophageal
(c) fundus
(d) body

3. Which one of the following is not found in the gastric juice?
(a) hydrochloric acid
(b) lipase
(c) intrinsic factor
(d) lysozyme

4. Bile is produced in the:
(a) liver
(b) pancreas
(c) stomach
(d) gallbladder

5. What is the serous membrane of the peritoneal cavity called?
(a) peritonitis
(b) peritoneum
(c) larynx
(d) oesophagus

6. Gingivitis is inflammation of the:
(a) stomach
(b) gums
(c) tongue
(d) pancreas

7. Peptic ulcer mainly occurs in the:
(a) oesophagus and the colon
(b) small intestine and the colon

(c) stomach and the duodenum

(d) jejunum and the rectum

8. If a patient has severe untreated diarrhoea, it may result in:

(a) severe water loss and dehydration

(b) poor absorption of proteins

(c) inflammation of the colon

(d) poor absorption of lipids

9. Proctitis is inflammation of the:

(a) rectum

(b) small intestine

(c) mouth

(d) duodenum

10. Colonoscopy is carried out to examine the:

(a) oral cavity

(b) stomach

(c) uterus

(d) colon

Answers: 1.c, 2.b, 3.d, 4.a, 5.b, 6.b, 7.c, 8.a, 9.a, 10.a, 5.d.

Test your knowledge

❷ Name the components of gastric juice.

❷ List the functions of the liver.

❷ Describe chemical and mechanical digestion.

❷ Is the gallbladder essential for the digestive process? Explain your answer.

❷ List the signs and symptoms of pancreatitis.

Glossary of terms

Absorption: The taking of nutrients from the gastrointestinal tract.

Anastomosis: Surgical joining of two parts.

Barium meal: Examination of the gastrointestinal tract using a contract medium; under X-ray control.

Bile: Alkaline fluid produced by the liver.

Chyme: Semisolid substance of the stomach.

Digestion: The breakdown of food stuff.

Duct: Tube.

Dyspepsia: Feeling of epigastric discomfort.

Elimination: To get rid off.

Endocrine: A ductless gland that secrets hormones into the blood stream.

Enzymes: Proteins produced by cells that speed up chemical reaction.

Eructation: The act of bringing up air from the stomach.

Exocrine: A gland that secrets hormones into ducts which carry the secretions to other sites.

Fibrous: Containing fibrous tissue.

Fistula: An abnormal opening from one organ to another.

Fundus: The upper portion of the stomach.

Gastroscopy: Examination of the gastrointestinal tract using a flexible gastroscope.

Glycogen: Excess glucose is stored as glycogen in the liver.

Intestine: Small and large bowel.

Large intestine: Colon; large bowel.

Mastication: Chewing, tearing and grinding of food.

Nucleotides: Subunit of nucleic acid.

Oesophagus: Gullet; food pipe.

Oliguria: Diminished urine production.

Oral cavity: Mouth.

Palate: Roof of the mouth.

Paralytic ileus: Absence of peristalsis movement.

Parenteral nutrition: The administration of nutrients other than the gastrointestinal tract, for example intravenously.

Peristalsis: Involuntary movement of the gastrointestinal tract.

Peritoneum: Serous membrane that covers the abdominal cavity.

Peritonitis: Inflammation of the peritoneum.

Pharynx: The throat.

Proctitis: Inflammation of the rectum.

Prostaglandins: Unsaturated fatty acids.

Ptyalin: Digestive enzyme; also known as salivary amylase.

Pyloric region: Funnel-shaped portion of the stomach.

Small intestine: Small bowel.

Stomach: The organ that received food from the oesophagus.

Terminates: Ends.

References

Burkitt, H.G., Quick, C.R.G. and Gatt, D. (2002). *Essential Surgery: Problems, Diagnosis and Management*, 3rd edn. Edinburgh: Churchill Livingstone.

Finlay, T. (1997). Making sense of parenteral nutrition in adult patients. *Nursing Times*, *93*(2), 35–36.

Hogan, M.A. and Hill, K. (2004). *Pathophysiology: Reviews and Rationals*. New Jersey: Prentice Hall.

Kozier, B., Erb, G., Berman, A. and Snyder, S.J. (2004). *Fundamentals of Nursing*. New Jersey: Pearson Prentice Hall.

Lemone, P. and Burke, K. (2004). *Medical and Surgical Nursing – Critical Thinking in Client Care.* New Jersey: Prentice Hall.

Mader, S.S. (2005). *Understanding Human Anatomy and Physiology*, 5th edn. Boston: McGraw Hill.

Marieb, E.N. and Hoehn, K. (2007). *Human Anatomy and Physiology*, 7th edn. San Francisco: Pearson Benjamin Cummings.

Miller, M., Crawshaw, A., Logan, L. and Paterson, R. (2006). Disorders of the gastrointestinal system, liver and biliary tract. In: Alexander, M.F., Fawcett, J.N. and Runciman, P.J. (eds) *Nursing Practice: Hospital and Home – the Adult*, 3rd edn. Edinburgh: Churchill Livingstone.

Nursing and Midwifery Council (2005). *Guideline for Record and Record Keeping*. London: NMC.

Paradiso, C. (1999). *Pathophysiology*, 2nd edn. Philadelphia: Lippincott.

Russell, P. (1999). Social behaviour and professional interaction. In: Hogston, R. and Simpson, P.M. (eds) *Foundations of Nursing Practice*. London: MacMillan.

Silverthorn, D.U. (1998). *Human Physiology: An Integrated Approach*. Edgewood Cliffs, NJ: Prentice Hall.

Shier, D., Butler, J. and Lewis, R. (2004). *Holes Human Anatomy and Physiology*, 10th edn. London: McGraw Hill.

Waugh, A. and Grant, A. (2006). *Ross and Wilson: Anatomy and Physiology*. Edinburgh: Churchill Livingstone.

Wynsberghe, D.V., Noback, C.R. and Carola, R. (1995). *Human Anatomy and Physiology*, 3rd edn. New York: McGraw Hill.

Chapter 12

Nutrition and associated disorders

Muralitharan Nair

KEY WORDS

- Anabolism
- Proteins
- Triglycerides
- Micronutreients

- Catabolism
- Vitamins
- Fatty acids
- Glycogen

- Carbohydrates
- Lipid
- Macronutrients
- Gluconeogenesis

Test your prior knowledge

- List the complications of obesity and undernutrition.
- What are micro- and macronutrients?
- What is the body's main energy source?
- List all the fat-soluble vitamins.

Learning outcomes

On completion of this section, the reader will be able to:

- Discuss the roles of carbohydrates, proteins and fats.
- List the micro- and macronutrients.
- Describe the role of micro- and macronutrients.
- List some of nutritional assessment tools.

Introduction

Nutrition is a vital component for human existence. An adequate intake of **nutrients** is essential for the survival of the body systems. Nutrients such as **proteins**, **carbohydrates**, **lipids** and **vitamins**, found in foodstuff are used by the body for energy production, growth and repair. The digestive organs (see Chapter 11) play a vital role in ingestion, absorption, transportation and elimination. When individuals do not receive sufficient nutrients, their body systems do not function efficiently. Food substances can be divided into **macronutrients** and **micronutrients**.

This chapter discusses the roles of micro- and macronutrients, identifies different types of food sources and nutritional requirements of the body, and outlines government recommendations (Department of Health, 2003) with regards to nutritional intake and nutritional disorders such as obesity and undernutrition. Nutritional assessment tools and their importance in clinical practice will be discussed. Nurses play a vital role in ensuring that the nutritional needs of the patient are met. Thus in the hospital, the key responsibilities of the nurse include nutritional assessment of the patient on admission, managing mealtimes, for example, providing privacy for the patient, ensuring that they are not disturbed during mealtimes and maintaining an accurate record of the patient's nutritional intake.

Macronutrients

Macronutrients are organic compounds required in relatively large quantities for normal physiological functions of the body. 'Macro' means large; thus macronutrients are nutrients needed in large quantities. Macronutrients include:

- carbohydrates
- proteins
- lipids
- alcohol

Carbohydrate

Carbohydrate is an organic compound that contains carbon, hydrogen and oxygen molecules. It makes up the body's main source of energy and is required in large quantities. Carbohydrates are mainly found in starchy foods (such as grain and potatoes), fruits, pasta and cereals. Other sources of carbohydrates are found in vegetables, beans and nuts but in lesser quantities. One gram of carbohydrate provides approximately 4 kcal/g of energy (Green and Jackson, 2006). Calories are units of energy found in food and drinks. The body burns calories to produce energy and any excess is stored as fat. In nutrition, values are given for the actual amount of kilocalories in food but commonly known as calories.

$$1000 \text{ calories } = 1 \text{ kcl}$$

Carbohydrates are divided into three groups:

- Monosaccharides – also known as simple carbohydrate found in food sources, for example, glucose (found in fruit, sweet corn and honey), fructose (fruit sugar) and galactose (produced from lactose – sugar in milk).
- Disaccharides – are obtained from sucrose (glucose and fructose), lactose (glucose and galactose) and maltose (glucose).
- Polysaccharides – also known as complex carbohydrates are found in grains and root vegetables.

Carbohydrates are broken down and converted into glucose by the digestive enzyme amylase found in the saliva and pancreas, which the cells utilise to produce energy. An individual may consume more carbohydrate than the body requires and as a result may have an excess of glucose in the system. The excess glucose is then converted to **glycogen** or fat (Lemone and Burke, 2004). Glycogen is stored in the liver and muscle cells and fat is stored in adipose tissue.

The body's capacity to maintain blood glucose levels is achieved by a variety of hormones; the two key hormones are **insulin** and **glucagon**. Both these hormones are produced by the pancreas and secreted into the blood stream. Insulin secretion is increased after a meal has been eaten and the main function of insulin is to transport glucose into the cells for energy production. In the absence of a carbohydrate meal and when the level of blood glucose is low, glucagon stimulates the liver to convert stored glycogen into glucose (a process called **glycogenolysis**). Thus, the important role of these hormones is to regulate blood glucose levels. However, glucose can be made available by the liver from non-carbohydrate sources such as proteins and fats through a process called **gluconeogenesis** (Jenkins *et al.*, 2007).

Proteins

Protein was the first nutrient to be identified as an important part of a living cell. It is mainly composed of carbon, hydrogen and oxygen. Proteins are highly complex molecules composed of amino acids. Amino acids are simple compounds containing carbon, hydrogen, oxygen, nitrogen, some sulphur and other elements such as phosphorus, iron and cobalt (Jenkins *et al.*, 2007). Amino acids link together to form chains called peptides.

Most foods contain at least some protein. Some good sources of protein include meat, fish, eggs, nuts and seeds, pulses, soya products (tofu, soya milk and textured soya protein such as soya mince), cereals (wheat, oats, and rice), eggs and some dairy products (milk, cheese and yoghurt). Approximately, 1 g of protein yields 4 kcal/g of energy (Simpson, 1999).

Different foods contain different proteins, each with their own unique amino acid composition. The proportions of essential amino acids in foods may differ from the proportions needed by the body to make proteins. Dietary proteins with all the essential amino acids in the proportions required by the body are said to be high-quality proteins. Therefore, the proportion of each of the essential amino acids in foods containing protein determines the quality of that protein.

Proteins are essential for growth and repair. They play a crucial role in virtually all biological processes in the body. All enzymes and many of the hormones are proteins and are vital for the body's function. Muscle contraction, immune protection and the transmission of nerve impulses are all dependent on proteins. Proteins found in the skin and bone provide structural support. The body uses carbohydrate and fat for energy, but when there is excess dietary protein or inadequate dietary fat and carbohydrate, protein is used to produce energy. Excess protein may also be converted to fat and stored in adipose tissue.

One important difference between proteins, carbohydrates and lipids is that a healthy individual can exclude carbohydrate from the diet without much ill effect – lipid, maybe excluded for a short while; however, daily protein intake is vital for bodily function. The lifespan of proteins vary: some last for a few minutes while others a few months. At the end of the lifespan the protein is broken down into amino acids and these are stored and reused in protein synthesis.

Lipids

Lipid is a term generally used for fats and oils and they are insoluble in water. The dietary lipids are derived from animal (visible fat on meat) and plant sources, milk and milk products such as cream, butter, cheese and nuts (Mann and Skeaff, 2007). Approximately 97% of natural lipids are **triglycerides** which consist of **fatty acids**. The fatty acid is common to most lipids. There are three types of fatty acids: saturated fatty acids, monounsaturated fatty acids and polyunsaturated fatty acids. Bender and Bender (2003) report that 1 g of fat yields approximately 9 kcal/g and provides 40% of energy intake. Fats and oils in food are mainly in the form of triglycerides.

Lipids are essential for:

- lubrication of food to facilitate swallowing
- transportation of fat-soluble vitamins such as A, D, E and K
- **synthesis** of steroid hormones such testosterone and oestrogen
- transportation of lipid-soluble drugs such as nicotine and caffeine
- biological membranes such as cell membranes and **organelle** membranes
- energy production

Some digestion of fats begins in the stomach with the aid of the digestive enzyme gastric lipase into free fatty acids. The fat is mixed with other nutrients and is passed into the duodenum. Once the contents of the stomach reaches the duodenum, the hormone cholecytokinin is released which stimulates the release of bile from the gallbladder and pancreatic lipase. Fats are then further broken and absorbed from the gastrointestinal tract (Wardlaw *et al.*, 2004).

The absorbed lipids are transported by units called **lipoproteins** (see Figure 12.1). There are five types of lipoproteins:

- chylomicrons
- very low density lipoproteins
- intermediate density
- low density (50% cholesterol, 25% protein)
- high density (20% cholesterol, 40–45% protein)

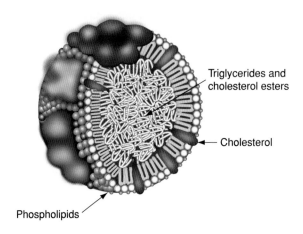

Figure 12.1 A lipoprotein.

Alcohol

Alcohol is a substance that is considered as a nutrient and a drug that affects brain function (Truswell, 2007). It also contains carbon, hydrogen and oxygen and yields approximately 7 kcal/g of energy; it has a high calorie content, which when consumed in great volume could result in obesity. Moderate intake of alcohol is associated with increased levels of high density lipoprotein which is useful in protecting the heart against heart disease. Excessive intake could result in diseases, for example, cirrhosis of the liver, stroke, heart disease, cancer of the oesophagus and other alcohol-related problems such as antisocial behaviour and road traffic accident (Peate, 2007).

Alcohol is measured in units and each unit of alcohol is equal to 8 g of pure alcohol. Department of Health (1995) recommends that men can consume 3–4 units of alcohol per day and women 2–3 units of alcohol per day.

Micronutrients

Micronutrients are organic compounds required in small quantities for the normal physiological functions of the body. They include chemical elements such as hydrogen, nitrogen and carbon, minerals and vitamins, for example, A, B group, C, D, E and K.

Vitamins

Vitamins are organic (carbon-based) substances essential for growth and cellular function. They are required in small quantities and are absorbed from the diet and altered by the body. There are two types of vitamins:

- fat-soluble
- water-soluble

Vitamins A, D, E and K are fat-soluble vitamins and they circulate in the blood stream; any excess is stored in adipose tissue and used when the levels are low in the blood stream. As these vitamins are stored, it is not essential to take these vitamins daily in the diet. In a healthy individual, fat-soluble vitamin supplements could lead to toxicity. Water-soluble vitamins B group and C circulate freely throughout the body and are not stored (except vitamins B_{12} and B_6). Excess of these vitamins is excreted in the urine and not stored in the body. Toxicity from these vitamins is less likely and the individual will need a daily intake of these vitamins in the diet. See Table 12.1 for a summary of the vitamins, food source and their functions.

Minerals

Minerals are essential nutrients for body function, for healthy teeth and bones; they function as **buffers**, components of **coenzymes** and form approximately 5% of body weight. Minerals are synthesised by the body such as vitamin D or mainly obtained from food sources. Sodium, potassium and calcium form the positive ions while sulphur and phosphorus form the negative ions. Some of these minerals are:

- calcium (Ca^2)
- iron (Fe)
- magnesium (Mg)
- phosphorus (P)
- potassium (K)
- sodium (Na)
- sulphur (S)
- zinc (Zn)

These minerals are essential for:

- strong bones and teeth
- controlling body fluids between **intracellular** and **extracellular** fluid compartments
- turning food into energy

The requirement of minerals varies – an ill person may require more minerals for body function than a healthy individual. A sick patient or a pregnant woman will require more minerals than they would normally need as a result of increased demand for body function. See Table 12.2 for a summary of the functions of minerals.

Nutritional requirements

Department of Health (1991) reports that nutritional requirements vary according to health status, activity pattern and growth. For example, an elderly person's energy requirement is not the same as a baby or a young adult. During the growth spurt period there is more demand for energy. The energy demand also depends on the activity the individual is engaged in. An athlete who is training will require more energy than a person who is not undertaking any activity and a patient recovering from surgery or illness will need more energy during the period of recovery.

Fat-soluble vitamins	Food sources	Functions
Vitamin A	In meat as retinol In vegetables as carotenoids	Good vision in dim light Growth and immunity
Vitamin D	Synthesis by ultraviolet rays of the sun. Some found in eggs, milk and fish	To maintain calcium level Normal growth, bone and teeth formation
Vitamin E	Green vegetables, eggs, nuts, whole grains and plant oils	Antioxidant Maintains immune system
Vitamin K	Found in leafy vegetables and milk	Important in blood clotting
Water-soluble vitamins	Food sources	Functions
Vitamin B_1 (thiamine)	Found in a variety of food sources such as liver, pork products, green beans, sunflower seeds and whole grain	Essential for growth and carbohydrate metabolism
Vitamin B_2 (riboflavin)	Milk, milk products, eggs and meat	Involved in citric acid cycle
Vitamin B_3 (niacin)	Tuna, peanuts, mushrooms, chicken and turkey	Involved in glycolysis
Vitamin B_6 (pyridoxine)	Liver, kidneys, meat, poultry and fish	Involved in amino acid metabolism
Biotin	Whole grain, nuts and eggs	Synthesis of nucleic acid and fatty acid
Vitamin B_5 (pantothenic acid)	Meat, milk and vegetables	Involved in glucose production from lipids and amino acids
Folate (folic acid)	Grain products, leafy vegetables and liver	Synthesis of nucleic acid
Vitamin B_{12}	Meat, poultry, seafood and eggs	Production of red blood cells
Vitamin C (ascorbic acid)	Fruits and vegetables	Synthesis of collagen, important component of tendons, blood vessels and bone

Adapted from Seeley *et al.* (2006).

Table 12.1 Summary of vitamins and their functions

Minerals	Functions
Calcium (Ca^2)	For healthy teeth and bone formation, blood clotting, nerve conduction and muscle function
Iron (Fe)	Production of red blood cells and energy production
Magnesium (mg)	Bone formation, muscle and nerve function
Phosphorus (P)	Teeth and bone formation
Potassium (K)	Muscle and nerve function
Sodium (Na)	Nerve and muscle function and maintains osmotic pressure
Sulphur (S)	Components of hormones, vitamins and proteins
Zinc (Zn)	Essential for enzyme function, carbon dioxide transport and protein metabolism
Selenium (Se)	Antioxidant properties

Adapted from Seeley *et al.* (2006).

Table 12.2 Minerals and their functions

Nutritional disorders

Learning outcomes

On completion of this section, the reader will be able to:

■ List some of the common disorders of nutrition.

■ Describe the pathophysiological processes related to nutritional disorders.

■ Outline the nursing care and interventions related to the disorders described.

Obesity

The term *obesity* is used when a person has excess amount of adipose tissue in relation to body mass and when the BMI is over 30 kg/m^2. Overweight refers to an increase in weight in relation to the individual's height and when the BMI is between 25 and 29.9 kg/m^2. The overweight may be due to an increase in adipose tissue or due to an increase in muscle mass. For example, a bodybuilder may be very lean and muscular but weigh more than others of same height. Thus, a bodybuilder may be considered as overweight as a result of an increased muscle mass but not fat.

Box 12.1 Some complications of obesity

■ Heart disease
■ Diabetes mellitus
■ Vascular disease
■ Respiratory disease
■ Hypertension
■ Bowel cancer
■ Deep vein thrombosis
■ Varicose veins
■ Cerebrovascular accident

Omari and Caterson (2007) report that obesity and overweight are very common and affect most parts of the world despite numerous health education and interventions. **Obesity** increases with age and it is much more common among the lower socioeconomic groups and the number is escalating (World Health Organization, 2003). The estimated cost of obesity to the nation is £3.3–£3.7 billion per year and of obesity plus overweight £6.6–£7.4 billion (House of Commons Health Committee, 2004). Obesity is an excessive accumulation of fat cells (adipose tissue) for an individual's height, weight, gender and ethnicity to such an extent that obesity could lead to health problems (Truswell, 2007). The fat may settle on the abdominal region (apple-shaped), hips or thighs (pear-shaped). One useful tool for calculating obesity is **body mass index** (BMI). The formula for BMI is as follows:

$$BMI = \frac{\text{weight (kg)}}{\text{height (m)}^2}$$

An individual with a BMI between 19 and 24.9 kg/m^2 is of normal weight, 25–29.9 kg/m^2 is considered overweight and people with a BMI of over 30 kg/m^2 are considered obese (Simpson, 1999). Obesity could reduce life expectancy and lead to complications (see Box 12.1).

Aetiology of obesity

Both hereditary and environmental factors have been associated with obesity which includes physiological, psychological and cultural influences (Jebb, 1997). Some of the causes include:

■ endocrine disorders such as hypothyroidism (under active thyroid) and Cushing's syndrome
■ familial history
■ depression as a result of, for example, bereavement
■ low physical activity and intake of high calorie diet
■ high consumption of alcohol
■ stress which may result in the person overeating
■ low esteem
■ steroid therapy

Signs and symptoms of obesity

Most practitioners use the BMI assessment tool to identify if a person is overweight or obese.

- BMI between 25 and 29.9 kg/m^2 is overweight
- BMI between 30 and 39.9 kg/m^2 is obese
- BMI over >40 kg/m^2 and above is extremely obese
- visible body fat accumulation on hips, waist and thighs
- increased abdominal girth
- increased weight
- waist–hip ratio

Screening tools for nutritional assessment

The following tools may be used to determine the level of obesity:

- BMI to identify excess adipose tissue but needs to be interpreted with caution as it is not a direct measure of adiposity (National Institute for Health and Clinical Excellence, 2006a)
- malnutrition universal screening tool (MUST) to determine nutritional status (Malnutrition Advisory Group, 2003)
- **anthropometry** measurements may be carried out to measure skinfold thickness
- clinical assessment of the patient
- biochemical tests are carried out to assess nutrient levels, for example protein, nitrogen and lipids

Nursing care of the patient with obesity

Patients with obesity often suffer from psychological problems such as depression, low self-esteem, social stigma and reduced mobility (Thomas, 1998). The nurse will need to be sensitive to the patient's feelings when providing care. The nurse should assist the patient to identify the cause of obesity and offer advice on preventative measures such as dieting and exercise (Alexander *et al.*, 2006).

Advice on diet and healthy eating (see Figure 12.2) should be offered as recommended by the Department of Health (British Nutrition Foundation, 2003). Food sources rich in saturated fat should be avoided and a diet low in calories and a high intake of fruits and vegetables is advocated. It has been estimated that eating at least five portions of a variety of fruit and vegetables per day could reduce the risk of death from chronic diseases such as heart disease, stroke and cancer by up to 20% (Department of Health, 2000). Encourage the patient to have their weight checked weekly and to keep a record.

The patient should be encouraged to take regular exercise for weight reduction. Unless contraindicated, British Nutrition Foundation Task Force (1999) recommends 30 minutes exercise such as walking, cycling or swimming for at least five times per week under the supervision of the practice nurse. The level of activity should be gradually increased to the level the patient can tolerate. The patient should be encouraged to participate in group activities such as Weight Watchers Club which could help them to lose weight. The aim is to ensure that energy output is greater than energy intake (see Figure 12.3) and this may be achieved through exercise and dieting. An individual may put on weight if the energy intake is more than energy expenditure.

Pharmacological interventions for the treatment of obesity

Currently, two medicines have been recommended by National Institute for Health and Clinical Excellence (2006b) and they are:

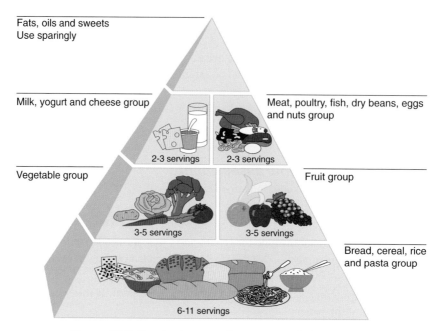

Figure 12.2 Food groups and recommended portions.

- orlistat – reduces gastrointestinal absorption of fatty acids, cholesterol and fat-soluble vitamins and increasing faecal fat elimination
- sibutramine – blocks the reuptake of serotonin and noradrenaline in the brain

These medicines are not recommended for all obese patients, only for patients with a BMI of 30 kg/m^2 and above and should be prescribed in concurrence with advice on diet, physical activity and lifestyle changes.

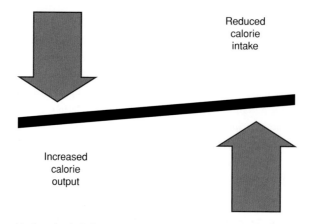

Reduced calorie intake – Increased calorie output = Weight loss

Figure 12.3 Energy balance.

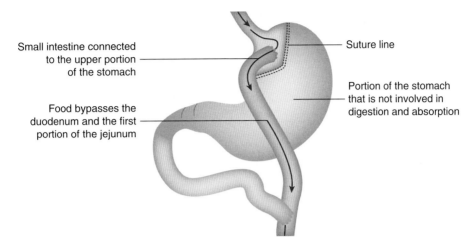

Small intestine connected to the upper portion of the stomach

Food bypasses the duodenum and the first portion of the jejunum

Suture line

Portion of the stomach that is not involved in digestion and absorption

Figure 12.4 Gastric bypass surgery.

Surgery

Surgery may be offered to some patients when dieting and exercise have not been successful in reducing their weight (Peate, 2007). Surgical procedures such as gastric bypass (Roux-en-Y connection) may be carried out to limit the quantity of food the individual can eat each time (see Figure 12.4).

Malnutrition

Malnutrition is a general term used to define undernutrition as a result of inadequate food intake, dietary imbalance or overnutrition from excess consumption of food. In clinical practice, malnutrition is regarded as undernutrition and overnutrition.

Undernutrition refers to the inability to meet the body's need for nutrition and energy. It could result from low intake of nutrients, high calorie demand of the body and poor absorption of nutrients from the gastrointestinal tract, for example as a result of stomach cancer. Undernutrition can be detrimental to health and if untreated could result in severe complications such as infection, severe weight loss, multisystem failure (see Box 12.2) and death.

Carbohydrates and fats are the main energy source of the body. When dietary intake is not sufficient to meet the energy requirements of the body, stored glycogen, body protein and fats are used to produce energy (Lemone and Burke, 2004). In a severe state of undernutrition, the body uses fat reserve and converts it into fatty acid and **ketones** which provide energy for the brain. As the disease process progresses, body mass is reduced and there is a reduction in energy expenditure. Alexander *et al.* (2006) report that undernutrition is often associated with patients and identified several possible factors:

■ stress as a result of hospital admission
■ pain as a result of surgery or chronic disease may reduce appetite
■ presentation and the taste of hospital food may not be to the patient's taste
■ unfamiliar environment
■ hospital meal times may not be suitable for the patient

Box 12.2 Some complications of undernutrition

- Tremors
- Impaired coordination
- Drowsiness
- Cardiovascular problems, for example enlarged heart
- Amenorrhoea
- Hypotension
- Constipation
- Muscle wasting
- Enlarged liver
- Susceptible to infection
- Low basal metabolic rate
- Severe weight loss

Signs and symptoms of undernutrition

- BMI between 17 and 18.5 kg/m^2 – mild undernutrition
- BMI between 16 and 17 kg/m^2 – moderate undernutrition
- BMI less than 16 kg/m^2 severe malnutrition
- severe muscle wasting
- wrinkled skin observed in patients with **marasmus**
- distended abdomen observed in patients with **kwashiorkor**
- swollen ankles observed in patients with kwashiorkor

Aetiology of undernutrition

Causes of undernutrition include:

- elderly people living on their own
- socioeconomic factors, for example poverty, isolation
- patients who suffer from osteo and rheumatoid arthritis
- unconscious patients
- chronic disease such as cardiovascular and renal disease
- ill fitting dentures and periodontal disease
- stomatitis or candida
- loss of appetite, for example, as a result of chemotherapy treatment and excessive alcohol consumption

Screening tools

- clinical assessment of the patient
- MUST to determine nutritional status (Malnutrition Advisory Group, 2003)
- body mass index
- anthropometry measurements

Nursing care of the patient with undernutrition

Prior to planning care, a full nursing assessment of the patient should be undertaken which should include a physical assessment, nutritional assessment, past nursing and medical history and any problems the patient may present with that could result in undernutrition. Nursing assessment may include the following:

- changes in dietary habit
- physiological problems such as swallowing difficulties that may have an effect on nutritional intake
- psychological problems, for example depression as a result of bereavement
- socioeconomic factors such as lack of finance that may affect purchasing and cooking of food
- cultural and religious beliefs of the patient

With the patient's consent the information gathered may be shared between the nurse and the other members of the MDT including the dietitian in order to plan optimum care.

The patient should be encouraged to keep a food diary of the quantity of food and fluids consumed each day. Weigh the patient daily (same time and wearing the same clothing) to ensure that the patient is gaining weight. The weight should be recorded and documented. Offer advice on the type of food to purchase that is nutritious and healthy. When giving advice, the nurse needs to consider the patient's preferences and their cultural and religious beliefs. If necessary information on oral supplements, for example, ensure plus should be offered; it is the nurse's role to ensure that the patients take the supplement as prescribed. For patients who may find these drinks unacceptable due to high milk content, they may prefer fruit-flavoured supplements such as Enlive or Fortijuice (MeReC Bulletin, 1998). The dietitian will be able to give advice on the appropriate supplement for the patient to take. Advice on supplements should be offered in accordance with the National Institute for Health and Clinical Excellence (2006c) recommendations and guidelines on nutritional support in adults.

Encourage the patient to take at least 180 mL of water every hour to prevent dehydration and infection – fluid is essential for effective body function. Educate the patient about the importance of taking adequate fluid. Maintain an input and output chart and ensure that all care givers are aware of the importance of maintaining an accurate fluid balance chart. Any significant changes in fluid balance should be reported immediately for prompt action, for example commencement of an intravenous infusion if the patient is dehydrated. Conversely, excessive fluid overload could result in heart or kidney failure.

When presenting food to the patient, the nurse needs to ensure that it is presented in an attractive manner as poorly presented food can be unappetising and the patient may refuse to eat the food. The quantity of food offered each mealtime should be related to the amount the patient can consume. Large portions of food should be avoided as it may be unattractive and unappetising for the patient. Mealtimes should be planned with the patient's relatives in order to make eating a pleasurable and social activity. It is the role of the nurse to ensure that the nutritional needs of the patient are met as recommended in Essence of Care (Department of Health, 2003).

The nurse needs to be aware that elderly patients who are on bed rest as a result of ill health are prone to developing complications such as decubitus ulcers (pressure ulcers), chest infection or urinary tract infection. Good nutrition is essential for growth and tissue repair. In the undernourished patient, loss of muscle mass and adipose tissue increases the risk of developing pressure ulcers and the most affected areas are the ankle, shoulder blades, sacrum and the elbows. Observe the pressure areas every 2 hours

Box 12.3 Some indications for enteral feeding

- Following major surgery such as **gastrectomy**
- Oesophageal stricture
- Carcinoma of the oesophagus
- Carcinoma of the mouth
- Coma following head injury
- Gastrointestinal **fistula**
- **Dysphagia** following cerebrovascular accident
- Patients who are confused and reluctant to eat
- Severe burns
- Inflammatory bowel disease

Adapted from Alexander *et al.* (2006).

for early signs of pressure ulcer developing, for example inflammation that is and to take appropriate action such as re-positioning the patient (Peate, 2005). The nurse will need to adhere to local policies and guidelines in the prevention of pressure ulcers.

Encourage passive and active movements of limbs in bed to improve circulation and prevention of complications such as deep vein thrombosis and infection. Deep breathing exercises should be encouraged to prevent complications such as chest infection should be encouraged.

Enteral nutrition

To facilitate **enteral** nutrition, a tube is inserted directly into the gastrointestinal tract and the patient is fed a liquid diet through the tube. Enteral feeding is used to supplement oral intake or if the patient is unable to take nutrition orally (see Box 12.3). Say (2005) reports that there are three types of enteral feeding:

- Nasogastric (NG) tube feeding involves the insertion of a nasogastric tube via the nasopharynx into the stomach. This procedure is normally carried out by a registered nurse or medical staff.
- Nasojejunal (NJ) tube feeding involves the insertion of a tube via the nasopharynx and the stomach into the jejunum. Insertion of the NJ tube is carried out by medical staff using endoscopy and is confirmed in place radiologically.
- Percutaneous endoscopic gastrostomy (PEG) or jejunostomy (PEJ) involves the insertion of a tube into the stomach through the abdominal wall. This procedure is carried out by the medical staff surgically.

Nursing care of the patient with enteral feeding

Nurses should ensure that patients receiving enteral feeding are monitored regularly for complications, for example breathlessness and abdominal distension, and their viral signs recorded every 2 hours. They should ensure that the enteral feeding tube is correctly positioned before commencing each feed. Nurses should adhere to local policies, guidelines and the National Institute for Health and Clinical Excellence (2006c) recommendations in the management and care of the patient with enteral feeding.

Nurses need to ensure that the patient who is receiving an enteral feed will need full nursing care such as oral and nasal hygiene, washing hands before administering the feed and documenting all the care given as per NMC guidelines (Nursing and Midwifery Council, 2005).

Parenteral nutrition

Parenteral nutrition is the direct infusion of a solution into a vein when the patient cannot be nourished with oral or enteral feeding. The solution contains all essential nutritional requirements (macro- and micronutrients) for the body including fluid replacement. It is a specialised method of feeding which requires specialist nursing care. The patient receiving parenteral nutrition in the community will need coordinated support from the district nurse, specialist nutrition nurse, dietitian, pharmacist and the GP (National Institute for Health and Clinical Excellence, 2006c). The patient receiving parenteral nutrition is at risk of developing complications such infection, fluid overload, heart failure, electrolyte imbalance, respiratory and renal complications. It is not the remit of this chapter to include this specialist care. Further in-depth discussion regarding the special care of patients receiving parenteral nutrition can be found elsewhere, for example Dougherty and Lister (2004).

Conclusion

Nutrition plays a vital role in body function and maintaining homeostasis. Nutrients are classified as macro- and micronutrients. The macronutrients include carbohydrates, proteins and fats, while micronutrients are vitamins and minerals. These nutrients are primarily obtained from the diet and are absorbed from the gastrointestinal tract after digestion. Macronutrients are primarily for energy production whilst micronutrients promote growth and development.

Obesity and undernutrition are two major global and national concerns (Wardlaw et al., 2004). In the UK, the estimated cost of obesity and nutrition is approximately £6.6–£7.4 billion pounds per year. Obesity is both a medical condition and a lifestyle disorder. Undernutrition is becoming increasingly prevalent as the elderly population is increasing. Some elderly people and children are more prone to undernutrition as a result of illness or due to socioeconomic factors.

The role of the nurse is varied as regards to nutritional care. The responsibilities include preventing undernutrition in patients and offering health education and support relating to obesity and undernutrition. It is the nurse's responsibility to prevent and highlight nutritional problems and to take prompt action to prevent complications such as heart failure, renal disease, constipation and even death.

Multiple choice questions

1. Macronutrients are composed of:
(a) fats, carbohydrates and proteins
(b) fats, vitamins and proteins
(c) proteins, carbohydrates and minerals
(d) proteins, carbohydrates and vitamins

2. Micronutrients are composed of:
(a) carbohydrates, fats and minerals
(b) vitamins and proteins
(c) vitamins and minerals
(d) minerals and fats

3. Gluconeogenesis is:
(a) glucose obtained from vitamins
(b) glucose obtained from non-carbohydrate sources
(c) glucose obtained from fruits
(d) glucose obtained from vegetables

4. Glycogenolysis is the conversion of:
(a) proteins to triglycerides
(b) carbohydrates to glucose by insulin
(c) protein to glucose
(d) stored glycogen to glucose

5. Lipoproteins are transport units for:
(a) carbohydrates
(b) proteins
(c) glucose
(d) lipids

6. Fat-soluble vitamins are:
(a) A, D, E and K
(b) B groups and folate
(c) Vitamin C and folate
(d) Vitamin C and folate

7. A patient with a BMI 25–30 kg/m^2 is:
(a) of normal weight
(b) overweight

(c) obese

(d) underweight

8. Marasmus is:

(a) malnutrition as a result of vitamin deficiency

(b) malnutrition as a result of fat deficiency

(c) malnutrition as a result of protein and carbohydrate deficiency

(d) malnutrition as a result of mineral deficiency

9. The main energy source of the body are:

(a) vitamins and minerals

(b) proteins and fats

(c) carbohydrates and vitamins

(d) carbohydrates and fats

10. Enteral feeding is used:

(a) in patients who have not teeth

(b) in patients who are obese

(c) to administer medication if the patients refuse to take the medication

(d) to supplement oral intake

Answers: 1.a, 2.c, 3.b, 4.d, 5.d, 6.a, 7.b, 8.c, 9.d, 10.d.

Test your knowledge

❖ Explain the roles of carbohydrate, protein and fats.

❖ Explain the terms macro- and micronutrients.

❖ List the fat-soluble vitamins and describe their functions.

❖ List the possible causes of obesity and undernutrition.

❖ How are lipids transported in the body?

Glossary of terms

Anthropometry: Assessment tool used to measure skinfolds.

Body mass index: Tool for calculating body mass.

Buffer: A chemical substance which will allow a slight change in pH when acid or base is added to the solution.

Carbohydrates: Organic compounds such as starch and sugar that make up body's main source of energy.

Coenzyme: A molecule that binds to an enzyme and is essential for its activity, but is not permanently altered by the reaction.

Dysphagia: Difficulty in swallowing.

Enteral: Through the gastrointestinal tract.

Extracellular: Outside the cell.

Fatty acids: Composed of carbon chemically bonded together.

Fistula: An abnormal opening from one organ to another.

Gastrectomy: Removal of the stomach surgically.

Glucagon: Hormone produced by the pancreas.

Gluconeogenesis: Production of glucose from non-carbohydrate sources.

Glycogen: Formed from glucose and mainly stored in the liver.

Glycogenolysis: Conversion of glycogen into glucose.

Intracellular: Inside the cell.

Ketones: Products of fat metabolism.

Kwashiorkor: Protein-deficiency malnutrition.

Lipids: Energy-rich organic compounds essential for cell structure and function.

Lipoproteins: Transport units for lipids with proteins.

Macronutrients: Nutrients that provide energy.

Marasmus: Protein- and carbohydrate-deficiency malnutrition.

Micronutrients: Vitamins and minerals.

Nutrients: Chemical components of foods.

Obesity: Excess of body fat.

Organelles: Small proteins found inside the cell.

Proteins: Organic nitrogenous compounds essential as building material for growth and repair.

Synthesis: Production.

Triglycerides: Major form of lipids in the body.

Undernutrition: Failing health as a result of inadequate nutrient.

Vitamins: Organic compounds essential for physiological functions of the body.

References

Alexander, M.F., Fawcett, J.N. and Runciman, P.J. (2006). *Nursing Practice: Hospital and Home – the Adult*, 3rd edn. Edinburgh: Churchill Livingstone.

Bender, D.A. and Bender, A.E. (2003). *Nutrition: A Reference Handbook*. Oxford: Oxford University Press.

British Nutrition Foundation (2003). Health eating: A whole diet approach. In: Alexander, M.F., Fawcett, J.N. and Runciman, P.J. (eds) *Nursing Practice: Hospital and Home – the Adult*. Edinburgh: Churchill Livingstone.

British Nutrition Foundation Task Force (1999). Obesity. In: Alexander, M.F., Fawcett, J.N. and Runciman, P.J. (eds) *Nursing Practice: Hospital and Home – the Adult*. Edinburgh: Churchill Livingstone.

Department of Health (1991). *Dietary Reference Values for Food Energy and Nutrients for the United Kingdom*. Report of the Panel on Dietary Reference Values of the Committee on Medical Aspects of Food Policy. London: HMSO.

Department of Health (1995). *Sensible Drinking: The Report of an Inter-Department Working Group*. London: HMSO.

Department of Health (2000). *The NHS Plan*. London: Department of Health.

Department of Health (2003). *The Essence of Care: Patient-Focused Benchmarks for Clinical Governance*. London: The Stationary Office.

Dougherty, L. and Lister, S. (2004). *The Royal Marsden Hospital Manual of Clinical Nursing Procedures*. Oxford: Blackwell Science.

Green, S. and Jackson, P. (2006) Nutrition. In: Alexander, M.F., Fawcett, J.N. and Runciman, P.J. (eds) *Nursing Practice: Hospital and Home – the Adult*, 3rd edn. Edinburgh: Churchill Livingstone.

House of Commons Health Committee (2004). *Obesity. Third Report of Session 2003–04*, Vol. 1. London: The Stationary Office.

Jebb, S.A. (1997). Aetiology of obesity. *British Medical Bulletin*, 53(2), 264–285.

Jenkins, G.W., Kemnitz, C.P. and Tortora, G.J. (2007). *Anatomy and Physiology from Science of Life*. New Jersey: John Wiley and Sons.

Lemone, P. and Burke, K. (2004). *Medical and Surgical Nursing: Critical Thinking in Client Care*. New Jersey: Prentice Hall.

Malnutrition Advisory Group (2003). *The MUST Report. Nutritional Screening of Adults: A Multidisciplinary Responsibility*. London: British Association for Parenteral and Enteral Nutrition.

Mann, J. and Skeaff, M. (2007). Lipids. In: Mann, J. and Truswell, A.S. (eds) *Essentials of Human Nutrition*, 3rd edn. Oxford: Oxford University Press.

MeReC Bulletin (1998). Oral nutritional support (Part 2): Nutritional supplements. *MeReC Bulletin*, 9, 33–36.

National Institute for Health and Clinical Excellence (2006a). *Obesity: Guidance on the Prevention, Identification, Assessment and Management of Overweight and Obesity in Adults and Children*. London: NICE.

National Institute for Health and Clinical Excellence (2006b). *Treatment for People Who Are Overweight or Obese*. London: NICE.

National Institute for Health and Clinical Excellence (2006c). *Nutrition Support in Adults – Nutrition Support in Adults: Oral Nutrition Support, Enteral Tube Feeding Parenteral Nutrition*. Clinical Guideline 32. London: NICE.

Nursing and Midwifery Council (2005). *Guidelines for Record and Record Keeping*. London: NMC.

Omari, A. and Caterson, I.D. (2007). Overweight and obesity. In: Mann, J. and Truswell, A.S. (eds) *Essentials of Human Nutrition*, 3rd edn. Oxford: Oxford University Press.

Peate, I. (2005). Mobility and movement. In: Peate, I. (ed) *Compendium of Clinical Skills for Student Nurses*. London: Whurr Publication.

Peate, I. (2007). *Men's Health – the Practice Nurse's Handbook*. Chichester: John Wiley and Sons.

Say, J. (2005). Eating and drinking: Nutrient and fluid replacement for health. In: Peate, I. (ed) *Compendium of Clinical Skills for Student Nurses*. London: Whurr Publication.

Seeley, R.R., Stephens, T.D. and Tate, P. (2006). *Anatomy and Physiology*, 7th edn. Boston: McGraw Hill.

Simpson, P.M. (1999). Eating and drinking. In: Hogston, R. and Simpson, P.M. (eds) *Foundation of Nursing Practice*. London: McMillian.

Thomas, D. (1998). Managing obesity: The nutritional aspects. *Nursing Standard*, 12(18), 49–55.

Truswell, S. (2007). Alcohol. In: Mann, J. and Truswell, A.S. (eds) *Essentials of Human Nutrition*, 3rd edn. Oxford: Oxford University Press.

Wardlaw, G.M., Hampl, J.S. and DiSilvestro, R.A. (2004). *Perspectives in Nutrition*, 6th edn. Boston: McGraw Hill.

World Health Organization (2003). *Nutrition. Controlling the Global Obesity Epidemic*. Geneva: WHO.

Chapter 13

The endocrine system and associated disorders

Carl Clare

KEY WORDS

- Hormones
- Homeostasis
- Receptors
- Up-regulation
- Down-regulation
- Negative Feedback
- Hypothalamus
- Calorigenic effect
- Glucagon
- Corticosteroids
- Hyposecretion
- Hypersecretion

Test your prior knowledge

- Name one organ of the endocrine system and one hormone it releases.
- What is the treatment for hypothyroidism?
- Name the two major types of diabetes.

Introduction

The endocrine system is the name given to a collection of small organs that are scattered throughout the body, each of which releases hormones (Marieb and Hoehn, 2007). **Hormones** are chemical substances that are released into the blood, by the endocrine system, and have a physiological control over the function of cells or organs other than those that created them (Guyton and Hall, 2006). The purpose of each hormone varies but the primary role of most hormones is to maintain **homeostasis** (that is keeping a normal physiological balance in the body). Endocrine-releasing organs can be split into three main categories (Marieb and Hoehn, 2007):

■ **Endocrine glands** – these are organs whose sole function is the production and release of hormones. The pituitary, thyroid, parathyroid and adrenal glands are all examples of this category.
■ Organs that are not pure glands but contain relatively large areas of hormone-producing tissue – examples of these are the pancreas, the hypothalamus and the gonads.
■ Other tissues and organs also produce hormones – areas of hormone-producing cells are found in the wall of the small intestine, the stomach, the kidneys and the heart.

The organs and their position in the body can be seen in Figure 13.1. Each of these organs will typically have a rich vascular (blood vessel) network and the hormone-producing cells within them are arranged into cords and branching networks around this supply (Marieb and Hoehn, 2007). This arrangement of blood vessels and hormone-producing cells ensures that hormones enter into the blood rapidly and are then transported throughout the body.

Hormones

There are a great number of hormones produced by the endocrine system and they each have very different effects and affect different cells and organs in the body. The major bodily processes that hormones influence or regulate are reproduction, growth and development, mobilising the bodies'

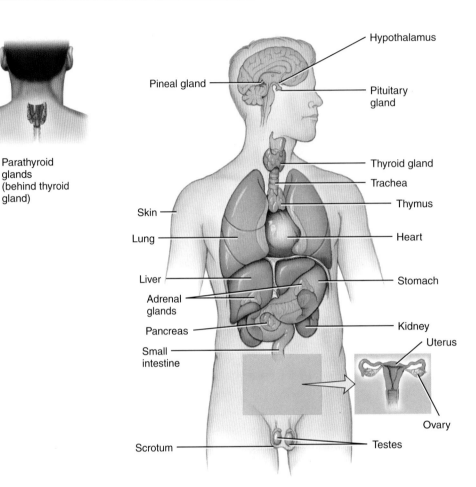

Figure 13.1 Position of the endocrine glands.

defence mechanisms against stressors, maintaining normal levels of electrolytes, water and nutrients in the body, and the regulation of cellular metabolism and energy (Marieb and Hoehn, 2007). Hormones are generally made from either **amino acids** (most) or cholesterol (the **steroid hormones**). As hormones are released into the blood stream they are carried throughout the body but they do not affect all cells. In order for a hormone to have an effect on a cell the cell must have **receptors** for that particular hormone. Cells that have receptors for a particular hormone are known as the **target cells** for that hormone (Guyton and Hall, 2006). Some hormones are very specific and thus receptors are only found on specific cells (for instance, adrenocorticotropic hormone), whereas thyroid hormone affects nearly every cell in the body.

Receptors for a hormone are proteins that are sited either on the cell wall or inside the cell. The exact location of a receptor depends on the type of hormone that the receptor is for (Marieb and Hoehn, 2007). Amino acid-based hormones cannot cross the cell membrane and therefore their receptors are found on the cell wall; activation of these receptors leads to the activation of secondary messenger systems within the cell. The steroid hormones can cross the cell membrane because they are small and lipid-soluble and thus their receptors are found within the cell itself. One exception is thyroid hormone, which is very small and can diffuse easily across the cell membrane into the cell (Marieb and Hoehn, 2007).

The activation of a target cell depends on the blood levels of the hormone, the number of receptors on the cell and the affinity of the receptor for the hormone. Changes in all three of these factors can happen relatively quickly in response to a change in stimuli. Changes in the number of receptors are known as up-regulation and down-regulation (Guyton and Hall, 2006).

- **Up-regulation** is the creation of more receptors in response to high circulating levels of a hormone. Thus, the cell becomes more responsive to the presence of the hormone in the blood.
- **Down-regulation** is the reduction in the number of receptors and is often caused by the exposure of a cell to prolonged periods of high circulating levels of a hormone. Thus, the cell becomes less responsive (desensitised) to a hormone which protects the cell from over-responding to continued high levels of that hormone.

Hormones can have a very powerful effect even at low concentrations and thus it is essential that the released hormones are disposed of efficiently. Some hormones are rapidly broken down within their target cells; most are inactivated by the liver or the kidneys and then excreted in the urine, but small amounts are excreted in the faeces (Guyton and Hall, 2006).

The control of hormone release

The creation and release of most hormones is commenced by an external or internal **stimulus**; further creation and release is then regulated by a **negative feedback system** (Figure 13.2). Thus, the influence of a stimulus, from inside or outside the body, leads to hormone release; following this some aspect of the target organ function then inhibits further reaction to the stimulus and thus further release of the hormone by the organ.

An example of a negative feedback system is the release of insulin by the pancreas. Insulin is released by the pancreas in response to rising levels of glucose, amino acids or fatty acids in the blood. The effect of insulin is to reduce these levels, thus reducing the stimulus for further insulin release.

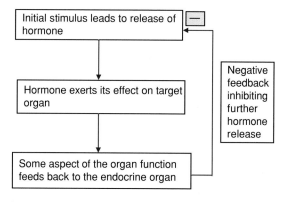

Figure 13.2 Control of hormone release by the negative feedback system.

The initial stimulus for the release of a hormone is usually one of three types, although some organs respond to multiple stimuli (Marieb and Hoehn, 2007).

Humoral

A response to changing levels of certain ions and nutrients in the blood. For instance, the release of parathyroid hormone is stimulated by falling blood levels of calcium ions.

Neural

A response to direct nervous stimulation. Only a few endocrine organs are directly stimulated by the nervous system. Increased activity in the sympathetic nervous system directly stimulates the release of catecholamines (adrenaline and noradrenaline) from the adrenal medulla.

Hormonal

A response to hormones released by other organs. Hormones that are released in response to hormonal stimuli are usually rhythmical in their release (that is the levels rise and fall in a specific pattern). Many of the hormones released from the anterior pituitary gland are released in response to releasing and inhibiting hormones from the hypothalamus.

Summary

- ■ **Hormones** are chemicals that are released into the blood stream.
- ■ Hormones are released by **glands** and other organs.
- ■ A hormone's effect on its **target cell** is through **receptors**, which are found in the cell wall or contained in the cell itself.
- ■ The stimulus for a hormone's release can be changing levels of **ions** or nutrients in the blood, direct stimulation by the nervous system or in response to other hormones.
- ■ Further control of hormone release is regulated by a **negative feedback** system.

The physiology of the endocrine glands

The hypothalamus and the pituitary gland

The pituitary gland is a pure endocrine gland that is located in the brain just below the hypothalamus. It is about the size and shape of a pea on a stalk. The pituitary stalk (**infundibulum**) connects the pituitary gland to the **hypothalamus** and contains both nerve fibres and blood vessels (Figure 13.3). The direct link between the hypothalamus and the pituitary gland is essential as it allows direct hypothalamic control of the release of the pituitary hormones.

Anatomically, the pituitary gland is split into two sections (Marieb and Hoehn, 2007). The posterior lobe (the **neurohypophysis**) is mostly made up of nerve fibres and nerve endings that have their origin in the hypothalamus; it stores two hormones that are created in the **hypothalamus** and are then transported down the nerve fibres in the stalk (the **hypothalamic–hypophyseal tract**) and stored in the nerve endings (Marieb and Hoehn, 2007). The anterior pituitary gland (the **adenohypophysis**) consists of glandular tissues. Whilst the anterior pituitary gland receives no direct neural link from the hypothalamus it does

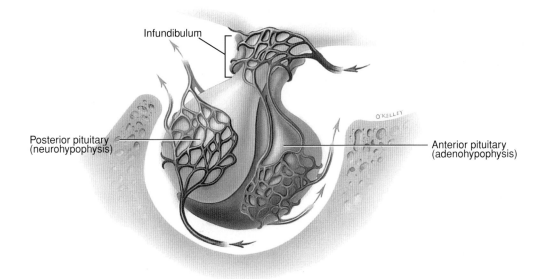

Figure 13.3 The pituitary gland.

receive its blood supply directly from the hypothalamus through the **pituitary portal system**. This blood supply is an essential component in the control of the release of hormones from the anterior pituitary gland as it transports inhibiting and releasing hormones created by the hypothalamus to the anterior pituitary gland (Table 13.1).

Growth hormone (somatotropin) stimulates most body cells to increase in size and divide; however, its major targets are the bones and skeletal muscle. Growth hormone also has several other effects including increasing the cellular uptake of amino acids to be used in the building of proteins. The secretion of growth hormone is regulated by two hypothalamic hormones: **growth hormone-releasing hormone** (GHRH) and **growth hormone-inhibiting hormone** (GHIH). It is usually released in a diurnal cycle (related to the pattern of day and night) and is found at its highest level about an hour after the onset of sleep.

Thyroid-stimulating hormone (TSH or thyrotropin) is released from the anterior pituitary gland in response to exposure of the gland to **thyrotropin-releasing hormone** (TRH) from the hypothalamus. The effect of TSH is to stimulate activity in the thyroid gland. The release of TSH is regulated by the exposure of the anterior pituitary gland to TRH and the blood levels of thyroid hormones.

Adrenocorticotropic hormone (ACTH or corticotropin) stimulates the cortex of each adrenal gland to release **corticosteroid** hormones. The release of ACTH usually follows a diurnal rhythm with the peak being in the morning just after rising (Marieb and Hoehn, 2007). The release of ACTH is stimulated by corticotropin releasing hormone (CRH) from the hypothalamus; however, other triggers for release include fever, trauma and other stressors (Marieb and Hoehn, 2007).

The **gonadotropins** is the collective name for **follicle-stimulating hormone** (FSH) and **luteinising hormone** (LH) (Marieb and Hoehn, 2007). The release of both hormones is regulated by the secretion of **gonadotropin-releasing hormone** from the hypothalamus. In the adult, FSH stimulates the production

Hypothalamus	Anterior pituitary gland	Target organ or tissues
Growth hormone releasing factor	Growth hormone	Many
Growth hormone release inhibiting factor	Growth hormone (inhibits release)	Many
Thyroid-releasing hormone	Thyroid-stimulating hormone	Thyroid gland
Corticotropin-releasing hormone	Adrenocorticotropic hormone	Adrenal cortex
Prolactin-releasing hormone	Prolactin	Breasts
Prolactin-inhibiting hormone	Prolactin (inhibits release)	Breasts
Gonadotropin-releasing hormone	Follicle-stimulating hormone Luteinising hormone	Gonads

Table 13.1 The hormones of the hypothalamus and the anterior pituitary gland

of gametes (sperm or egg) and in females it regulates ovulation in conjunction with LH. Luteinising hormone promotes the production of gonadal hormones in both males and females (Marieb and Hoehn, 2007).

Prolactin stimulates milk production in the breasts and is controlled by releasing and inhibiting hormones produced by the hypothalamus. Prolactin-inhibiting hormone is produced in high levels in men, whereas in women the production of the releasing and inhibiting hormones varies depending on the amount of oestrogen in the blood.

Two hormones are released from the posterior pituitary gland: **oxytocin** and **antidiuretic hormone** (ADH). Oxytocin has an effect on uterine contraction in childbirth and is responsible for the 'let down' response in breastfeeding mothers (the release of milk in response to suckling). In men and non-pregnant women, it plays a role in sexual arousal and orgasm (Marieb and Hoehn, 2007).

The primary role of ADH (vasopressin) is to prevent wide swings in the water balance of the body. Osmoreceptors in the hypothalamus monitor the concentration of dissolved ions in the blood (and therefore water levels). An increase in the concentration of dissolved ions leads to an increase in ADH release from the posterior pituitary gland. The main target of ADH is the renal tubules in the kidneys causing them to increase the amount of reabsorption of water from the urine and back into the blood (thus decreasing urine output and increasing blood volume). A decrease in blood pressure also stimulates ADH release.

The thyroid gland

The thyroid gland is a butterfly-shaped gland located in the front of the neck on the trachea just below the larynx (Marieb and Hoehn, 2007). The thyroid gland is made up of hollow, spherical, follicles which contain thyroglobulin molecules with attached iodine molecules (Marieb and Hoehn, 2007); the thyroid hormone is created from this. One unique factor of the thyroid gland is its ability to create and store large amounts hormone; this can be up to 100 days of hormone supply (Guyton and Hall, 2006). The thyroid gland releases two forms of **thyroid hormone**: thyroxine (T_4) and triiodothyronine (T_3), both of which require iodine for their creation. However, T_4 is the primary hormone released by the thyroid gland; this is then converted into T_3 by the target cells (Marieb and Hoehn, 2007).

Thyroid hormone affects virtually every cell in the body, except the adult brain, the spleen, the testes, the uterus and the thyroid gland itself (Marieb and Hoehn, 2007). In the target cells, thyroid hormone stimulates enzymes that are involved with glucose oxidation. This is the **calorigenic effect** and its overall effects are an increase in basal metabolic rate, an increase in oxygen consumption and an increase in the production of body heat. Thyroid hormone also has an important role in the maintenance of blood pressure as it stimulates an increase in the number of receptors in the walls of blood vessels (Marieb and Hoehn, 2007).

The control of the release of thyroid hormone is mediated by a negative feedback system which involves the hypothalamus and cascades through the pituitary gland (Figure 13.4).

Increased levels of T_4 in the blood inhibit the release of TRH from the hypothalamus, thus reducing the stimulation for the release of TSH from the anterior pituitary gland. The effect of TSH on the thyroid gland is to promote the release of thyroid hormone into the blood; therefore, a reduction in TSH reduces the release of T_3 and T_4. A reduced level of T_4 in the blood reduces the negative feedback and thus there is an increase in the release of TRH which leads to an increase in thyroid gland function. Conditions that increase the energy requirements of the body (such as pregnancy or prolonged cold) also stimulate the release of TRH from the hypothalamus and therefore lead to an increase in blood levels of thyroid hormone. In these situations, the stimulating conditions override the normal negative feedback system (Marieb and Hoehn, 2007).

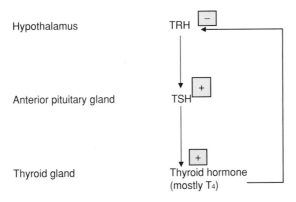

Figure 13.4 The negative feedback control of thyroid hormone production.

The parathyroid glands

The **parathyroid glands** are tiny glands normally located on the back (posterior) of the thyroid gland. There are usually two pairs of glands, but the precise number varies and some patients have been reported to have up to four pairs (Marieb and Hoehn, 2007). The parathyroid glands release **parathyroid hormone** (PTH) which is the single most important hormone for the control of the calcium balance in the body (Marieb and Hoehn, 2007). Physiologically, calcium is important in the transmission of nerve impulses, is involved in the muscle contraction and is also required in the creation of clotting factors in the blood.

The release of PTH by the glands is controlled by the blood levels of calcium; a reduced calcium level stimulates the release of PTH and an increased calcium level inhibits its release. PTH increases blood levels of calcium by its action on three target areas in the body (Marieb and Hoehn, 2007):

- **Bones** – PTH stimulates the activity of **osteoclasts** to digest some of the bone and release calcium into the blood.
- **Kidneys** – PTH increases reabsorption of calcium.
- **Intestines** – PTH increases the absorption of calcium in the intestines by activating vitamin D (which is required for the absorption of calcium in the gut).

The adrenal glands

The adrenal glands are two pyramid-shaped glands that lie on top of each of the kidneys (Marieb and Hoehn, 2007). Each of the adrenal glands is structurally and functionally two glands in one. The inner core of each of the adrenal glands is called the **adrenal medulla**; this is surrounded by the much larger **adrenal cortex** (Figure 13.5). Both the medulla and the cortex secrete different hormones and respond to different stimuli.

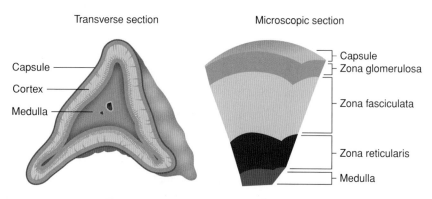

Figure 13.5 Anatomy of an adrenal gland.

The adrenal medulla

The adrenal medulla secretes adrenaline and (to a lesser extent) noradrenaline in response to stimulation by the sympathetic nervous system. Although adrenaline and noradrenaline are essential for normal bodily functioning, the role of the adrenaline and the noradrenaline secreted by the adrenal medulla is not essential and serves only to intensify the effects of sympathetic nervous stimulation (Marieb and Hoehn, 2007).

The adrenal cortex

The adrenal cortex is functionally separated into three different zones (Figure 13.5), each of which creates at least one steroid hormone (hormones made from cholesterol known collectively as the **corticosteroids**):

- **zona glomerulosa** – produces the **mineralocorticoids**
- **zona fasciculata** – produces the **glucocorticoids**
- **zona reticularis** – this zone is also involved in the production of **glucocorticoids** but also produces small amounts of adrenal sex hormones (the **gonadocorticoids**)

(Marieb and Hoehn, 2007).

Mineralocorticoids are hormones whose primary function is the regulation of **electrolyte** concentrations (especially potassium and sodium) in the blood. Several mineralocorticoid hormones are known; however, **aldosterone** is the most potent and accounts for 95% of all the mineralocorticoid hormones secreted (Marieb and Hoehn, 2007). The effect of aldosterone on the body is to reduce the excretion of sodium in the urine by regulating the reabsorption of sodium from the urine in the distal portion of the renal tubules. Aldosterone also has an effect on the body levels of water and several other ions (including potassium, bicarbonate and chloride) as their regulation is coupled to the regulation of sodium in the body. The stimulus for the release of aldosterone is primarily related to the blood concentrations of sodium (Na^+) and potassium (K^+), blood pressure (BP) and blood volume. Increased concentrations of potassium, reduced blood concentrations of sodium and a reduction in blood pressure and/or blood volume all stimulate the release of aldosterone, whilst the opposite inhibits release (Figure 13.6).

There are several mechanisms that regulate the release of aldosterone. The primary control mechanism is the production of **angiotensin II** by the **renin angiotensin system**. However, in response to a severe, non-specific stressor hypothalamic release of CRH stimulates the increased release of ACTH. This increase in ACTH stimulates a slight increase in the release of aldosterone leading to a slight increase in blood volume and pressure which will help to ensure the adequate delivery of oxygen and nutrients to the tissues (Marieb and Hoehn, 2007).

The **glucocorticoid** hormones influence the metabolism of most body cells and are also involved in providing resistance to stressors and promoting the repair of damaged tissues. They also suppress the immune system and inflammatory processes of the body (Saladin, 2004), hence their use in the treatment of inflammatory conditions such as asthma and arthritis. The glucocorticoids include **cortisol** (hydrocortisone), cortisone and corticosterone; however, only cortisol is secreted in any significant amounts (Marieb and Hoehn, 2007). Cortisol is normally released in a rhythmical pattern, with most being released shortly after the person gets up from sleep and the lowest amount being released just before, and shortly after, sleep commences. Cortisol release is promoted by ACTH from

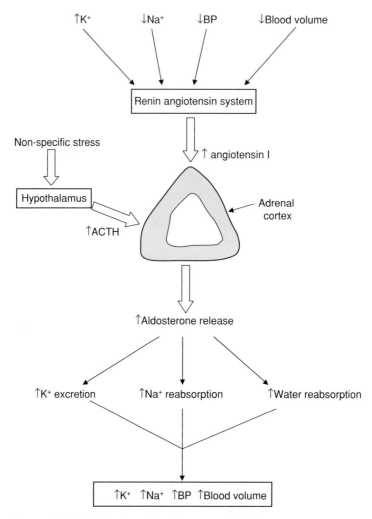

Figure 13.6 Mechanisms for the control of aldosterone secretion.

the anterior pituitary gland; increasing levels of cortisol act on both the hypothalamus and the pituitary gland inhibiting further release of both CRH and ACTH in a negative feedback system. However, this negative feedback system is overridden by acute physiological stress (for instance, trauma, infection or haemorrhage). The increase in sympathetic nervous system activity in response to an acute stress triggers greater CRH release and thus there is a significant increase in subsequent cortisol production (Figure 13.7).

The effect of cortisol on the body is to promote **gluconeogenesis** (the formation of glucose from fats and proteins), the release of fatty acids into the blood and the breakdown of stored proteins to create amino acids for tissue repair (Marieb and Hoehn, 2007). Cortisol also enhances the **vasoconstrictive** effect of adrenaline in the control of **vascular tone**. Thus, cortisol helps to enable the body to respond to stressors of various types.

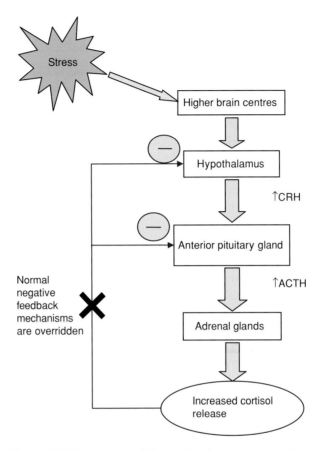

Figure 13.7 Response of the endocrine system to stress.

The pancreas

Located partially behind the stomach the pancreas is a mixed gland containing both endocrine and exocrine gland cells. The majority of the gland is made up of acinar cells; these cells produce an enzyme-rich fluid that is secreted into the small intestines and aids the digestion of food. Scattered amongst the acinar cells are pancreatic islets otherwise known as the **islets of Langerhans** (Fox, 2008). Each one of these islets is a collection of at least three major endocrine cell types, each cell type producing a different hormone (Saladin, 2004):

- **Alpha cells** create the hormone **glucagon**.
- **Beta cells** are the most numerous of the cells and they create **insulin**.
- **Delta cells** release somatostatin, a hormone that inhibits the release of glucagon and insulin.

Both insulin and glucagon are involved in the control of the blood levels of glucose but they have directly opposite effects. **Glucagon** promotes the breakdown of **glycogen**, stored in the liver, into glucose (**glucongenolysis**); it also promotes the synthesis of glucose from fatty acids and amino acids (**gluconeogenesis**) and the release of the newly created glucose from the liver into the blood stream

(Marieb and Hoehn, 2007). Thus, the major effect of glucagon is to raise glucose levels in the blood. The stimuli for the release of glucagon are decreased blood levels of glucose and increased blood levels of amino acids (for instance, after a protein-rich meal).

Insulin reduces the blood glucose levels and plays a role in the breakdown of protein and in the metabolism of fat (Marieb and Hoehn, 2007). The target cells of insulin are virtually every cell in the body, especially the skeletal muscle cells (but not the brain, the liver and the kidneys). The effect of insulin on these cells is to promote the transport of glucose across the cell membrane into the cell body. Insulin also activates and promotes the enzyme systems within the cell to metabolise glucose to create **adenosine triphosphate** (ATP), the basic fuel of body cells (Fox, 2008). Once the energy needs of the cells are met, insulin promotes the conversion of the remaining glucose into glycogen and in the **adipose tissues** it promotes the conversion of glucose into fat molecules and the subsequent storage of these fat molecules in the cells (Marieb and Hoehn, 2007). Finally, insulin promotes amino acid uptake by the muscle tissue and the creation of proteins from these amino acids. The release of insulin is stimulated by a rise in glucose levels in the blood, or increased blood levels of amino acids and fatty acids.

As the effect of each of these two hormones leads to the conditions that stimulates the release of the other hormone (for instance, as insulin reduces the blood levels of glucose so the stimulus for the release of glucagon is increased) insulin and glucagon release is constantly being adjusted. The overall effect is to try to maintain homeostasis by preventing large swings in blood glucose.

Disorders of the endocrine system

Learning outcomes

On completion of this section, the reader will be able to:

- Describe the potential impact of hypopituitarism on the endocrine system.
- Describe the symptoms of disorders of the thyroid gland.
- Explain the need for close monitoring and observation of the patient suffering from an adrenal crisis.
- Discuss the role of the nurse in the management of diabetes.

General considerations for nursing patients with an endocrine condition

Regardless of the particular endocrine condition they have all patients share a need for psychological support and information, as will their relatives and significant others (Department of Health, 2001a). Patients will require information on the particular disorders that they are suffering from and the signs and symptoms that they can expect the condition to manifest. Providing the patient with a clear understanding will:

- Reduce anxiety as to what the future may hold.
- Allow the patient to attribute signs and symptoms to their condition rather than enduring them.
- Give the patient control of their health and illness.

- Enable the patient to monitor their own disease and report deviations that may be attributed to a worsening condition or poor control.
- Encourage compliance with treatment regimes.

The pituitary gland

Hypopituitarism is the inability of the pituitary gland to produce enough hormones for normal bodily functioning (Schneider *et al.*, 2007). It can be caused by disorders of the pituitary gland itself or the reduction of hypothalamic releasing hormones due to a disorder of the hypothalamus, thus reducing the stimuli for pituitary gland activity (see Figure 13.8).

In adults, the majority of patients will have a deficit in more than three pituitary hormones (Prabhakar and Shalet, 2006) whereas in children, multiple pituitary hormone deficiencies are rare (Lamberts *et al.*, 1998). The most common cause of hypopituitarism is a tumour of either the pituitary gland or the hypothalamus, or a tumour in the same region that is putting pressure on the pituitary gland (Schneider *et al.*, 2007). Other causes include genetic causes, and increasingly the role of trauma to the brain has been recognised (for instance, stroke, trauma or radiation therapy of the brain). If a tumour is identified

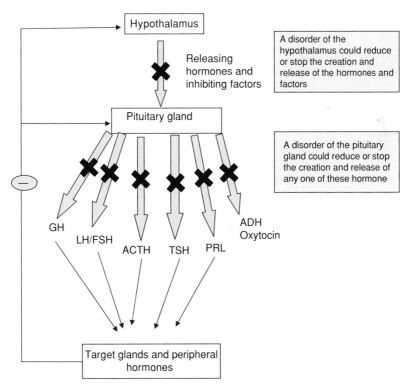

Figure 13.8 Causes of hypopituitarism and its effects on hormone release. GH, growth hormone; LH, luteinising hormone; FSH, follicle-stimulating hormone; ACTH, adrenocorticotropic hormone; TSH, thyroid-stimulating hormone; PRL, prolactin; ADH, antidiuretic hormone.

and surgically removed then normal pituitary functioning may be returned; however, if destruction of pituitary gland tissue has occurred, or the cause is not reversible, the condition is chronic and lifelong.

The signs and symptoms of hypopituitarism are related to the pituitary hormones that are deficient and their effect on target organs and tissues. In patients who have hypopituitarism that is caused by a tumour there may be additional signs and symptoms caused by the tumour pressing on other structures in the same area of the brain, for instance visual disturbances and headaches (Prabhakar and Shalet, 2006). The treatment for the symptoms of hypopituitarism is to replace the hormones that are not being produced. This can either be a direct replacement of pituitary hormones such as growth hormone or replacement of the hormones normally created by a target organ (for instance, thyroxine replacement therapy if TSH production is reduced). The signs and symptoms that patients may exhibit due to a reduction in the relevant target organ activity is dealt with in the associated sections of this chapter.

Diabetes insipidus is a condition where ADH production and release is reduced (for example, due to head injury) leading to an excessive urine output. A conscious patient can compensate for this increased output by drinking more to replace the fluids passed out as urine. An unconscious patient who may be at risk of diabetes insipidus, for instance following head injury, requires close monitoring of their urine output. In the event of a reduction in ADH production the patient would pass large amounts of urine and rapidly dehydrate. The patient should be catheterised and the urine output monitored and recorded at regular intervals; in the event of increased urine output an unconscious patient cannot replace the excess fluid and would require intravenous fluids, close monitoring of fluid balance and observation for the signs of dehydration.

The thyroid gland

Disorders of the thyroid gland are the most common endocrine disorder encountered in the community setting (Larson *et al.*, 2000). Disorders of the thyroid gland can be classified as either **hypersecretion** of thyroid hormones (excessive thyroid gland activity – hyperthyroidism) or **hyposecretion** of thyroid hormones (reduced thyroid gland activity – hypothyroidism). Thyroid disorders can be divided into two categories:

- Primary – due to a disorder of the thyroid gland itself.
- Secondary – alterations in thyroid function due to an increase or decrease in the production of either TRH from the hypothalamus or TSH from the pituitary gland.

The diagnosis of a disorder of the thyroid gland is often delayed as the signs and symptoms are vague and diverse, and in the elderly many signs and symptoms may be attributed to age (Larson *et al.*, 2000). The introduction of simple laboratory tests for blood levels of the thyroid hormones has now made the diagnosis much easier but delays in diagnosis are still common (Larson *et al.*, 2000). The most useful tests for thyroid disease are the analysis of blood levels of TSH and **free T$_4$**. The expected findings of these tests in clinical thyroid disease are detailed in Table 13.2.

Hyperthyroidism

Excessive production of thyroid hormone is commonly due to **Graves' disease**, an **autoimmune** disorder where autoimmune antibodies mimic the effect of pituitary TSH, thus stimulating the excessive release of thyroid hormone (Cooper, 2003). Other causes include thyroid cancer, **thyroid nodules** (usually

	TSH	Free T$_4$
Hyperthyroidism	Reduced	Normal or elevated
Hypothyroidism	Elevated	Normal or reduced

Table 13.2 Common laboratory test findings in the diagnosis of thyroid disease

non-cancerous), viral **thyroiditis**, postpartum thyroiditis and patients taking iodine-containing drugs (such as amiodarone) (Cooper, 2003). The signs and symptoms of hyperthyroidism are related to the increased levels of thyroid hormone (see Box 13.1).

The long-term effects of hyperthyroidism can include cardiovascular disease and **osteoporosis** (Boelaert and Franklyn, 2005). In pregnancy, hyperthyroidism has been linked with higher rates of miscarriage, premature labour, **eclampsia** and low birth weight of the baby (Cooper, 2003).

Treatments for hyperthyroidism are:

- Surgery to remove part or all of the thyroid gland (rarely used except in the case of the surgical removal of thyroid tumours).
- Radioactive iodine: this treatment relies on the fact that the most active cells in the thyroid gland will take up the most iodine and thus be destroyed. Radioactive iodine is contraindicated in pregnancy.
- Antithyroid drugs (ATDs), these reduce thyroid hormone production but do not damage the gland. However in common with all drugs, ATDs have associated side effects and are poorly tolerated in the long-term (Larson *et al.*, 2000).
- Symptomatic relief of tachycardia, palpitations, tremors and nervousness can be gained from the use of beta-blocking drugs such as atenolol.

Box 13.1 Signs and symptoms of hyperthyroidism

- Nervousness, restlessness, fatigue, insomnia
- **Tachycardia, palpitations** (atrial fibrillation is common in the elderly)
- Shortness of breath
- Weight loss despite an increased appetite, frequency of passing stools, nausea, vomiting
- Muscle weakness, tremors
- Warm, moist flushed skin
- Fine hair
- Staring gaze, **exophthalmia**
- **Goitre**
- Heat intolerance

Box 13.2 Endocrine emergency: thyroid storm

Thyroid storm is most common in patients with undiagnosed or poorly managed hyperthyroidism; it is due to the effect of high blood levels of thyroid hormone in association with increased sympathetic nervous system activity. There are several known causes of thyroid storm, including emotional or physical trauma and stress (Noble, 2006).

The patient exhibiting thyroid storm will be **hyperthermic** (temperature over 40°C), tachycardic (commonly **atrial fibrillation** is found on ECG monitoring), agitated and confused, and may be vomiting or have diarrhoea.

Patients in thyroid storm require close observation and monitoring in a critical care area. The temperature should be reduced by active cooling; intravenous fluids will be required as the patient will rapidly dehydrate, and the tachycardia may require control with beta-blocking drugs (Gardner and Greenspan, 2004). Control of thyroid function and the reduction of circulating thyroid hormone is also normally required.

The role of the nurse in the management of hyperthyroidism is related to the alleviation of signs and symptoms, the provision of education and support, and monitoring of the patient for any deterioration of the condition (Walsh, 2002).

- Anxiety management is essential and the use of beta-blockers should not be ignored. Psychological support and a calm environment are required to prevent exacerbation of nervousness.
- Provision of a well-ventilated cool environment and an electric fan will help the patient to remain comfortable.
- Encouraging regular fluid intake in patients who are perspiring excessively.
- The patient will be fatigued but will find it difficult to rest. The provision of a comfortable environment may aid relaxation and sleep.
- The nurse should be watchful for the potential onset of a thyroid storm (see Box 13.2) especially in the newly diagnosed or patients awaiting definitive treatment. Regular monitoring of vital signs and patterns of patient activity/mental state should be carried out.

Hypothyroidism

The causes of hypothyroidism are diverse and include treatment for hyperthyroidism (especially radioactive iodine therapy), radiation therapy of the neck and drugs such as amiodarone and lithium (Larson *et al.*, 2000). However, the most common cause of hypothyroidism is **Hashimoto's thyroiditis** (an autoimmune disorder). As with hyperthyroidism the signs and symptoms of hypothyroidism are varied and it affects virtually every bodily system (Box 13.3). However, the development of the symptoms of hypothyroidism is often slow due to the fact that the thyroid gland stores a large amount of thyroid hormone that is released despite the inability of the gland to produce more.

In pregnancy, hypothyroidism has been linked to recurrent miscarriages and preterm labour; it is also suspected that untreated maternal hypothyroidism has an effect on the development of the fetus including the pituitary gland and is linked to reduced IQ in the child (Boelaert and Franklyn, 2005).

The treatment of hypothyroidism is lifelong thyroxine replacement therapy (Larson *et al.*, 2000). In the first months of commencing thyroxine therapy patients will require regular blood tests to ensure

Box 13.3 Signs and symptoms of hypothyroidism

- Confusion, lethargy, memory loss, depression
- Bradycardia, enlarged heart (cardiomegaly), pericardial effusions
- Constipation, weight gain
- Muscle cramps, myalgia (generalised muscle aches), stiffness
- Dry cool skin
- Brittle nails
- Coarse hair, hair loss
- Oedema of hands and eyelids
- Cold intolerance
- Vacant expression

that a suitable blood level is achieved and the dose may need to be altered several times during this period (Larson *et al.*, 2000). Once a suitable dose has been found patients will require yearly blood tests to ensure that their needs have not changed; over-replacement of thyroid hormone is one of the leading causes of hyperthyroidism, but can be avoided and is easily rectified. Monitoring of **concordance** with replacement therapy and the use of strategies to encourage and maintain concordance are essential as many patients are reluctant to take long-term thyroxine therapy (Crilly, 2004). Patients should be counselled as to the possible side effects of thyroid replacement therapy, including temporary hair loss (Roberts and Ladenson, 2004). Patients should be given information regarding the need for adherence to the replacement therapy and what to do in the event of prolonged gastrointestinal disturbance that prevents taking oral medications. Acute illness or trauma may precipitate myxedemic coma (Box 13.4) and patients must be made aware of the need to seek medical help. Caution must be exercised in commencing thyroxine therapy in patients with known **ischaemic heart disease**, these patients are usually commenced on a lower dose and this is then slowly increased, as giving the patient the full replacement dose may worsen the symptoms of angina or even precipitate a **myocardial infarction** (Boelaert and Franklyn, 2005). Elderly patients are also usually commenced on a lower dose and

Box 13.4 Endocrine emergency: myxedemic coma

Myxedemic coma is the end stage of untreated hypothyroidism (Gardner and Greenspan, 2004). This may be due to the previously unrecognised hypothyroidism or the patient stopping replacement therapy; often the crisis is brought on by an underlying illness or trauma. If untreated, it will eventually result in the death of the patient.

The patient in myxedemic coma will be **hypothermic**, **bradycardic** and have a slow, shallow respiratory rate. Blood tests will usually identify low blood levels of sodium and glucose as well as low blood levels of thyroid hormone.

Patients suffering from myxedemic coma require admission to an intensive care unit for close monitoring, intubation and ventilation and intravenous replacement of thyroxine, and will require a fluid restriction to avoid further diluting the sodium levels in the blood.

their replacement requirements may be lower than those of a younger patient (Larson *et al.*, 2000). Elderly patients in the community may also require regular nursing checks to ensure concordance with replacement therapy and monitoring of their symptoms (especially as relatives or carers may attribute symptoms to old age rather than thyroid disease).

The parathyroid glands

Prior to the discovery of the parathyroid glands, patients undergoing surgery for removal of the thyroid gland often suffered from hypoparathyroidism as the glands were removed with the thyroid. The patient would subsequently suffer from **parasthaesia**, **tetany** and seizures due to the reduced availability of calcium (Potts, 2005). With the discovery of the parathyroid glands and the reduction of surgery for thyroid disorders this outcome is now rare. Hypoparathyroidism due to the destruction of the parathyroid gland is now largely due to autoimmune syndromes. These patients require calcium and vitamin D replacement therapy to ensure the availability of calcium for normal muscle functioning.

Hyperparathyroidism (excessive production of parathyroid hormone) is most commonly due to an **adenoma** (a benign tumour) and is most common in women (Marx, 2000). These patients have raised blood levels of calcium, calcium in the urine and a decreased bone mass; they may also exhibit subtle signs of fatigue and muscle weakness. The current treatment for hyperparathyroidism is the surgical removal of the overactive glands, but many patients remain asymptomatic, as the condition progresses slowly (if at all) and monitoring of parathyroid function is all that is required (Marx, 2000).

The adrenal glands

Excessive release of the corticosteroids is rare but is normally due to a pituitary **tumour** increasing the release of ACTH; the most common cause of raised blood levels of the glucocorticoids is their therapeutic use in inflammatory conditions (such as asthma and arthritis). Patients with high levels of glucocorticoids in the blood show the signs and symptoms of **Cushing's disease** (Aron *et al.*, 2004). These patients are commonly obese, with the main distribution of fat being around the face (moon facies), neck (buffalo hump), trunk and abdomen. Relative to the central obesity the patients' arms and legs are often thin and spindly and the patient may report muscle weakness. The patient will often have thin, easily bruised skin, and may report slow wound healing or frequent fungal infections; the majority of female patients will report increased hair growth on the face. Osteoporosis is common and back pain is the most common presenting symptom (Aron *et al.*, 2004). The majority of patients with Cushing's disease will exhibit some signs of psychological disturbance, for instance **euphoria**, mood swings, irritability, poor memory and difficulty in concentrating; disturbance of sleep patterns is common. The long-term effects of persistently high levels of glucocorticoids in the blood include **hypertension**, cardiovascular disease, susceptibility to infection and the development of steroid induced diabetes. The treatment of Cushing's disease is to remove or destroy the tumour (Aron *et al.*, 2004) or reduction of the doses of glucocorticoid treatment where possible.

Adrenal insufficiency (the reduced production and release of corticosteroids from the adrenal glands) is divided into two types (Arlt and Allolio, 2003):

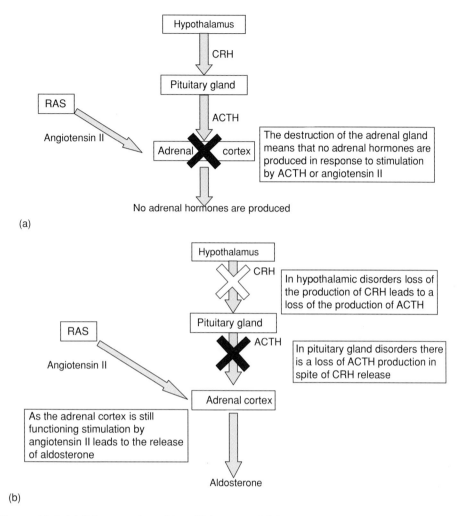

Figure 13.9 (a) Primary adrenal insufficiency and (b) secondary adrenal insufficiency.

■ Primary adrenal insufficiency (Addison's disease) due to a disorder of the adrenal glands (Figure 13.9a). The leading cause of Addison's disease is autoimmune **adrenalitis**; other causes include tuberculosis, and fungal infection in immunosuppressed patients (such as HIV/AIDS or therapeutic suppression of the immune system).

■ Secondary adrenal insufficiency (Figure 13.9b). This is most commonly due to the sudden cessation of glucocorticoid therapy; however, tumours of the hypothalamic–pituitary region and their treatment are also a cause of secondary adrenal insufficiency.

The signs and symptoms of primary adrenal insufficiency are related to the lack of both glucocorticoid hormones and mineralocorticoid hormones (in secondary adrenal insufficiency the release of mineralocorticoid hormones is preserved as it is under the control of the renin angiotensin system and thus symptoms related to a lack of aldosterone are not present). In the event of destruction of the adrenal

Box 13.5 Signs and symptoms of adrenal insufficiency

- Fatigue, lack of stamina, loss of energy
- Reduced muscle strength
- Increased irritability
- Nausea
- Weight loss
- Muscle and joint pain
- Abdominal pain
- Low blood pressure
- Women may report a reduction in or loss of libido due to the lack of adrenal sex hormones

Primary adrenal insufficiency only:

- Symptoms related to the loss of aldosterone production, including dehydration, **hypovolaemia** (with possible **postural hypotension**), low blood levels of sodium and raised blood levels of potassium.
- Hyperpigmentation of the skin due to the stimulation of skin receptors by increased levels of ACTH. This can show as a darkening of the creases of the skin (e.g. in the palms, knuckles and oral mucosa), vitiligo (pale patches of skin) or an overall darkening of the skin (similar to a sun tan).

glands (primary adrenal insufficiency) the loss of the adrenal medulla is not associated with clinically important symptoms as the role of the medullary hormones (adrenaline and noradrenaline) is to magnify the effect of sympathetic nervous system activity which remains intact (Arlt and Allolio, 2003). The signs and symptoms of adrenal insufficiency (Box 13.5) are vague and thus the majority of patients will exhibit signs and symptoms for up to a year before diagnosis (Arlt and Allolio, 2003); however, a proportion will present as an acute adrenal crisis, which is often precipitated by trauma or infection (Box 13.6).

Box 13.6 Endocrine emergency: adrenal crisis

Adrenal (or Addisonian) crisis is an acute life-threatening event often precipitated by an acute traumatic event, fever or other serious illness. Patients present with severe **hypotension** resistant to standard therapies such as **inotropes**, hypovolaemic shock, acute abdominal pain, vomiting, fever, **hypoglycaemia**, **hyponatraemia** and **hyperkalaemia** (Aron *et al.*, 2004).

Treatment of an adrenal crisis requires close monitoring of a patient including blood pressure monitoring, cardiac monitoring for potential **arrhythmias** caused by the high potassium levels in the blood, intravenous hydrocortisone to replace the depleted levels of corticosteroids and intravenous fluids to replace volume. Normal saline is the usual fluid used as it will also replenish the reduced blood levels of sodium. Intravenous glucose may be required and depending on the levels of potassium in the blood therapies to reduce these levels may be commenced (for instance, **diuretics** to promote the excretion of potassium from the kidneys).

Patients who have been taking high-dose glucocorticoid therapy (such as prednisolone) are at risk of developing temporary adrenal gland **atrophy**; if the therapy is stopped suddenly they can present with the signs and symptoms of adrenal insufficiency and even an acute adrenal crisis. Therefore, all patients taking glucocorticoid therapy should never stop their medication suddenly and should carry a 'steroid treatment card' at all times. A reducing dose of glucocorticoids is required to allow for the recovery of the adrenal glands to their full function (British Medical Association/Royal Pharmaceutical Society of Great Britain, 2007).

The treatment of adrenal insufficiency is the replacement of glucocorticoid hormones with oral hydrocortisone in two to three daily doses. In primary adrenal insufficiency, replacement of the mineralocorticoid hormones is also required; this is achieved by the administration of oral fludrocortisone once a day. However, the quality of life of patients with adrenal insufficiency is often reduced, even with optimum replacement therapy, and patients report fatigue, a lack of energy, depression and anxiety (Arlt and Allolio, 2003).

Patients with permanent adrenal insufficiency (primary or secondary) will require education on the management of their replacement therapy (Arlt and Allolio, 2003). Adrenal crises are often the result of a patient not increasing their replacement therapy in response to physical stressors (such as strenuous exercise, trauma, infection or fever). Patients admitted to hospital for a surgical procedure will require either intravenous or intramuscular hydrocortisone prior to surgery to prevent the onset of a crisis. In the event of persistent diarrhoea and vomiting, preventing the patient from taking their normal oral medications, hydrocortisone may be administered by intramuscular injection and increasingly patients and their significant others are doing this themselves. Patients are often supplied with an emergency injection kit (hydrocortisone for intramuscular injection, needles and syringes) for the immediate management of an acute traumatic event or illness, and both the patient and their significant others should be trained in its use and their training and knowledge regularly refreshed (Kenward and White, 2003). It is strongly recommended that all patients with adrenal insufficiency wear a medical alert talisman (typically a bracelet or necklace).

The pancreas

Hypersecretion of insulin is very rare, and the vast majority of patients presenting with increased blood levels of insulin will be due to the over-administration of insulin in the management of diabetes mellitus (Marieb and Hoehn, 2007).

Diabetes mellitus (diabetes) is a group of disorders characterised by raised blood levels of glucose (World Health Organization, 2006). There are two main types of diabetes: type 1 diabetes and type 2 diabetes; however, the signs and symptoms of the two types are similar (Box 13.7).

The signs and symptoms of diabetes are related to the high levels of glucose in the blood and the inability of the cells to utilise glucose due to a lack of insulin production or resistance to the effect of insulin in the body. Glucose is excreted by the renal tubules into the urine and this leads to increased urine production due to the **osmotic** effect of the glucose (water is drawn into and retained in the urine by the high levels of glucose). Thus, body levels of water are depleted and the subsequent development of chronic thirst. The inability of the cells to use glucose as a primary fuel source leads to the metabolism of fats and amino acids and thus weight loss. Furthermore, the utilisation of fats and amino acids as fuel in the cells leads to the production of **ketones** (which are strong acids); these are excreted in the

Box 13.7 Signs and symptoms of diabetes

◼ High blood glucose levels
◼ Glucose in the urine
◼ Ketones in the urine
◼ Frequency in passing urine (including waking at night)
◼ Thirst
◼ Increased appetite (usually type 1 only)
◼ Weight loss (usually type 1 only)
◼ Fatigue
◼ Abdominal pain

Type 2 diabetes can often be asymptomatic and only diagnosed on **opportunistic screening** or as a chance finding whilst the patient is being investigated or treated for other medical problems.

urine and as they are negatively charged they carry sodium and potassium ions with them leading to electrolyte imbalance, a sign of which is abdominal pain (Marieb and Hoehn, 2007). Eventually, these processes can lead to an acute life-threatening hyperglycaemic event (Box 13.8).

Type 1 diabetes

Type 1 diabetes develops most commonly in childhood or early adulthood and comprises about 15% of the total incidence of diabetes in the UK; however, the rate of type 1 diabetes is increasing, particularly in children less than 5 years of age (Department of Health, 2001b). Type 1 diabetes is normally caused by autoimmune destruction of the beta cells of the pancreas and is therefore associated with a severe reduction in, or complete loss of, insulin production (Daneman, 2006).

The treatment of type 1 diabetes is the replacement of insulin, normally by subcutaneous injection, although alternative methods of administration (including inhaled insulin, nasal administration of insulin and oral insulin) are currently under investigation (Gomez-Perez and Rull, 2005). Care must be taken to ensure that the insulin administered is balanced by a sufficient intake of food (particularly carbohydrates as sugars are quickly used in the body) to avoid low blood sugar levels (**hypoglycaemia**). Profound hypoglycaemia leads to the patient becoming mentally agitated, possibly aggressive, often the patient will be sweating profusely and will look pale. If sufficient insulin has been taken the patient will eventually become comatose and may die. Conscious patients may be given a sugary snack or drink and some form of carbohydrates; the patient will then require monitoring of their blood glucose until the crisis has passed. Unconscious patients require immediate medical assistance and the administration of an intramuscular injection of glucagon and potentially intravenous glucose (Kearney and Dang, 2007).

Type 2 diabetes

This is the most common form of diabetes and is traditionally thought to be a disease of people over the age of 40. Overall the number of patients developing type 2 diabetes is increasing and this increase is occurring across all age ranges, including in adolescents and young adults (Department of Health,

---

Box 13.8 Endocrine emergency: hyperglycaemia

Patients with either type 1 or type 2 diabetes are at risk of developing life-threatening hyperglycaemia (Kearney and Dang, 2007).

Hyperosmolar hyperglycaemic state (HHS) is commonly associated with older patients with type 2 diabetes. The onset is usually over days to weeks and it may be the first indication that a patient is suffering from type 2 diabetes. HHS is characterised by a very high blood glucose (>33.3 mmol/L and often over 50 mmol/L), dehydration and confusion but the absence of significant levels of ketones and therefore no **acidaemia** (reduced blood pH). Dehydration occurs due to excessive urine output and low blood levels of sodium and potassium are common.

Diabetic ketoacidosis (DKA) is associated with type 1 diabetes and has a rapid onset (normally less than 24 hours). Patients present with hyperglycaemia (but usually not more than 40 mmol/L due to the rapid onset of DKA), **ketosis** (ketones in the blood), acidaemia, dehydration and reduced blood levels of sodium and potassium. The characteristic 'pear drop' or 'acetone' smell to the breath of a patient with DKA is produced by the excess of ketones in the blood.

The management of both HHS and DKA is similar and is aimed at replacing the lost fluid, reducing the blood glucose and correcting electrolyte imbalances. Large amounts of intravenous fluids are given (typically 1–1.5 L in the first hour), and potassium is usually added to subsequent fluids after the initial rapid fluid resuscitation. Low-dose intravenous insulin is commenced to slowly reduce the blood glucose and the patient is closely monitored, including regular assessment of vital signs, blood glucose and electrolytes (Kearney and Dang, 2007).

2001b). The reasons for this increase are probably related to lifestyle factors, including the increase in the rates of obesity, overeating (particularly sugary foods) and a lack of exercise (Stumvoll *et al.*, 2005).

Type 2 diabetes is normally characterised by the development of resistance to the effects of insulin in the tissues, and a reduction in the ability of the beta cells to increase the production of insulin in response to this increased **insulin resistance** in the body (Stumvoll *et al.*, 2005). The resulting high blood levels of glucose leads to damage of the beta cells, thus further reducing the production of insulin. The treatment of type 2 diabetes varies depending on the severity of the condition. In some patients, weight reduction, increased exercise and reduced food intake can resolve the raised blood sugar levels. However, once the beta cell damage has occurred the need for medications is increased. Current drug therapies for type 2 diabetes (**oral hypoglycaemics**) target several aspects of the disease including reducing glucose production by the liver, enhancing insulin output from the pancreas or increasing the sensitivity of the muscle, fat and liver cells to the effects of insulin thus reducing insulin resistance (Nathan *et al.*, 2006). Increasingly, a role is being seen for the use of insulin in type 2 diabetes.

Patients with both type 1 and type 2 diabetes will have similar educational needs in terms of their personal control of their diabetes. The aim of nursing management is to alleviate the symptoms of diabetes, optimise the control of blood glucose levels and thus prevent long-term complications (Nair, 2007). Nursing interventions include:

- Advice on appropriate diet; current advice emphasises the need for a healthy, balanced, diet. This includes reducing the amount of sugar and fat that is eaten, increasing the intake of fruit, vegetables, and substituting wholemeal bread and pastas for refined products such as white bread.
- Encouraging regular physical activity. However, strenuous exercise can reduce blood glucose levels and exercise regimes should be agreed with appropriate health care staff.

Box 13.9 Focus on diabetic foot ulcers

Excluding accidents, diabetes is the leading cause of lower limb amputations in the UK (Department of Health, 2001b); patients with diabetes have a 12–25% lifetime risk of developing a foot ulcer (Cavanagh *et al.*, 2005).
 The causes of diabetic foot ulcers are neuropathic, ischaemic or a mixture of both:

- Neuropathic – the reduced sensation in the feet of patients with peripheral neuropathy means that they are often unaware of the mechanical stresses being placed on their feet due to poorly fitting footwear or trauma (such as standing on a sharp object).
- Ischaemic – the reduced peripheral circulation in patients with long-term complications leads to easily damaged skin with a reduced ability to heal in response to damage.

Not all diabetic foot ulcers become infected, but when they do the patients' limb, and sometimes life, can be in danger as the wound does not heal rapidly and infection can spread easily due to the reduction in the delivery of white blood cells to the peripheral tissues.
 The treatment of diabetic foot ulcers may require surgical **debridement** of the wound to remove dead tissue which is a host for bacteria; appropriate wound dressings and antibiotics may also be necessary. Relief of pressure on the ulcer is critical to the success of treatment and referral to a **podiatrist** will be required for continued foot care and assessment for pressure-relieving shoes (Falanga, 2005).

- Advice and support for weight loss if required. Weight loss in overweight patients improves the control of diabetes as inactivity and obesity are strongly linked to insulin resistance (Stumvoll *et al.*, 2005).
- Advice and support on stopping smoking. Patients with diabetes have an increased risk of vascular diseases (including heart disease and stroke), and smoking further increases this risk.
- Education on how to monitor blood glucose levels using capillary blood glucose monitoring or urinalysis (as appropriate).
- The use and administration of medications, such as insulin injection techniques and adjusting insulin doses.

Poor control of diabetes often leads to **hyperglycaemia** and is associated with a range of long-term complications including blindness or reduced vision, peripheral **neuropathy**, renal failure, cardiovascular disease, **peripheral artery disease** and foot ulcers (Box 13.9).

Conclusion

This chapter has introduced the physiology of both normal and disordered endocrine functioning and the treatment of the related disorders. The endocrine system has a wide and varied role in the maintenance of normal bodily functioning. Disorders of any of the endocrine organs can produce a variety of signs and symptoms and may even lead to a life-threatening crisis. The nurse has a crucial role in the detection of endocrine conditions, the monitoring of disease progression and treatment effects, and the prevention and treatment of endocrine emergencies. Most patients with an endocrine disorder will take responsibility for the management of their own condition and it is essential that they are given appropriate advice and support. In order to carry out these roles the nurse must have a good understanding of the physiology and treatment of the endocrine disorders.

Multiple choice questions

1. The parathyroid gland is important in the control of which ion in the body?
(a) sodium
(b) calcium
(c) potassium
(d) all of the above

2. Production of thyroid hormone is primarily stimulated by:
(a) a neural stimulus
(b) an external stimulus
(c) a hormonal stimulus
(d) a negative feedback system

3. The hypothalamus secretes which of the following hormones?
(a) thyroid-stimulating hormone
(b) cortisol
(c) thyroid releasing hormone
(d) the gonadocorticoids

4. The release of ACTH from the anterior pituitary gland stimulates which endocrine organ(s)?
(a) adrenal glands
(b) thyroid gland
(c) parathyroid glands
(d) pancreas

5. The calorigenic effect of thyroid hormone refers to which of these effects?
(a) increased oxygen use in the cells
(b) increased heat production
(c) increased basal metabolic rate
(d) all of the above

6. A patient who reports constantly feeling cold, depressed and lethargic may be suffering from which endocrine disorder?
(a) hypothyroidism
(b) hyperthyroidism
(c) diabetes insipidus
(d) hypoparathyroidism

7. The presence of glucose and ketones in the urine indicates:
(a) hypoglycaemia

(b) hyperglycaemia

(c) adrenal crisis

(d) hypopituitarism

8. Patients with type 2 diabetes mellitus commonly manage their condition with:

(a) insulin

(b) mineralocorticoids

(c) oral hypoglycaemics

(d) iodine

9. Patients experiencing an adrenal crisis will require:

(a) restricted fluids

(b) hydrocortisone injection

(c) glucagon injection

(d) kidney dialysis

10. The most common cause of the thyroid disorders is:

(a) cancer

(b) pregnancy

(c) trauma to the neck

(d) autoimmune

Answers: 1.b, 2.c, 3.c, 4.a, 5.d, 6.a, 7.b, 8.c, 9.b, 10.d.

Test your knowledge

❷ What is the most common endocrine disorder in the community care setting?

❷ Why are patients with ischaemic heart disease started on lower doses of thyroxine?

❷ What is the difference between primary and secondary adrenal insufficiency?

❷ What is the function of glucagon in the regulation of blood glucose?

❷ Why should patients never suddenly stop taking steroid therapy?

Glossary of terms

Acidaemia: A state of relative acidity of the blood.

Adenoma: A tumour of any gland tissue (usually benign).

Adenosine triphosphate: A compound of an adenosine molecule with three attached phosphoric acid molecules.

Adrenalitis: Inflammatory condition of the adrenal glands.

Amino acids: Chemical compound that is the basic building blocks of proteins and enzymes.

Arrhythmia: A disorder of the normal heart beat.

Asymptomatic: Lacking in symptoms.

Atrial fibrillation: An arrhythmia of the atria of the heart – often presenting as a fast, irregular, heart beat.

Atrophy: A reduction in size or activity.

Autoimmune: Immune response to the bodies' own tissues.

Benign: Non-cancerous.

Bradycardic: Having a slow heart beat (usually defined as less than 60 beats per minute).

Concordance: Current term for the patient's adherence to a prescribed treatment.

Debridement: Removal of damaged tissues and cells.

Diuretics: Class of drugs that increase urine output.

Eclampsia: A condition presenting in pregnancy that is characterised by high blood pressure, fits and even coma.

Electrolytes: A group of chemical elements or compounds that includes sodium, potassium, calcium, chloride and bicarbonate.

Endocrine: Used to refer to groups of cells that secrete hormones into the blood.

Euphoria: An exaggerated state of well-being.

Exocrine: Used to refer to groups of cells that secrete substances through a duct into a vessel (such as into the intestines).

Exopthalmia: Excessive protrusion of the eyeballs.

Free T_4: Refers to thyroxine, in the blood, that is not bound to proteins.

Gland: Refers to any organ in the body that secretes substances not related to its own, internal, functioning.

Glycogen: A carbohydrate (complex sugar) made from glucose.

Goitre: Pronounced swelling of the neck.

Homeostasis: The state of balance of the internal environment of the body.

Hormone: Chemical substance that is released into the blood, by the endocrine system, and has a physiological control over the function of cells or organs other than those that created it.

Hyperglycaemia: High blood levels of glucose.

Hyperkalaemia: High blood levels of potassium.

Hypersecretion: High rate of secretion.

Hypertension: High blood pressure.

Hyperthermic: High body temperature.

Hypoglycaemia: Low blood levels of glucose.

Hyponatraemia: Low blood levels of sodium.

Hyposecretion: Low rate of secretion.

Hypotension: Low blood pressure.

Hypothermic: Low body temperature.

Hypovolaemia: Low levels of fluid in the circulation.

Inotropes: A class of drugs used to increase the blood pressure in the critically ill.

Insulin resistance: A condition where the usual body reaction to insulin is reduced.

Ion: An atom or group of atoms that carry an electrical charge.

Ischaemic heart disease: Condition of the heart related to a lack of oxygen reaching the heart muscle.

Ketosis: Ketones in the blood.

Malignant: Invasive, has a tendency to grow and may spread to other parts of the body.

Myocardial infarction: Death of an area of heart muscle due to an interruption of the blood supply to the affected area.

Neuropathy: Inflammation and degeneration of the nerves.

Opportunistic screening: Testing a patient for particular diseases or conditions, at a point in time they are accessing health care for other reasons.

Oral hypoglycaemics: Group of drugs used in the treatment of diabetes that are taken by mouth and reduce the blood sugar level.

Osmotic: The movement of water through a semipermeable barrier from an area of low concentration of a chemical to an area of high concentration of a chemical.

Osteoclasts: A type of cell that breaks down bone tissue and thus releases the calcium used to create bones.

Osteoperosis: Condition characterised by reduced bone density and an increased risk of fractures.

Palpitations: A feeling of pounding or racing of the heart.

Parasthaesia: Abnormal nerve sensations such as pins-and-needles, tingling or burning.

Peripheral artery disease: Disease of the arteries of the legs.

Podiatrist: Health care professional who specialises in the diagnosis and treatment of disorders of the feet (also known as chripodist).

Postural hypotension: Inability of the body to maintain an adequate blood pressure when the person rises from sitting or lying to standing too rapidly. Usually characterised by dizziness or fainting if the person rises too quickly to a standing position.

Tachycardia: Fast heart beat (usually defined as above 100 beats per minute).

Tetany: Prolonged muscular spasms.

Thyroiditis: Inflammatory condition of the thyroid gland.

Thyroid nodule: Growth of thyroid tissue or fluid-filled cyst of the thyroid tissue.

References

Arlt, W. and Allolio, B. (2003). Adrenal insufficiency. *The Lancet*, *361*(9372), 1881–1893.

Aron, D.C., Findling, J.W. and Tyrrell, J.B. (2004). Glucocorticoids and adrenal androgens. In: Greenspan, F.S. and Gardner, D.G. (eds) *Basic and Clinical Endocrinology*, 7th edn. London: Lange Medical Books/McGraw-Hill, pp. 362–413.

Boelaert, K. and Franklyn, J.A. (2005). Starling review: Thyroid hormone in health and disease. *Journal of Endocrinology*, *1*(187), 1–15.

British Medical Association/Royal Pharmaceutical Society of Great Britain (2007). *British National Formulary*, 53rd edn. London: British Medical Association/Royal Pharmaceutical Society of Great Britain.

Cavanagh, P.R., Lipsky, B.A., Bradbury, A.W. and Botek, G. (2005). Treatment for diabetic foot ulcers. *The Lancet*, *366*(9498), 1725–1735.

Cooper, D.S. (2003). Hyperthyroidism. *The Lancet*, *362*(9382), 459–468.

Crilly, M. (2004). Correspondence: Thyroxine adherence in primary hypothyroidism. *The Lancet*, *363*(9420), 1558.

Daneman, D. (2006). Type 1 diabetes. *The Lancet*, *367*(9513), 847–858.

Department of Health (2001a). *The Expert Patient: A New Approach to Chronic Disease Management in the 21st Century*. London: Department of Health.

Department of Health (2001b). *National Service Framework for Diabetes: Standards*. London: Department of Health.

Falanga, V. (2005). Wound healing and its impairment in the diabetic foot. *The Lancet*, *366*(9498), 1736–1743.

Fox, S.I. (2008). *Human Physiology*, 10th edn. London: McGraw-Hill.

Gardner, D.G. and Greenspan, F.S. (2004). Endocrine emergencies. In: Greenspan, F.S. and Gardner, D.G. (eds) *Basic and Clinical Endocrinology*, 7th edn. London: Lange Medical Books/McGraw-Hill, pp. 867–892.

Gomez-Perez, F.J. and Rull, J.A. (2005). Insulin therapy: Current alternatives. *Archives of Medical Research*, *36*(3), 258–272.

Guyton, A.C. and Hall, J. (2006). *Textbook of Medical Physiology*, 11th edn. Philadelphia: Elsevier Saunders.

Kearney, T. and Dang, C. (2007). Diabetic and endocrine emergencies. *Postgraduate Medical Journal*, *83*(976), 79–86.

Kenward, D. and White, K.G. (2003). Correspondence: Adrenal insufficiency. *The Lancet*, *362*(9383), 579–580.

Lamberts, S.W.J., DeHerder, V.W. and Van Der Lely, A.J. (1998). Pituitary insufficiency. *The Lancet*, *352*(9122), 127–134.

Larson, J., Anderson, E.H. and Koslawy, M. (2000). Thyroid disease: A review for primary care. *Journal of the American Academy of Nurse Practitioners*, *12*(6), 226–232.

Marieb, E.N. and Hoehn, K. (2007). *Human Anatomy and Physiology*, 7th edn. San Francisco: Pearson Benjamin Cummings.

Marx, S.J. (2000). Hyperparathyroid and hypoparathyroid disorders. *New England Journal of Medicine*, *343*(25), 1863–1875.

Nair, M. (2007). Nursing management of the person with diabetes mellitus. Part 2. *British Journal of Nursing*, *16*(4), 232–235.

Nathan, D.M., Buse, J.B., Davidson, M.B. *et al.* (2006). Management of hyperglycaemia in type 2 diabetes: A consensus algorithm for the initiation and adjustment of therapy. *Diabetes Care*, *29*(8), 1963–1972.

Noble, K.A. (2006). Thyroid storm. *Journal of PeriAnesthesia Nursing*, *21*(2), 119–125.

Potts, J.T. (2005). Starling review. Parathyroid hormone: Past and present. *Journal of Endocrinology*, *187*(3), 311–325.

Prabhakar, V.K.B. and Shalet, S.M. (2006). Aetiology, diagnosis and management of hypopituitarism in adult life. *Postgraduate Medical Journal*, *82*(966), 259–266.

Roberts, C.G.P. and Ladenson, P.W. (2004). Hypothyroidism. *The Lancet*, *363*(9411), 793–803.

Saladin, K.S. (2004). *Anatomy and Physiology. The Unity of Form and Function*, 3rd edn. London: McGraw-Hill.

Schneider, H.J., Aimaretti, G., Kreitschmann-Andermahr, I., Stalla, G. and Ghigo, E. (2007). Hypopituitarism. *The Lancet*, *369*(9571), 1461–1470.

Stumvoll, M., Goldstein, B.J. and van Haeften, T.W. (2005). Type 2 diabetes: Principles of pathogenesis and therapy. *The Lancet*, *365*(9467), 1333–1346.

Walsh, M. (2002). Caring for a person with a disorder of the endocrine system. In: Walsh, M. (ed) *Watson's Clinical Nursing and Related Sciences*, 6th edn. London: Balliere Tindall, pp. 561–610.

World Health Organization (2006). *Fact Sheet No 312 Diabetes*. Geneva: World Health Organization.

Chapter 14

The reproductive systems and associated disorders

Ian Peate

KEY WORDS

- Reproduction
- Hormones
- Cancer
- Genitalia

- Ovulation
- Menstruation
- Self esteem
- Puberty

- Prostaglandins
- Fertility
- Risk
- Reproductive tracts

Test your prior knowledge

- Describe the menstrual cycle.
- What are the functions of the prostate gland?
- How can issues associated with the reproductive tract impinge on an individual's self-esteem?

Learning outcomes

On completion of this section, the reader will be able to:

- Describe the main functions of the male and female reproductive tracts.
- List the organs of the female and male reproductive tracts.
- Discuss the normal functions of male and female reproductive tracts.
- Discuss the normal and abnormal pathophysiological changes that can occur in association with the male and female reproductive tracts.
- Outline the nursing care of people who have problems associated with the reproductive tract.

Introduction

Reproduction of the human species is a complex activity that requires a series of integrated anatomical and physiological events. The physiological and anatomical aspects of the reproductive tract are predominately associated with procreation; the psychological and social aspects of reproduction are also important, as too is the pleasure that is often provided by the reproductive organs. Ill health in relation to the reproductive tract can result in loss of life, acute and chronic illness combined with physical and emotional distress.

The way an individual expresses themselves is a key aspect of reproductive health and this is often bound up in attitudes (the person's attitudes as well as the nurse's attitudes). Social norms and cultural upbringing will also impact on an individual's reproductive health; sexuality and sexual health are also closely linked to reproductive health.

This chapter provides an outline of the male and female reproductive tracts. A number of reproductive-related conditions and their associated nursing care are discussed.

Reproductive health

Reproductive health (a complex term) should be a right for all men and women and is a component of overall health throughout the life cycle regardless of the way the person chooses to express their sexuality; it is also an essential feature of human development. Reproductive health is defined by the United Nations (1994) as:

> A state of physical, mental, and social well-being in all matters relating to the reproductive system at all stages of life. Reproductive health implies that people are able to have a satisfying and safe sex life and that they have the capability to reproduce and the freedom to decide if, when, and how often to do so. . .

It is evident from this definition that individuals have rights; these rights are enshrined in UK and International Law. People have the right under the Human Rights Act 1998 (article 8) to the right to respect for private and family life. Reproductive health also includes the reproductive processes and functions necessary to reproduce.

There have been a number of groundbreaking developments and the introduction of new technologies over the recent years that are associated with reproduction; it could be suggested that these innovations have been in response to the national and global incidence of subfertility. For some members of our society having children and bringing up a family are important aspects of their lives and for those who experience fertility problems, this can be devastating, denying them their opportunity to realise their aspirations and hopes.

Reproductive health will also take into account issues associated with sexual health and personal relationships. The role of the nurse is multifaceted and one aspect of this role is to act as a health educator, promote good reproductive health, prevent ill health and support people who may experience problems. In order to care for a person or people who have reproductive health issues, and to be able to assess and plan care in an effective manner, the nurse must be familiar with the anatomy and physiology of the reproductive tract.

The pelvis

The male and female pelve (singular pelvis) differ, with the female pelvis being wider and more shallow than the male pelvis, the reason for this is so that the baby at childbirth can pass through it. The thickness of the bones of the pelvis also differs in the male and female. The female pelvic bones are thinner and more delicate than the male.

Generally, the pelvis is a ring of bone that supports the weight of the upper body. It can be described as a basin-shaped cavity. The bones of the pelvis are:

- the innominate bones
- the sacrum
- the coccyx

There are two innominate bones and both are made up of:

- the ilium
- the pubic bone
- the ischium

Towards the front of the pelvis (anteriorly) the bones join at the symphysis pubis. The sacrum and the coccyx come together at a joint that is moveable (inferiorly) – the sacrococcygeal joint (Thibodeau and Patton, 2007). Strong connective tissues (ligaments) join the pelvis to the sacrum at the base of the spine. Large nerves and muscle pass through the pelvis, and there are a number of digestive and reproductive organs housed in the pelvis. See Figure 14.1 for an illustration of the female pelvis.

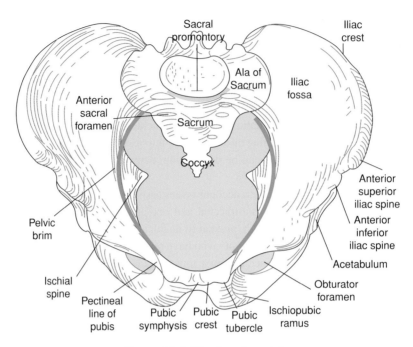

Figure 14.1 The female pelvis.

The female reproductive tract

Female external genitalia

The external genitalia are also known as the accessory structures of the female reproductive tract, which are external to the vagina. Collectively, they are known as the vulva or pudendum and consist of:

- mons pubis
- prepuce
- clitoris
- labia majora
- labia minora
- urethral orifice
- vagina
- Bartholin's glands

The aspects of the external genitalia are demonstrated in Figure 14.2.

There is a soft mound of fatty tissue covering the symphysis pubis at the front of the vulva – the **mons pubis**; post puberty this area is covered with pubic – hair. The **labia majora** extend to both sides of the vulva and are covered with pubic hair – these are two longitudinal prominent folds of tissue. The outer surface of the labia majora are covered by a thin layer of skin containing hair follicles, sweat

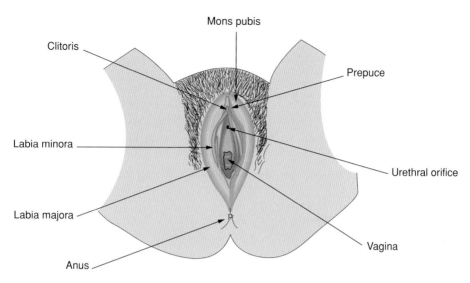

Figure 14.2 The female external genitalia (also known as the pudendum or vulva).

and sebaceous glands, and the inner surfaces are smoother, without pubic hair and contain a larger number of sebaceous follicles. Both labia majora and minora are protective structures protecting the inner structures of the vulva. Two soft folds of skin make up the **labia minora** within the labia majora and are situated either side of the opening of the vagina. The labia minora join close to the **prepuce**; these then cover the **clitoris** (the vulval vestibule) and extends backwards enclosing the urethral and vaginal orifices (Waugh and Grant, 2006). Connective, fatty and elastic tissues are what chiefly comprise the labia minora; there are no sweat glands or hair follicles as seen in the labia majora, but there are, however, sebaceous glands present. The size and colour of the labia minora will change in response to sexual stimulation.

The clitoris (a sexual organ) is situated where the labia meet near the anterior folds of the labia minora; it is situated above the urethral and vaginal orifices. The clitoris is composed of erectile tissue; it is a small rounded area enclosed in fibrous membranes in layers; it is homologous to the penis and it originates embryologically from the same tissue that forms the penis.

The clitoris becomes enlarged, erect and sensitive during sexual stimulation; the clitoris initiates and elevates sexual tension levels, and functions solely to bring about sexual pleasure. It is possible for female orgasm to occur when the clitoris is stimulated.

The **Bartholin's glands** are situated slightly below and to the left and right to the opening of the vagina (Marieb, 2007). As the female becomes sexually aroused, these glands secrete lubrication in the form of mucus; it is suggested that this can facilitate intercourse and allows for sexual stimulation; however, the exact purpose is not fully understood. The secretions are known to contain pheromones; these are chemicals that can trigger a natural behavioural response in another person. Usually, the Bartholin's glands cannot be felt (palpated); however, in the event of obstruction, cyst formation can occur and the cysts may become infected resulting in abscess formation. It must be noted that not all Bartholin's cysts are the result of an infection.

The fundus	The thick muscular region that is situated above the insertion of the fallopian tubes
The body (sometimes called the corpus)	The main aspect of the uterus joined to the cervix by an **isthmus** of tissue
The cervix	This is the narrower lower segment of the uterus, with an external **os** extending into the vagina

Table 14.1 The three main aspects of the uterus

Female internal genitalia

The four organs of the female reproductive tract will be discussed:

- fallopian tubes
- ovaries
- vagina
- uterus

The uterus is said to be a dense, muscular, pear-shaped hollow organ and is approximately 7.5 cm long. It is situated deep in the pelvic cavity located between the urinary bladder and the rectum; it also touches sigmoid colon and the small intestines. The uterus has three main parts (see Table 14.1). Figure 14.3 provides an illustration of the uterus.

The cavity of the uterus is continuous (**laterally**) with the lumen of the fallopian tubes and narrows as it reaches the cervix, it creates a triangular, pear shape. The size of the uterus varies amongst women; during pregnancy, the uterus changes the size, shape, structure and position (Meredith *et al.*, 2006).

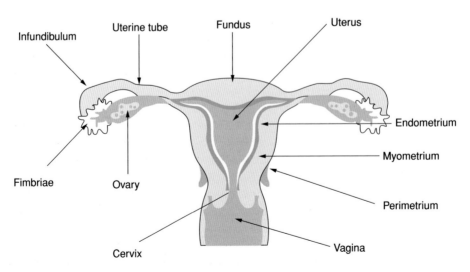

Figure 14.3 The uterus and associated structure.

The perimetrium	This layer is the peritoneum and fascial outer layer; it supports the uterus within the pelvis. Sometimes this is called the parietal peritoneum
The myometrium	This layer is the middle layer and is composed of smooth muscle. The muscles in the myometrium stretch during pregnancy to allow for the growing fetus and contract during labour. After delivery the myometrium contracts further to expel the placenta and to control blood loss
The endometrium	This is the inner lining of the uterus and has a mucus lining. The surface is continuous with the vagina and the uterine tubes. During menstruation the layers of the endometrium **slough** away from the inner layer. During the menstrual cycle the endometrium thickens and becomes rich with blood vessels and glandular tissue

Table 14.2 The three distinct layers of the uterus

Postpartum, it usually returns to its normal shape and size within 6–8 weeks. The uterus has three layers (see Table 14.2 and Figure 14.3).

A direct route exists from the vagina through the cervix, uterus and the fallopian tubes to the peritoneum as there is an opening of the uterus near the fundus into the **lumen** of the fallopian tubes.

The cervix (a Latin word for neck) is the lower constricted segment of the uterus; it is conical in shape and is a little wider in the middle than it is at the lower or upper ends; it joins to form the upper aspect of the vagina (see Figure 14.4).

The ectocervix is the aspect of the cervix that projects into the vagina and has an epithelial surface. The opening of the cervix is known as the external **os** and opens to the endocervical canal; the canal terminates at the internal **os**. The cervix provides a channel for discharge of the menstrual fluid; it secretes secretions to assist in the transport of semen; during labour, it dilates to allow the passage of the fetus.

The fallopian tubes (also known as the salpinges) are two fine tubes that lead from the ovaries into the uterus and they range from 8 to 14 cm long (Marieb, 2007). Collectively, the fallopian tubes, ovaries and support tissues are known as the adnexa. The key functions of the fallopian tubes are to provide a site for fertilisation and transport of the ovum to the uterus; this allows sperm and ova to meet for fertilisation in the tube. The ova are transported along the tube by the action of **cilia** and **peristalsis**. The fallopian tubes terminate at or near one ovary becoming a structure called the fimbria (see Figure 14.3).

The egg-producing organs are called the ovaries; they are the size and shape of a large almond and the two of them are situated on either side of the uterus. As well as being the reproductive organs they are also endocrine glands. The ovaries are homologous to the testes in the male.

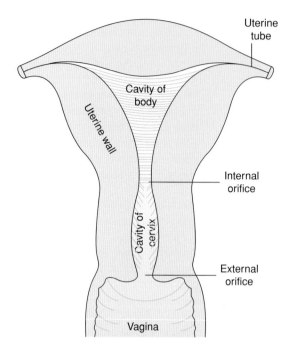

Figure 14.4 The cervix – ectocervix, internal **os** and external **os**.

When a girl is born, each ovary will contain approximately 200 000–400 000 follicles – these are all the eggs that she will ever possess; the follicles are the shells of each egg. As the girl reaches puberty, the number of follicles will gradually decline, i.e. at puberty the number is between 100 000 and 200 000, and as the woman ages the number of follicles will continue to decline.

As the girl reaches puberty she begins to ovulate – her first menstruation is termed as the menarche (Sutherland, 2001). Ovulation is the release of a ripe, mature egg from the ovaries every month until the menopause, a term used to describe the cessation of the menstrual cycle. Ovulation occurs as the body prepares the woman to become pregnant. If pregnancy does not occur, the woman has a menstrual period and the cycle begins again. The cycle is complex and is under the control of reproductive hormonal system.

The menstrual cycle

The cycle begins when a gland in the brain (the pituitary gland) releases a hormone called follicle-stimulating hormone (FSH); this hormone causes approximately 20 eggs to begin to grow and mature in the ovaries. The eggs grow within the follicle (its own shell) and FSH causes the follicle to produce oestrogen, and as the levels of oestrogen (another hormone) increase FSH production is stopped. The number of follicles produced monthly is limited to only one egg containing follicle that will continue to grow and mature, the others die off (Marieb, 2007; Porth, 2005).

The next stage in the cycle occurs when the egg becomes mature; at this stage the pituitary gland then produces another hormone called luteinising hormone (LH), and this hormone causes the follicle

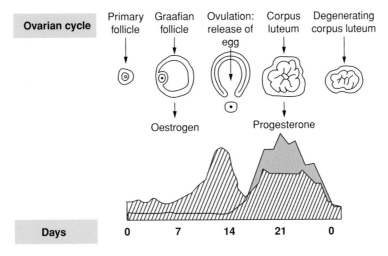

Figure 14.5 The menstrual cycle (ovarian).

to burst and the egg is released from the ovary. The follicle is now empty and becomes known as the corpus luteum; oestrogen continues to be produced by the corpus luteum and it then begins to produce another hormone called progesterone (Hubbard and Mechan, 1997; Thibodeau and Patton, 2007). The role of progesterone at this stage is to begin to prepare the uterus to receive a fertilised egg.

The lining of the uterus (the endometrium) responds to the effects of oestrogen and progesterone and starts to thicken, resulting in a soft, nourishing environment for the fertilised egg. Implantation occurs as a result of the two hormones and the egg attaches itself to the endometrium. When implantation is successful, the egg then begins to divide by meiosis, forming cells and tissues that will eventually become a human being. See Figure 14.5 for a diagrammatic representation of the ovarian aspect of the menstrual cycle.

If fertilisation fails to occur (and there are many reasons why) then the egg will pass into the uterus and dissolves. When the hormone production slows down, the endometrial lining begins to break down and **sloughs** off; this then passes through the cervix and vagina and is known as menstruation. The menstrual cycle is said to begin from the first day of one menstrual period until the start of another one, that is on an average from 22 to 45 days (Carter and Lewen, 2005).

The female breast

The female breasts are usually considered as accessory organs of the reproduction and play a key role in nurturing the young when milk is produced. Structurally, the male breast is identical to the female breast but less prominent; male and female breasts develop embryologically from the same tissue (Marieb, 2007). Figure 14.6 demonstrates a cross-sectional view of the female breast.

The breast is composed of lobes. The lobes contain glandular tissue and fat; breasts are modified sweat glands that produce milk (lactation), and the hormone **prolactin** is produced by the pituitary gland at the end of pregnancy stimulating the glandular tissue to lactate (Marieb, 2007). The glandular tissue is further stimulated when the infant suckles at the breast resulting in contraction, transporting

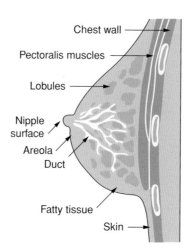

Figure 14.6 A cross-sectional view of the female breast.

the milk via the ducts to the nipple. The breasts are covered with skin and each breast contains a nipple surrounded by a pink to dark brown tissue called the areola. The areola contains a number of sebaceous glands. Marieb (2007) suggests that the role of sebum produced by the sebaceous glands is to reduce chapping and cracking of the skin of the nipple.

During the menstrual cycle, some women may experience changes in their breasts; they may become enlarged and tender. In the premenstrual period in response to the increasing levels of oestrogen and progesterone the breasts may enlarge and become tender or nodular. After menstruation this growth reverts.

Menstrual disorders

Some women may experience problems with their menstrual cycle and this can include:

- irregular periods
- excessive pain
- excessive bleeding

This aspect of the chapter addresses some of these problems.

Diseases of the reproductive tract

On completion of this section, the reader will be able to:

- Discuss the normal and abnormal pathophysiological changes that can occur in association with the male and female reproductive tracts.
- Outline the nursing care of people who have problems associated with the reproductive tract.

Dysmenorrhoea

Dysmenorrhoea is defined as the pain that occurs during menstruation (McQueen, 2006). During the menstrual cycle, the women may experience pain in the abdomen, and the pain can be so severe that it can impinge on her ability to perform the activities of daily living such as going to work; often it is because the woman is unable to carry out her activities of daily living that she may seek help. Jones (2004) states that approximately 40–50% of menstruating women experience dysmenorrhoea and that it is the most common cause of absenteeism amongst young women.

Prior to the period beginning the breasts may feel large and ache. Some pain during the menstrual period is normal but extreme pain is not; women can experience pain prior to and during the menstrual period, and it tapers off towards the end of the period. The pain can be sharp, intermittent or a dull ache and is felt predominantly in the pelvic region/lower abdomen; it may also be felt in the back and thighs and can be described as 'dragging'. The abdomen may become distended and can be tender to touch, and constipation can occur. The woman experiences severe blood loss and can become incapacitated. Two types of dysmenorrhoea have been described:

- primary dysmenorrhoea
- secondary dysmenorrhoea

Primary dysmenorrhoea

This refers to menstrual pain that is a result of physiological activities of menstruation accompanied with muscle contraction. Wright and Solange (2003) suggest that this type of pain exists in women who are otherwise healthy. Women in the younger age bracket (late teens to early 20s) experience primary dysmenorrhoea more than older women do. Procter *et al.* (2002) suggest that the duration of pain is usually between 8 and 72 hours.

Secondary dysmenorrhoea

In contrast to primary dysmenorrhoea, secondary dysmenorrhoea is attributed to some form of organic pelvic disease (underlying pelvic pathology). In secondary dysmenorrhoea, there is evidence of an underlying disease process or some form or structural abnormality within or outside of the uterus. Secondary dysmenorrhoea is uncommon before the age of 25 years (Rees, 2003). The most common cause is due to endometriosis.

Risk factors

Increased risk is associated with those who are in the younger age group and if they have a past medical history that is listed in Box 14.1.

Pathophysiology

Excessive levels of **prostaglandin** are closely related to dysmenorrhoea, and prostaglandins are produced by the uterus during the menses. Prostaglandins are released during menstruation due to the breakdown of the endometrial cells and the release of their contents. The increased production of prostaglandins that the uterus produces results in intense uterine contractions (uterine hypercontractility); the uterus can go in to spasm and the muscle (the endometrium) becomes **ischaemic** producing

Box 14.1 Medical conditions associated with increased risk

- Early age of menarche
- **Nulliparous**
- Obesity
- Cigarette smoking
- Alcohol consumption
- Family history of dysmenorrhoea
- Pelvic infection (i.e. pelvic inflammatory disease)
- History of (or current) sexually transmitted infection
- Endometriosis
- Leiomyomas
- Use of an intrauterine device

Source: Adapted from Heffner and Schust (2006), Andrews and Steele (2005) and Cotton *et al.* (2003).

uterine pain that is similar to the pain experienced in angina (see Chapter 5). The excessive amount of prostaglandin can also cause the women to experience:

- nausea
- vomiting
- diarrhoea
- faintness
- headache
- lower backache

The reason why some women produce excessive prostaglandin is unknown (Linhart, 2007); prostaglandins have been found to be much higher in those women with excessive menstrual pain as opposed to those who feel moderate to no pain. Andrews and Steele (2005) point out that there may be other causes of dysmenorrhoea, for example congenital abnormalities, and these may need to be investigated. Table 14.3 outlines the differences between primary and secondary dysmenorrhoea.

Diagnosis

Diagnosis is made by taking a full nursing and medical history from the woman. The nurse should pay particular attention to the type of pain the woman describes, the duration and what (if any) remedies she uses to alleviate the pain.

Diagnosis may be confirmed by:

- ultrasound
- hysterosalpingogram
- laparoscopy
- laparotomy

	Primary dysmenorrhoea	Secondary dysmenorrhoea
Age at symptom onset	Adolescence	Mid- to late 20s
Pain at other times of menstrual cycle	First 2–3 days of period	Persists beyond first 2–3 days of period
Other types of pain?	No	Dyspareunia

Source: Adapted Mazza (2004).

Table 14.3 Primary and secondary dysmenorrhoea – distinctions

Nursing care and management

Controlling the pain associated with dysmenorrhoea is a primary nursing intervention. Medications such as those that include non-steroidal anti-inflammatory drugs (NSAIDs) such as ibuprofen, mefenamic acid and naproxen are very effective in the treatment of the pain that is associated with dysmenorrhoea. NSAIDs are able to inhibit the synthesis of prostaglandin (Andrews and Steele, 2005). The nurse must be aware that some patients are unable to take NSAIDs as they have the ability to cause:

- gastrointestinal bleeding
- nephrotoxicity
- nausea
- vomiting
- dyspepsia
- headache

It must also be remembered that these drugs are contraindicated in patients who have:

- aspirin-induced asthma
- peptic ulcer
- renal disease
- clotting disorders

NSAIDs in this context are used to prevent pain rather than acting as an analgesic and the woman should be told that she should take the NSAID as soon as she knows that the period is imminent or as soon as the bleeding begins; the medication should be taken on regular basis for the first 1–3 days of the period as they prevent pain.

The oral contraceptive pill according to Mazza (2004) is an effective first-line agent for the treatment of primary dysmenorrhoea when NSAIDs have failed (Wolf and Schumann, 1999). In those women where the oral contraceptive pill or NSAIDs do not work (and this may be in approximately 10–20%), transdermal glyceryl trinitrate patches may be of benefit (Jones, 2004). The patches (containing glyceryl trinitrate) can cause relaxation of uterine contractions (French, 2005).

Second-line treatment such as oral contraceptives may be effective in treating primary dysmenorrhoea as they have the potential to block ovulation and reduce blood flow to the uterus. Another prostaglandin inhibitor is vitamin E. The aim of treatment in secondary dysmenorrhoea is to identify and correct the underlying organic cause. The options available may include surgical intervention and/or pharmacological intervention.

As stated, the treatment of secondary dysmenorrhoea will depend on identifying the underlying cause. Pelvic inflammatory disease (PID) is a cause of secondary dysmenorrhoea, and if this is the case then the PID should be treated to relieve the symptoms associated with secondary dysmenorrhoea.

There are a number of non-pharmacological treatments that may help the women. Transcutaneous electrical nerve stimulation (TENS) can help with or without pharmacological analgesics (Procter *et al.*, 2002). Acupuncture may be of value; however, there is insufficient evidence to determine the effectiveness of acupuncture in reducing pain.

In rare cases surgical intervention may be required for some women. Hysterectomy according to Walgrove (2001) can be a success in the terms of relieving women of their presenting symptoms. Rosevear (2002) suggest that this is preformed once childbearing is complete.

Some women may find comfort in the use of a hot water bottle. Exercise can have the effects of releasing endogenous endorphins – these are the bodies' own analgesic (Cassidy, 2001).

Amenorrhoea

Amenorrhoea, the absence of periods which can occur:

■ prior to the menarche
■ after the menopause
■ during pregnancy
■ postoperatively
■ posttreatment

Primary amenorrhoea occurs prior to the menses happening and secondary amenorrhoea occurs when menstruation has previously taken place but has stopped for at least 6 consecutive months in a woman who has had regular periods (McIver *et al.*, 1997).

The most common cause of secondary amenorrhoea is pregnancy. Other causes according to the Royal College of Obstetricians and Gynaecologists (2003) include:

■ polycystic ovary syndrome
■ hypothalamic causes – and these are due to excessive weight loss (anorexia) or excessive exercise
■ hyperprolactinaemia – an elevated level of **prolactin** in the blood, in women this may be caused a **prolactinoma**
■ contraception – contraceptive pill and depot injection

Diagnosis

The nurse must undertake a full nursing, medical and menstrual history, including:

■ sexual history in order to rule out pregnancy
■ family history to determine if there are any genetic abnormalities
■ the presence of any associated illness such as hypothyroidism, diabetes mellitus
■ emotional upsets
■ changes in body weight
■ increase in exercise
■ drug history, for example contraceptive pill/injection, chemotherapy
■ previous surgery

In all women who present with amenorrhoea it may be advisable to perform a pregnancy test. In secondary amenorrhoea, a number of blood tests may be carried out in order to assess levels of hormones such as, FSH, LH as well assessment of thyroid function. **Prolactin** levels will also need assessment to determine if there is an evidence of hyperprolactinaemia. A pelvic ultrasound can demonstrate the presence of polycystic ovaries (enlarged ovaries), and magnetic resonance imaging (MRI) or computer tomography (CT) scans can identify pituitary tumour; if these are suspected a hysteroscopy may be required.

Nursing care and management

The role and function of the nurse is to provide the women with emotional as well as physical support, providing her with information that she is able to understand in order to make informed decisions about her treatment and treatment options. The nurse is ideally placed to discuss with the women lifestyle issues such as smoking and alcohol consumption, stress-reducing activities, providing information about diet and weight gain (if needed), and the balance between excessive and therapeutic levels of exercise. The woman may need support in relation to the perceived threat to her self-esteem and with concerns associated with fertility as a result of amenorrhoea. Explanations should be provided about the type of investigations that may be required and the reason why they are being performed. The treatment required will depend on the cause. Surgical intervention or hormone replacement therapy may be needed.

Menorrhagia

The term *menorrhagia* is defined as bleeding in excess of 80 mL (Andrews and Steele, 2005); on an average, women lose approximately 35 mL of blood with each period (Mazza, 2004); some people refer to menorrhagia as heavy periods. The heavy period can interfere with a woman's physical, social, emotional and/or material quality of life (National Institute for Health and Clinical Excellence (NICE), 2007a).

Diagnosis

A full nursing, medical and menstrual history will need to be undertaken by the nurse in order to offer the woman appropriate and effective treatment, the aim of any intervention should be to improve the woman's quality of life. Questions to be asked will include:

- How much bleeding occurs (how often are tampons/sanitary pads changed)?
- Are there any blood clots?
- How long do periods last?
- Does bleeding occur after sex?
- Is there any pelvic pain?
- Is there any bleeding between periods?
- Are there any other related symptoms?

A physical examination will need to be undertaken and this can include an internal examination as well as an external abdominal examination (palpation). The person carrying out the examination can identify, for example, if there are any indications of **fibroids**.

There are a variety of tests and investigations may be undertaken in order to determine why the woman is experiencing menorrhagia. Blood testing will determine if the women is anaemic or has a blood clotting disorder.

An ultrasound scan may be required as this may determine if there are any structural abnormalities. In some instances, a biopsy may be needed to exclude any potential disorders, for example endometrial cancer. If the ultrasound demonstrates that there are abnormalities (or it is inconclusive), then hysteroscopy can be performed to aid diagnosis or to determine the exact location of the fibroid.

Nursing care and management

If the ultrasound examination and the biopsy demonstrate that there are no obvious problems with the uterus, then a pharmacological approach to treatment may be considered. Table 14.4 outlines the different kinds of drugs that may be used in the treatment of menorrhagia. The woman must be provided with all the information she requires to make an informed decision; however, for some women hormonal contraception as a form of treatment may be unacceptable, for example she may have religious reasons for this or she wish to conceive. The woman may need to be treated with hormone replacement; she might also require other interventions such as counselling.

When the pharmacological approach fails or is unacceptable, surgical intervention may be recommended after the woman has been given the opportunity to review and agree any treatment decision. The nurse should ensure that sufficient time has been provided and appropriate support given to the women during the decision-making process. There are several interventions that need to be given consideration. Table 14.5 outlines the alternatives.

If surgical intervention is required, the woman (and her family) will need support; this can be physical and psychological support as well as socioeconomical support. The nurse is central when the coordination of services is required, and a coordinated multidisciplinary approach is advocated with the women at the centre of it.

The information provided to the woman must be provided in a format she understands, and it must also be relevant to her circumstances; this may mean that the information may need to be translated into her mother tongue. Information must point out the risks and benefits of the various treatments and procedures being offered, and opportunity must be provided for the woman to ask questions and it must be emphasised that she can if she wishes change her mind as well as her entitlement to a second opinion.

The male reproductive tract

The male reproductive tract is designed to produce spermatozoa and deposit it inside the female vagina; this contributes to reproduction. The spermatozoa are responsible for the fertilisation of the female egg. Unlike the female genitalia, male genitalia are found primarily outside of the body (see Figure 14.7).

Male genitalia

The penis and scrotum comprise the male external genitalia. Within the scrotal sac, a loose bag-like sac of skin, suspended by the spermatic cord in between the thighs, are the testes. They are approximately the size of a walnut – 4.5 cm long, 2.5 cm in breadth and 3 cm diameter; they feel smooth and move freely within the scrotal sac (Hubbard and Mechan, 1997). The testes are found outside of the abdominal cavity in the scrotum; however, they begin their development in the abdominal cavity and normally descend into the scrotal sac during the last 2 months of fetal development. The testes traverse the inguinal canal and inguinal rings and into the scrotum where they are suspended.

Drug	What it is?	How it works?	Possible unwanted effects	Comments
Levonorgestrel – a hormone	A small plastic device that is placed in the uterus, slowly releasing progestogen	The hormone prevents the lining of the uterus from growing too quickly	■ Irregular bleeding ■ Breast tenderness ■ Acne ■ Headaches ■ Amenorrhoea	This is also a contraceptive. First-line treatment
Tranexamic acid	Tablet format. The medication is taken from the start of the menstrual period for up to 4 days	Promotes clot formation within the uterus thus reduces the amount of bleeding	■ Indigestion ■ Headaches ■ Diarrhoea	If symptoms do not improve within 3 months, treatment should be stopped. Considered as second-line treatment
Non-steroidal anti-inflammatories (NSAIDs)	Tablet format. Medication to be taken from the start of the menstrual period or just before and until heavy bleeding stops	Prostaglandin production is reduced	■ Indigestion ■ Diarrhoea	If symptoms do not improve within 3 months, treatment should be stopped
Combined oral contraceptives	Pill format that contains the hormones progestogen and oestrogen. One pill is taken for 21 days then stopped for 7 days and the cycle is repeated	Prevents the menstrual cycle from occurring	■ Mood change ■ Headache ■ Nausea ■ Fluid retention ■ Breast tenderness	This is also a contraceptive. Considered as second-line treatment

Table 14.4 Drugs that may be used in the treatment of menorrhagia

(Continued)

Drug	What it is?	How it works?	Possible unwanted effects	Comments
Oral progesterone (norethisterone)	Tablets taken 2–3 times per day from the 5th to 26th day of the menstrual cycle	Prevents the lining of the uterus is from growing too quickly	■ Weight gain ■ Bloating ■ Breast tenderness ■ Headache ■ Acne	This is also a contraceptive. Considered as third-line treatment
Injected or implanted progesterone	The hormone progestogen is injected or implanted. The implant releases the hormone slowly for 3 years	Prevents the lining of the uterus is from growing too quickly	■ Weight gain ■ Bloating ■ Breast tenderness ■ Headache ■ Acne ■ Irregular bleeding ■ Amenorrhoea ■ Bone density loss can occur	This is also a contraceptive. Considered as third-line treatment
Gonadotrophin-releasing hormone analogue	An injection that stops the body producing oestrogen and progesterone	Prevents the menstrual cycle from occurring	■ Menopause-like symptoms (hot flushes, increased sweating, vaginal dryness)	Considered as third-line treatment

Source: Adapted NICE (2007b).

Table 14.4 (*Continued*)

Proposed surgical intervention	What it is?	Possible unwanted effects	Comments
Endometrial **ablation**: ■ Thermal balloon endometrial **ablation** (TBEA) ■ Impedance-controlled bipolar radiofrequency **ablation** ■ Microwave endometrial **ablation** (MEA) ■ Free fluid thermal **ablation**	A device is inserted in all techniques through the vagina and cervix into the uterus. When the device is in situ several methods can be used to heat the device, for example, by using radio energy microwaves. The purpose is to destroy the lining of the uterus	■ Vaginal discharge ■ Increased pain during the menstrual period ■ Infection	In some women the procedure may need to be repeated as the lining of the uterus can grow back. This procedure is not suitable if the woman wishes to become pregnant
Uterine artery embolisation (UAE)	This procedure aims to block blood supply to the uterus. Small particles are injected in to the blood vessels that take blood to the uterus with the aim of blocking any blood supply to fibroids in the expectation that they shrink	■ Vaginal discharge ■ Pain ■ Nausea ■ Vomiting	There may be need for further surgery. Women undertaking this procedure may be able to become pregnant
Myomectomy	Surgical removal of a fibroid can performed either through an abdominal incision or via the vagina. The vaginal route necessitates the use of a hysteroscope	■ Adhesions and as a result a possibility of pain and impaired fertility ■ Infection ■ Perforation of the uterus	Women undertaking this procedure may be able to become pregnant
Hysterectomy	There are two main methods of performing a hysterectomy – vaginally or abdominally. In total hysterectomy the uterus and cervix are removed, whereas in subtotal hysterectomy only the uterus is removed	■ Haemorrhage during or after surgery ■ Infection ■ Damage to adjacent organs, for example, bowel or urinary tract ■ Urinary/faecal dysfunction	Women wishing to undertake hysterectomy will not be able to become pregnant. Removal of the uterus means the women will no longer have a menstrual period

Table 14.5 Potential surgical treatments for women with heavy periods

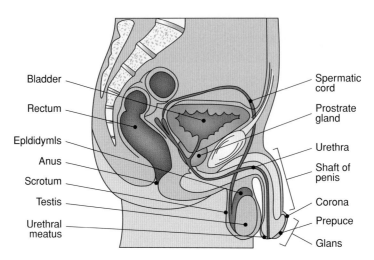

Figure 14.7 The male reproductive system.

It is normal for one testes to hang lower than the other. As the cremasteric muscle contracts the spermatic cord (to which it is attached) shorten and the testes moves up towards the abdomen; the result of this is that it provides the testes with more warmth. For proper development of sperm, the testes must be at a lower temperature than the body; this is the reason the testes are situated outside of the body.

The testes have two functions – to secrete the hormone testosterone, which is responsible for the development of the male secondary sex characteristics (deep voice, beard growth, body hair), as well as the function of the male reproductive system in the production of spermatozoa (Tortora and Grabowski, 2006). The testes are the essential organs of reproduction.

The composition of the testes, contained under a membranous shell, is glandular tissue that is composed of several lobules differing in size to their location. The lobule consists of approximately 660–1200 seminiferous tubules that are small convoluted structures, responsible for the production of sperm. The spermatozoa develop in different stages in different parts of the tubules. The tubules form sperm continuously; in a young man, sperm is produced at the rate of 120 million per day. The sperm travel from the seminiferous tubules to the rete testes, to the efferent ducts onwards to the epididymis where spermatogenesis takes place and newly created mature sperm cells are formed. Spermatogenesis is complex and according to Heffner and Schust (2006), this can be divided into three phases:

- mitotic proliferation to produce large number of cells
- meiotic division to produce genetic diversity
- maturation, preparing sperm for transit and penetration of the oocyte in the female tract

The sperm cells are then moved on to the vas deferens and expelled through the urethra as a result of rhythmic contractions.

Situated between the seminiferous tubules are cells called the Leydig cells, where testosterone and other androgens are formed. Box 14.2 provides details concerning physical changes in the male related to testosterone.

The penis is an external male reproductive organ, and within the penis is the urethra. The penis provides a route for the elimination of ejaculate and urine via the urethral orifice situated at the tip of the penis, the enlarged aspect is called the glans penis. The glans penis is homologous with the female **clitoris**.

Box 14.2 Some male changes related to testosterone

■ Increase in penile size
■ Enlargement of the scrotum
■ Growth in the size of the testes
■ Enlargement of the larynx and deepening of the voice
■ Increased muscle mass
■ Increase in basal metabolic rate
■ Increase in sebaceous glands
■ Thickening of the bones

The penis is made up of three columns of erectile tissue:

■ two corpora cavernosa
■ one corpus spongiosum

The end of the corpus spongiosum is the bulbous glans penis; the glans is covered with a thin layer of skin that allows for erection and in uncircumcised males the skin at the glans folds over on itself to form the **prepuce** or foreskin; the area where the foreskin is attached, underneath the penis, is called the frenulum, which is homologous with the female clitoral hood. The urethra, the terminal end of the urinary tract, lies on the tip of the glans and is known as the urethral meatus. Erection requires complex vascular activity – dilation of the arteries supplying blood to the penis and sympathetic nervous system activity.

The prostate gland is said to be approximately 2.5 cm in length and lies at the base of the urinary bladder surrounded by the upper part of the urethra (Marieb, 2007; Spark, 2000). The function of the prostate gland is not well understood. The gland is described as chestnut-shaped and is made up of 20–30 compound tubular–alveolar glands; these glands are embedded in a mass of smooth muscle and dense connective tissue. A thin milky fluid is secreted adding bulk to semen on ejaculation. Prostatic fluid accounts for approximately one-third of semen volume. During orgasm, sperm cells are transmitted from the urethra via the ejaculatory ducts that are situated in the prostate gland, and smooth muscle within the prostate gland contract during ejaculation helping to expel semen.

Male reproductive disorders

This aspect of the chapter discusses four common male reproductive tract disorders:

■ phimosis
■ paraphimosis
■ hydrocele
■ **benign** and **malignant** prostate cancer

It is not possible in chapter of this size to outline in depth all of the details associated with these disorders. The reader is advised to delve deeper into the subject area in order to gain more comprehensive insight into the care and management of men with reproductive tract disorders.

Phimosis

Phimosis occurs when the opening of the foreskin (or **prepuce**) is unable to be retracted behind the glans penis; the foreskin is too tight for retraction. Phimosis can be congenital or it can occur as result of infection, inflammation or trauma (Warshaw, 2007). Brewster *et al.* (2001) suggest that it is most frequently due to a condition known as balanitis xerotica obliterans (BXO), the cause of which is unknown. BXO (sometimes called lichen sclerosis) is a fibrosing condition resulting in thick (sclerosing) scaring of the skin of the penis, because of which the skin becomes discoloured.

Diagnosis

As the foreskin cannot be retracted this may result in poor hygiene and the man with phimosis may present with balanoposthitis. The glans penis becomes infected (balanitis); and the foreskin also becomes infected (posthitis); the patient may complain of itching and irritation, pain, discomfort, bleeding at sexual intercourse or masturbation, white discharge (smegma) and in some instances there may be dysuria and retention of urine due to restriction of the foreskin. Urethral stenosis and inflammation can also occur.

Nursing care and management

The nurse must carry out a holistic assessment of individual needs and provide appropriate health promotion activity by teaching the patient and reinforcing the need for good personal hygiene. If infection is present, then prescribed antibiotic therapy is the first line of treatment along with an antifungal preparation (if required); analgesia will also be required. Hot baths may also aid in reducing the swelling cause by infection. The nurse must ascertain if the man is sexually active; if this is the case, his partner may also require treatment; if a barrier method of contraception is not being used then the use of a condom for sexual intercourse should be advocated to prevent transmission of infection.

In severe cases of foreskin restriction, for example when urinary retention occurs, an emergency circumcision may need to be performed. Postcircumcision, the nurse must promote wound healing, a non-adherent dressing is required and patient education focusing on ways to reduce inflammation are required, the man should be taught how to perform personal hygiene. The penis should be bathed at least daily in warm soapy water and the non-adherent dressing reapplied in order to prevent clothing disturbing wound healing. The nurse should explain what the signs of infection are and the patient should be told that if excessive bleeding occurs he should contact his general practice or accident and emergency department. Sexual intercourse and masturbation should cease until after the wound has healed.

Paraphimosis

Conversely, paraphimosis occurs when the foreskin is retracted over the glans penis and forms a constriction near the base of the glans. The cause is usually related to failure of the foreskin to return to its usual position covering the glans penis after manipulation had occurred. The band of foreskin that is retracted becomes swollen and can cause compression of the blood vessels supplying the glans – as circulation is reduced, pain can occur. Downey (2000) suggests that paraphimosis can be classed as a medical emergency as gangrene of the penis can occur.

In an attempt to relieve the swelling cold compresses can be applied to the penis and the foreskin may be able to be manipulated back over the glans penis. Analgesia, oral and/or topical, can be applied to help with manipulation. If manipulation fails then a **dorsal** slit may be made in the foreskin, and circumcision may be advised at a later date as recurrence can occur.

When assisting those men who are unable to carry out the activities living independently, for example when assisting with personal hygiene and when performing catheter care, the nurse must ensure that the foreskin (in uncircumcised men) is fully retracted to cover the glans penis. This can also apply to those men who may be confused or those who have decreased sensation in the penis.

Hydrocele

A hydrocele occurs when there is collection of fluid in the membranous sac that surrounds the testes within the scrotum; typically a hydrocele appears **unilaterally**. A hydrocele can occur spontaneously and the cause may be unknown, or it can be the result of inflammatory conditions such as epididymitis or orchitis, inflammation of the epididymis or testes (respectively); trauma may also cause hydrocele. In some cases, the cause may be the result of a testicular tumour.

Diagnosis

A detailed nursing and medical history will need to be taken asking the patient about any recent injury or trauma, other medical conditions and his sexual history. The scrotum can swell to a considerable size and it is usually painless (**asymptomatic**), but the excessive swelling can cause discomfort. It becomes painful when the fluid surrounding the testes becomes infected. The patient may seek help because the size of the swelling can prevent him from enjoying and taking part in social activities such as swimming, running, walking and sexual activity. The swelling can progress and cause the blood supply to the testes to become compromised.

Examination of the contents of the scrotal sac reveals a dullness when the sac is percussed, the swelling feels smooth and is usually located in front of the testes. Differentiation between hydrocele and tumour can be verified by the use of illumination, i.e., a light source (transillumination) is used; a hydrocele allows the light to pass through whereas a tumour is dense and prevents this from occurring. Ultrasound may be required to determine if there is any underlying cause, for example testicular cancer.

Nursing care and management

Elevation of the scrotum by the wearing of a scrotal support may reduce the swelling. In most cases, however, the fluid will need to be drained off and a small **trocar** and cannula used to drain the fluid, as aspiration of the fluid carries with it the risk of infection. If the fluid is infected then the person will need prescribed antibiotics.

Hydrocelectomy (also known as hydrocele repair) is a surgical procedure that is used to correct a hydrocele; this can be performed with the patient attending the hospital on an outpatient basis. Postoperatively, the patient will be observed for any signs of haemorrhage, as there is a risk of infection, however, this is rare, and damage may occur to the spermatic vessels, which again this is rare.

Benign and malignant prostate cancer

As a man ages his prostate gland becomes larger, and as ageing progresses the gland atrophies and connective tissue accumulates; cancer of the prostate gland (**benign** and **malignant**) occurs slowly and as such the symptoms may occur over many years. This accumulation of connective tissue and **atrophy** is not usually due to cancer and when this occurs it is known as benign prostatic hyperplasia (BPH). BPH is the most common neoplastic growth in men; over 50% of men aged 60 years will have BPH and according to Thorpe and Neal (2003) not all of those men will have symptoms (they may be classed as **asymptomatic**).

Diagnosis

When symptoms are present they are the same for BPH and **malignant** prostate cancer and include:

- dysuria
- frequency of micturition
- urgency
- nocturia
- hesitancy

There may be a history of recurrent urinary tract infection and increasing urinary obstruction can cause back pressure leading to renal impairment. Acute urinary retention can occur if the prostate gland becomes enlarged and is further complicated if the gland is also infected (prostatitis). Pathological changes as a result of abnormal enlargement of the prostate gland or cell multiplication in either benign or malignant prostate cancer can occur; the key change is pressure caused by the enlarged gland on the prostatic urethra, which can (as discussed) lead to impeded urinary outflow (Kilstoff and Bonner, 2006). Over time urinary retention can impair urinary function and prostatic obstruction can result in:

- obstruction of the urethra
- **diverticulum** of the bladder
- **hydroureter**
- **hydronephrosis**
- infection
- renal failure

After a detailed nursing and medical history has been undertaken, diagnosis may be confirmed by digital rectal examination (DRE), transrectal ultrasound (TRUS), assessment of prostate-specific antigen (PSA) and other blood tests such as measurement of serum acid phosphatase.

Malignant cancer of the prostate gland can also cause the cells of the cancer to spread to other parts of the body (metastasise) and this occurs in particular to the bones as well as the lymph gland and lungs.

Care and management

The care and management of the man with prostate cancer is complex and will depend on the individual. There are a number of factors that must be given consideration and the nurse's role is to provide the man with the information he requires and in a format that he understands in order to make an informed decision. The staging of the cancer will reveal its size and how far it has spread. The treatment options for a cancer that is small and has not spread far will be different for a cancer that is large and has spread widely. The cells of the cancer are also examined under microscope (histology) and this then allows it to be graded. The more abnormal the cells, the higher the grade is likely to be; low-grade cancers usually spread more slowly. Other factors that need to be taken into account will include the age of the person and the results of the PSA, DRE and TRUS.

The following treatment options have been identified by Thorpe and Neal (2003), but it must be remembered that the treatment depends on the wishes of the individual person and if the cancer has spread or not:

- watchful waiting
- surgery
- laser therapy
- transurethral **ablation**
- transurethral microwave therapy
- **brachytherapy**

Chemotherapy, radiotherapy and hormone therapy are also considered, again depending on the individual person.

Surgical intervention may be required to remove the whole gland or the part of the gland that is causing the obstruction. The most common surgical procedure used for BPH is transurethral resection of the prostate gland (TURP). When TURP is performed a **cystoscope** is passed into the bladder to visualise the interior of the urinary bladder, a rectoscope is then passed and resection begins where small sections of the gland are chipped away removing the tissue that is compressing the urethra and the neck of the bladder.

Postoperatively, a three-way urethral catheter is in situ and the urinary bladder is continuously flushed out with a non-electrolyte solution to prevent blood clots from forming and the infusion of normal saline to irrigate the bladder. There are potential complications that can arise in association with surgery on the prostate gland, for example:

- haemorrhage
- infection
- clot retention
- deep vein thrombosis
- urethral stricture
- incontinence
- erectile dysfunction
- retrograde ejaculation

The nurse is required to ensure that the patient is kept pain free postoperatively; it is vital that a strict fluid balance is maintained and that catheter care is carried out making every effort to prevent infection. The patient should be encouraged to mobilise as soon as this is possible and his condition permits. If the patient is to be discharged home with his catheter in situ, he or she will need to be taught how to care for this, and referral will need to be made to the district nurse.

Conclusion

Reproduction of the human species is complex with the key function of the male and female reproductive tracts being associated with procreation. Whilst the physiological functions associated with reproduction are important, it is also essential that the nurse remembers that there is pleasure associated with the reproductive tract and that this component of a human being can also be important for a number of people.

This chapter has provided insight into the normal and abnormal anatomy and physiology as well as providing discussion on a number of pathological changes that may occur to both the male and female reproductive tracts. Emphasis has been placed on the provision of sound information provided in a format that the person understands in order to make complex decisions concerning treatment options and care pathways.

Multiple choice questions

1. The part of the internal lining of the uterus that is not shed during menstruation is:
(a) myometrium
(b) endometrium
(c) mesometrium
(d) endocardium

2. Prostate cancer is said to be:
(a) a disease of younger men
(b) a disease of both males and females
(c) a disease of older men
(d) a sexually transmitted infection

3. Nulliparous means:
(a) having given birth to twins
(b) having given birth to no children
(c) having given birth to triplets
(d) having given birth only to boys

4. Which of the following can be classed as a medical emergency?
(a) amenorrhoea
(b) paraphimois
(c) hydronephrosis
(d) hydroureter

5. The word cervix literally means:
(a) neck
(b) chest
(c) vagina
(d) fallopian tube

6. Why are the testes found outside of the body?
(a) to enhance sexual satisfaction
(b) to provide protection to the epididymis
(c) for the proper development of sperm
(d) to produce more sperm

7. What is a hydrocele?
(a) water in the knee joint
(b) excessive collection of water around the brain

(c) a collection of serous fluid in the scrotal sac

(d) presence of fluid in the lung

8. What is the correct term for removal of the uterus?

(a) oophorectomy

(b) myomectomy

(c) hysterectomy

(d) mastectomy

9. The fallopian tubes are also known as the:

(a) appendage

(b) pharynx

(c) salpinges

(d) os

10. What is a cystoscope?

(a) medication used in chemotherapy

(b) a type camera used to view the urinary bladder

(c) a type camera used to view the stomach

(d) a collection of fluid around the testes

Answers: 1.b, 2.c, 3.b, 4.b, 5.a, 6.c, 7.c, 8.c, 9.c, 10.b.

Test your knowledge

❷ List three causes of menstrual dysfunction.

❷ Explain how the nurse can improve the self-esteem of an individual who has experienced reproductive health problems.

❷ Explain how an enlarged prostate gland can cause difficulties with urinary output.

❷ Define the term *infertile* and list the possible causes.

❷ What advice would you give to a woman who is experiencing heavy and painful bleeding during her menstrual period?

Glossary of terms

Ablation: To destroy. Endometrial ablation, for example, means to destroy the layer of the cells that line the uterus.

Asymptomatic: Without symptoms.

Atrophy: Wasting away, a diminution in the size of a cell, tissue or organ.

Bartholin's glands: Two small round structures on either side of the vaginal opening. Secretion from these glands provide vaginal lubrication. The exact purpose of the fluid secreted is not fully understood.

Benign: Something that does not metastasise.

Brachytherapy: In prostate cancer, implantation of tiny radioactive seeds implanted under anaesthetic directly into the prostate gland.

Cilia: Small hair-like structures used to propel liquids.

Clitoris: A small body of tissue that is highly sexually sensitive, it is protected by the prepuce. Becomes enlarged and erect during sexual stimulation.

Cystoscope: A thin tube with a light and eye piece attached to it allowing the user to see the inside of the urinary bladder.

Diverticulum: A pouch or sac opening from a tubular or saccular organ, for example the urinary bladder.

Dorsal: Pertaining to the back, the rear aspect.

Dyspareunia: Pain with intercourse.

Fibroids: A non-cancerous growth in the uterus.

Hydronephrosis: An abnormal enlargement of the kidney that may be due to ureteral obstruction.

Hydroureter: Distension of the ureter with urine as a result of blockage.

Hysterosalpingogram: X-ray examination for the uterus and uterine tubes after radio-opaque dye has been injected.

Ischaemia: A low oxygen state. Usually, the result of and obstruction to the blood supply to tissues.

Isthmus: The main aspect of the uterus that is joined to the cervix by a neck of tissues.

Labia majora: The inner layers of the vulva thinner than the labia majora, protects the urethra, vagina and clitoris.

Labia minora: The outer lips of the vulva, covered with pubic hair containing sweat and sebaceous glands. Situated on either side of the vagina.

Laparoscopy: The passage of a laparoscope into the abdominal cavity via the abdominal wall to allow viewing of the cavity.

Laparotomy: A surgical procedure that requires an incision to be made into the abdomen.

Lumen: The space in the interior of a tubular structure such as the fallopian tubes.

Malignant: Tending to become progressively worse and to result in death.

Mons pubis: Also known as the mons veneris (Latin for the Hill of Venus, the Roman Goddess of love). Fatty tissue covering the symphysis pubis.

Nulliparous: Never having given birth.

Os: The mouth, a term applied to an opening in a hollow organ such as the cervix.

Peristalsis: A wave-like contraction.

Prepuce: In the female, it is also known as the clitoral hood. In the male, this is also known as the foreskin.

Prolactin: A hormone primarily associated with lactation. Secreted by the anterior pituitary gland.

Prolactinoma: A prolactin-producing tumour of the anterior pituitary gland, a slow-growing benign swelling.

Prostaglandin: A group of complex fatty acids present in the body acting messenger substances between cells. The effects of prostaglandin include the stimulation of smooth muscle, for example the uterus.

Slough: Dead tissue that has separated from the living structure.

Trocar: A sharp-pointed surgical instrument.

Unilateral: Affecting only one side as opposed to bilateral affecting both sides.

References

Andrews, G. and Steele, J. (2005). Common gynaecological problems. In: Andrews, G. (ed) *Women's Sexual Health*, 3rd edn. Edinburgh: Elsevier, pp. 513–546.

Brewster, S., Canston, D., Noble, J. and Reynard, J. (2001). *Urology: A Handbook for Medical Students*. Oxford: BIOS.

Carter, P.J. and Lewen, S. (2005). *Lippincott's Textbook for Nursing Assistants*. Philadelphia: Lippincott.

Cassidy, M. (2001). Dysmenorrhoea and puerperal pain. *The World of Irish Nursing*, July/August, 28–30.

Cotton, J., Jones, M. and Steggall, M. (2003). Nursing patients with sexual health and reproductive problems. In: Brooker, C. and Nicol, M. (eds) *Nursing Adult: The Practice of Caring*. Edinburgh: Mosby, pp. 705–769.

Downey, P. (ed) (2000). The penis and urethra. In: *Introduction to Urological Nursing*. London: Whurr, pp. 98–110.

French, L. (2005). Dysmenorrhoea. *American Family Physician*, 71(2), 285–291.

Heffner, L.J. and Schust, D.J. (2006). *The Reproductive System at a Glance*, 2nd edn. Massachusetts: Blackwell Publishing.

Hubbard, J. and Mechan, D. (1997). *The Physiology of Health and Illness with Related Anatomy*. Cheltenham: Stanley Thornes.

Jones, A.E. (2004). Managing the pain of primary and secondary dysmenorrhoea. *Nursing Times*, 100(10), 40–43.

Kilstoff, K. and Bonner, A. (2006). Renal health breakdown. In: Chang, E., Day, J. and Elliott, D. (eds) *Pathophysiology Applied to Nursing Practice*. Sydney: Mosby, pp. 169–199.

Linhart, J. (2007). Female reproductive problems. In: Monahan, F.D., Sand, J.K., Neighbors, M., Marek, J.F. and Green, C.J. (eds) *Phipps' Medical Surgical Nursing: Health and Illness Perspectives*, 8th edn. St. Louis: Mosby, pp. 1685–1720.

Marieb, E.N. (2007). *Human Anatomy and Physiology*, 4th edn. Menlo Park: Addison Wesley.

Mazza, D. (2004). *Women's Health in General Practice*. Edinburgh: Butterworth Heinemann.

Meredith, J., Battersby, S., Evans, M., Marsh, B. and Walker, A. (2006). *Oxford Handbook of Midwifery*. Oxford: Oxford University Press.

McIver, B., Romanski, S.A. and Nippoldt, T.B. (1997). Evaluation and management of amenorrhea. *Mayo Clinic Proceedings*, 72(12), 1161–1167.

McQueen, A.C.H. (2006). Disorders of the reproductive system and the breasts. In: Alexander, M.F., Fawcett, J.N. and Runciman, P.J. (eds) *Nursing Practice: Hospital and Home – the Adult*, 3rd edn. Edinburgh: Churchill Livingstone, pp. 253–356.

National Institute for Health and Clinical Excellence (2007a). *Heavy Menstrual Bleeding: NICE Clinical Guideline 44*. London: NICE.

National Institute for Health and Clinical Excellence (2007b). *Treatment and Care for Women with Heavy Periods*. London: NICE.

Porth, C.M. (2005). *Pathophysiology: A Concepts of Health States*, 7th edn. Philadelphia: Lippincott.

Procter, M.L., Smith, C.A., Farquhar, C.M. and Sones, R.W. (2002). *Transcutaneous Electrical Nerve Stimulation and Acupuncture for Primary Dysmenorrhoea. Cochrane Review*. Cochrane Library Issue 1. Chichester: Wiley.

Rees, M.C.P. (2003). Menstrual problems. In: Waller, D. and McPherson, A. (eds) *Women's Health*, 5th edn. Oxford: Oxford University Press, pp. 1–45.

Rosevear, S.K. (2002). *Handbook of Gynaecology Management*. Oxford: Blackwell.

Royal College of Obstetricians and Gynaecologists (2003). *Long Term Consequences of Polycystic Ovary Syndrome: Guidance Number 23*. London: RCOG.

Spark, R.F. (2000). *Sexual Health for Men: The Complete Guide*. Massachusetts: Perseus.

Sutherland, C. (2001). *Women's Health: A Handbook for Nurses*. Edinburgh: Churchill Livingstone.

Thibodeau, G.A. and Patton, K.T. (2007). *Anatomy and Physiology*, 6th edn. St. Louis: Mosby.

Thorpe, A. and Neal, D. (2003). Benign prostatic hyperplasia. *Lancet*, *361*(9366), 1359–1367.

Tortora, G.J. and Grabowski, S.R. (2006). *Principles of Anatomy and Physiology*, 11th edn. New York: Wiley.

Walgrove, H. (2001). Hysterectomy. *Nursing Standard*, *15*(29), 47–53.

Warshaw, M.K. (2007). Male reproductive problems. In: Monahan, F.D., Sand, J.K., Neighbors, M., Marek, J.F. and Green, C.J. (eds) *Phipps' Medical Surgical Nursing: Health and Illness Perspectives*, 8th edn. St. Louis: Mosby, pp. 1721–1749.

Waugh, A. and Grant, A. (2006). *Ross and Wilson Anatomy and Physiology in Health and Illness*, 10th edn. Edinburgh: Churchill Livingstone.

Wright, J. and Solange, W. (2003). *The Washington Manual of Obstetrics and Gynecology Survival Guide*. Philadelphia: Lippincott.

Wolf, L.L. and Schumann, L. (1999). CE forum: dysmenorrhoea. *Journal of the American Academy of Nurse Practitioners*, *111*(3), 125–132.

United Nations (1994). *International Conference on Population and Development*. Report of the International Conference on Population and Development: Cairo. New York: UN.

Chapter 15

Pain and pain management

Anthony Wheeldon

KEY WORDS

- Acute pain
- Chronic pain
- Neuropathy
- Opioid
- Ascending pain pathway
- Descending pain pathway
- Nociceptors
- Somatic pain
- Analgesia
- Gate control theory
- Non-opioid
- Visceral pain

Test your prior knowledge

- ❓ What is the difference between acute and chronic pain?
- ❓ How would you assess a patient's pain?
- ❓ List five non-pharmacological methods of pain control.

> ## Learning outcomes
>
> On completion of this section, the reader will be able to:
>
> - Describe the physiology of pain transmission and sensation.
> - Explain the difference between acute and chronic pain.
> - Discuss the impact of psychosocial issues on the individual with pain.
> - Explain the principles of the gate control theory of pain.

Introduction

Pain is an integral part of life. Everyone experiences it at various times throughout their lifetime; indeed, pain is the most common reason for an individual to seek medical advice (McCaffery and Beebe, 1994). Yet despite its prevalence, it remains difficult to define. One common definition states that 'Pain is whatever the experiencing person says it is, existing when he says it does' (McCaffery, 1979, p. 11). Pain is not only an unpleasant or uncomfortable sensation that occurs as a result of injury, strain or disease, it can also be an emotional experience unrelated to tissue damage. For example, pain is a term used to describe feelings relating to loss, grief and even unrequited love. Pain is also an individual and personal experience. The way someone expresses and deals with their pain will be determined by their culture, life experiences and personality.

Unresolved pain can have an adverse affect on the cardiovascular, the respiratory, the gastrointestinal, the neuroendocrine and the musculoskeletal systems. It can also promote anxiety and sleeplessness (Macintyre and Ready, 2001). The management of pain is often associated with the administration of **analgesia**; however, there are a wide range of non-pharmacological methods of pain control available. Because it is an emotional as well as physiological phenomenon the successful assessment and control of pain is reliant upon an individualised holistic plan of care, which utilises both pharmacological and non-pharmacological treatments.

The physiology of pain

The physiology of pain is complex and in some instances not fully understood. However, the generation of pain follows a basic three-step process. Firstly, an irritation or injury, such as a cut or burn, is detected in the **peripheral nervous system** by special nerve cells called **nociceptors**. A nerve impulse is then generated, sending a pain impulse towards the **central nervous system**. Finally, this message is received by the brain where the extent and significance of the irritation or injury is interpreted and pain is sensed (see Figure 15.1).

Nociceptors

Nociceptors are free nerve endings present in every tissue in the body, except for the brain. They are activated by noxious stimuli, of which there are three broad types – thermal, mechanical and chemical.

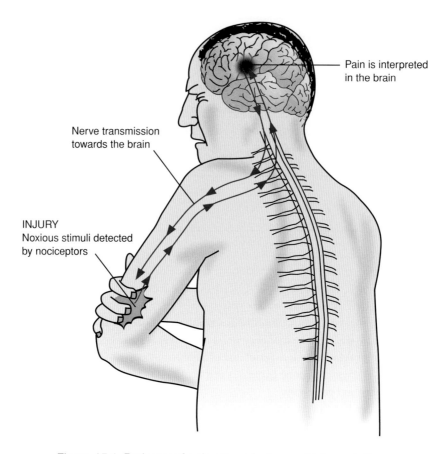

Pain is interpreted in the brain

Nerve transmission towards the brain

INJURY
Noxious stimuli detected by nociceptors

Figure 15.1 Pathway of pain transmission and interpretation.

As the name suggests thermal stimuli are sensations of severe heat or cold. Mechanical stimuli on the other hand are produced by tissue damage caused by trauma or disease (see Box 15.1). Chemical stimuli detect the presence of chemicals such as **histamine**, **kinins** and **prostaglandins** which are released as a result of tissue damage and inflammation. The actions of nociceptors are not clear; however, two types have been identified, polymodal nociceptors that detect mechanical, thermal and chemical stimuli and mechanoceptors, which sense intense mechanical stimuli only (Julius and Basbaum, 2001).

Box 15.1 Examples of mechanical nociceptor stimuli

- Damage to tissue due to trauma or minor injury
- Lack of blood flow and oxygen, i.e. **ischaemia** and **hypoxia**
- **Ulceration**
- Infection
- Nerve damage
- Inflammation

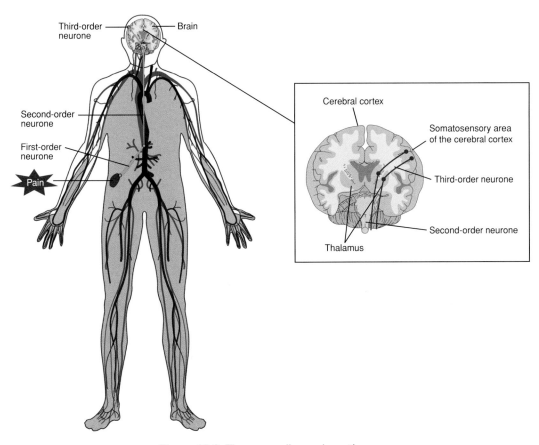

Figure 15.2 The ascending pain pathway.

The ascending pain pathway

Nociceptor stimulation leads directly to the transmission of a pain impulse along special **sensory fibres** towards the **thalamus** and **somatosensory cortex** within brain, where the severity and meaning of the pain is analysed. This line of communication is called the ascending pain pathway. It consists of three linked **neurones** called first-, second- and third-order neurones depending on their place in the pathway. The first-order neurones travel from the nociceptors to the spine, second-order neurones travel upwards through the spinal cord towards the thalamus in the brain and the third-order neurones run from the thalamus through the brain towards the somatosensory cortex, which is a section of the **cerebral cortex** (see Figure 15.2). The line of communication between the first-, second- and third-order neurones is maintained by a number of **neurotransmitters**, such as **substance P** and s**erotonin** (Mac Lellan, 2006).

The two first-order neurones responsible for the transmission of the pain impulse between the nociceptors and the spinal cord are A-delta (Aδ) fibres and C fibres. The speed of this transmission depends upon the diameter of the fibre and whether or not the fibre is **myelinated**. The **axons** of myelinated fibres are surrounded by a sheath of **myelin**, which electrically insulates them and increases the speed of nerve conduction (see Figure 15.3). Aδ fibres are thicker and are myelinated and therefore transmit pain impulses faster than C fibres, which are thinner and non-myelinated (see Table 15.1).

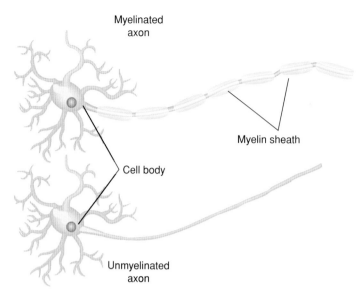

Myelinated
axon

Myelin sheath

Cell body

Unmyelinated
axon

Figure 15.3 Basic structure of myelinated and unmyelinated nerve fibres.

Pain is often described as having two phases referred to as *first* and *second pain*. *First pain* is described as a sharp or pricking pain, whereas *second pain* is the dull, burning or aching pain that follows. Aδ fibres are thought to receive input from mechanoceptors and also generate the *first pain* sensation. C fibres on the other hand are thought to receive input from polymodal nociceptors and are more likely to produce *second pain*. Pain impulses follow the same pathway as touch and mild heat and cold. The sensory fibres responsible for these sensations are A-beta (Aβ) fibres. Aβ fibres are myelinated and are thicker than both Aδ fibres and C fibres and therefore can transmit signals much faster. By stimulating Aβ fibres, by rubbing a mild injury, for example, the pain sensation may subside.

The first-order neurones enter the spinal cord at a location called the **dorsal horn** (see Figure 15.4). Here they **synapse** (connect) with second-order neurones, of which there are two types: nociceptive-specific (NS) and wide dynamic range (WDR) neurones. Both respond to noxious stimuli; however, WDR neurones also react to non-noxious input, such as those transmitted by Aβ fibres, i.e. touch, heat and cold. Both NS and WDR neurones cross over the spinal cord into **white matter** where they continue

Sensory fibre	Diameter	Myelinated	Speed of conduction
A-beta (Aβ) fibres	6–12 μm	Yes	35–75 m/s
A-delta (Aδ) fibres	1–5 μm	Yes	5–35 m/s
C fibres	0.2–1.5 μm	No	0.5–2 m/s

Table 15.1 Size and speeds of first-order sensory fibres

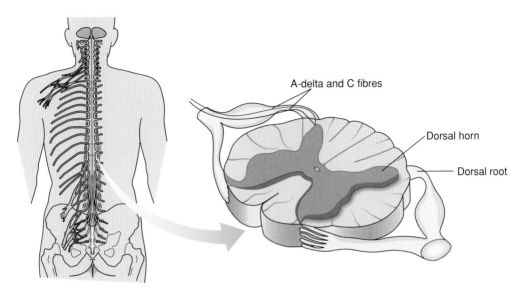

Figure 15.4 Cross section of the spinal cord. Note that both sides are identical.

to rise up the spinal cord towards the thalamus along a pathway called the **spinothalamic tract** (see Figure 15.5).

Pain interpretation

The spinothalamic tract ends at the thalamus, where second-order neurones meet third-order neurones. Third-order neurones travel through the brain towards the somatosensory cortex, a part of the brain that allows the individual to locate pain and describe it. As well as locating the pain the brain will also generate an emotional response, be it anger or distress or mild irritation. The area of the brain thought to influence this emotional response is the **limbic system** (see Figure 15.6). Often referred to as the 'emotional brain', the limbic system deals with feelings of pain, pleasure, affection and anger. An individual's response is not predictable as it is dependent upon their personality, life history and culture. The limbic system also evaluates the seriousness of the pain and helps the individual to remember why the pain occurred. Over time people learn to avoid painful stimuli, such as sharp objects and broken glass, and thus protect themselves from injury (Godfrey, 2005a). However, this protective element has its limits, for example individuals may deliberately expose themselves to potential injury and pain if it means rescuing a loved one from a perilous situation, i.e. from a house fire (Johnson, 2005).

Reflex arcs

Another protective element of the pain pathway is the **reflex arc**, which aims to reduce the level of tissue damage by forcing the body to move away from the source of injury very quickly, after stepping on a pin, for example. Pain only becomes pain when the brain has collected and interpreted the pain message generated by nociceptors. If the body had to wait until pain is sensed by the brain, more tissue damage would occur. Reflex arcs ensure that the foot will involuntarily move up and away from the pin

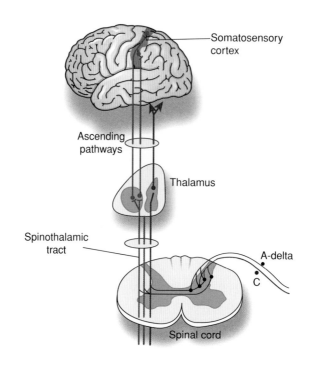

Figure 15.5 The spinothalamic tract.

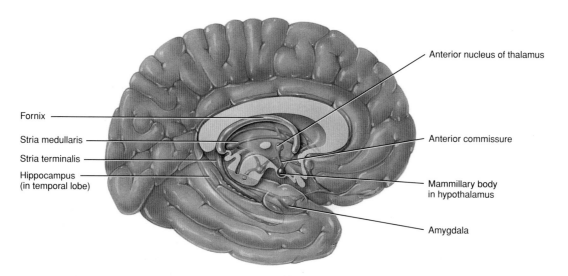

Figure 15.6 The limbic system.

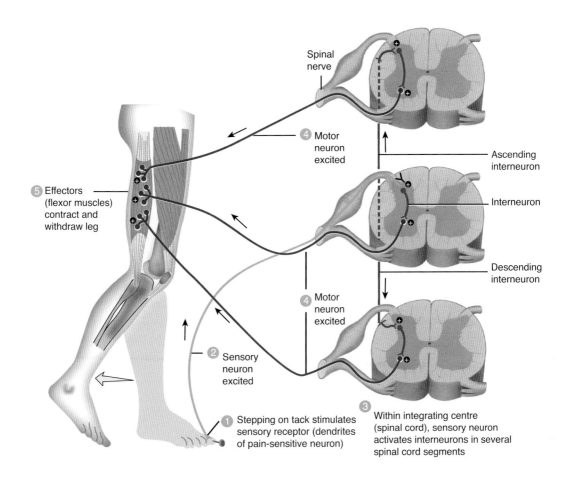

Spinal nerve

④ Motor neuron excited

Ascending interneuron

⑤ Effectors (flexor muscles) contract and withdraw leg

Interneuron

Descending interneuron

④ Motor neuron excited

② Sensory neuron excited

① Stepping on tack stimulates sensory receptor (dendrites of pain-sensitive neuron)

③ Within integrating centre (spinal cord), sensory neuron activates interneurons in several spinal cord segments

Figure 15.7 Example of a reflex arc, working in response to pain.

before pain is sensed. Reflex arcs work by collecting pain impulses from first-order neurones and then immediately sending impulses, via **interneurones**, along **motor nerves** towards skeletal muscle (see Figure 15.7).

Descending pain pathways

Descending pain pathways seek to inhibit the sensation of pain. They involve the release of special **neuropeptides** that have analgesic properties. They bind with **opiate receptors**, which are present throughout the central nervous system, and block the action of the neurotransmitter, substance P. Because of their analgesic effect these neuropeptides are often referred to as endogenous or natural **opiates**. There are three groups of endogenous opiate, **endorphins**, **enkephalins** and **dynorphins**, and there are four major categories of opiate receptor: mu (μ), kappa (κ), sigma (σ) and delta (δ). Levels of endorphins, enkephalins and dynorphins increase during periods of stress and pain. However, stimulation of opiate receptors also promotes feelings of euphoria and well-being and it is endogenous opiates such as endorphins that are associated with the pleasant sensations experienced during excitement, sexual activity and even exercise (Stranc, 2002).

Pain classification

Transient, acute and chronic pain

Pain is classified according to its duration. A short episode of pain, as a consequence of a stubbed toe or a cut finger, for example, is classified as *transient pain*. The injured individual, despite perhaps becoming momentarily upset, will consider the pain to be of no consequence and not seek medical attention. *Acute pain* is associated with a severe sudden onset; however, unlike transient pain it is prolonged and continues until healing begins. Acute pain is intense and can be an intolerable experience and in response areas of the brain seek to restore homeostasis and by initiating an **autonomic** response. The thalamus, the **hypothalamus** and the **reticular formation** (see Figure 15.8), for example promote **diaphoresis**, **tachycardia**, **hypertension** and **tachypneoa** in response to acute pain. The term *chronic pain* is used to describe pain that continues even though healing is complete. Although the pain may remain as intense

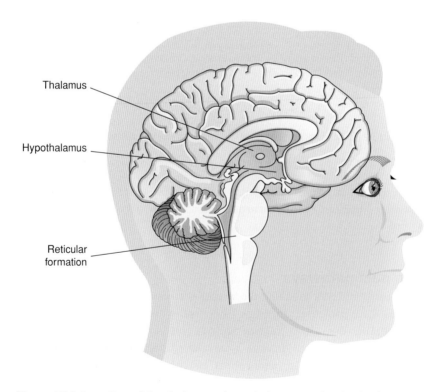

Figure 15.8 Location of the thalamus, hypothalamus and reticular formation.

as acute pain, there is little or no autonomic response. Acute pain is a symptom of an associated medical condition or injury. Chronic pain, on the other hand, exists after the injury or disease has ceased. For this reason chronic pain is often considered as a **syndrome** – a medical condition in its own right (Melzack and Wall, 1988).

Superficial and deep pain

Pain is categorised according to location and is often called *deep* or *superficial*. Superficial pain occurs due to nociceptor stimulation in the skin. Because there are large numbers of nociceptors in skin pain can be easily located. Acute superficial pain is often described as a sharp, pricking sensation (Gould and Thomas, 1997). Deep pain, on the other hand, is dull and prolonged. Deep pain can be either *somatic* or *visceral*. Somatic pain emanates from structures such as bones, muscles, joints and tendons. Visceral pain is produced when nociceptors in organs such as kidneys, stomach, gall bladder and intestines are stimulated. Unlike the skin these organs and others like them have far fewer nociceptors, and therefore it is often difficult for an individual to describe the exact location of their pain (Mac Lellan, 2006).

The pain experience

The term *pain threshold* is often used to describe an individual's response to pain, for instance a patient may be said to have a high or low pain threshold. Pain threshold is the point at which an individual will report pain. It is generally accepted that all humans have a similar pain threshold. People nonetheless express pain in a variety of ways. This is because the expression of pain is influenced by emotional state, personality, past experience, culture and social status rather than a personal pain threshold (Large *et al.*, 2002).

The limbic system, which processes emotional responses to pain, interacts closely with the **frontal lobes** which are responsible for cognitive thought. This would explain why people in acute pain may at times behave irrationally. Conversely, people can often control their emotions if pain occurs when it is socially unacceptable to cry out or complain (Marieb and Hoehn, 2007). The patient's state of mind also has an influence on pain intensity. Anxiety and depression, for example, have been shown to increase pain levels (Carr *et al.*, 2005). Whereas reducing anxiety levels through patient education can reduce pain (Lin and Wang, 2005).

An individual's attitude towards pain can also affect its intensity. Attitudes towards pain are often influenced by the meaning of the pain experience. For example, patients having undergone elective surgery report less pain than patients involved in sudden traumatic accidents. This may be because postsurgical pain may be viewed as a symptom of surgery and healing and therefore as something positive (Skevington, 1995). The meaning of pain can change and alter pain perception. For instance, mild abdominal pain may become severe when the individual learns that it may be something serious (Melzack and Wall, 1988). Past experiences are also a contributing factor. Patients who have been exposed to severe pain during a prior medical procedure may become anxious about future treatments and ultimately sense greater levels of pain. People also learn how to express and react to pain by observing those around them. A patient's attitude towards their pain may be influenced by the experiences of family members or their ethnicity and culture (Adams and Field, 2001).

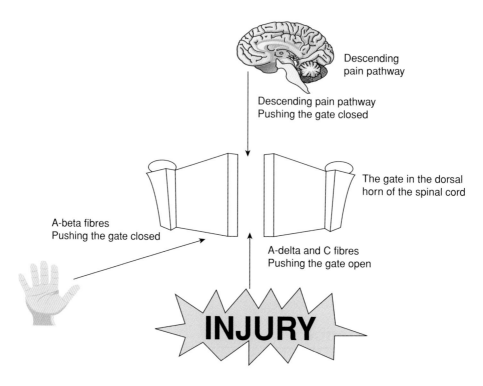

Figure 15.9 The gate control theory of pain.

Pain theories

Most pain theories acknowledge that the pain experience is both emotional and psychological. The *specificity theory* hypothesises that pain is experienced when specific nerve endings are stimulated. Information is then carried to a pain centre in the brain. It is the characteristics of the stimulus that determines the intensity of the pain, rather than the brain. *Pattern theory*, on the other hand, suggests that no separate system for pain sensation exists. Rather pain is interpreted by the brain when intense peripheral nerve stimulation occurs (Gould and Thomas, 1997). Such theories do not explain why pain can occur as a result of gentle stimulus, i.e. neuralgia, or when no tissue damage exists. Neither do they explain why two people with the same injury may experience different levels of pain. For this reason, Melzack and Wall's (1965) gate control theory is more widely accepted as the most important pain theory (Main and Spanswick, 2000).

Gate control theory of pain

The gate control theory of pain proposes that pain impulses must pass through a theoretical 'gate' at the dorsal horn of the spinal cord before ascending towards the brain (see Figure 15.9). Pain messages from Aδ and C fibres will push open the gate. However, the actions of Aβ fibres and the descending pain pathway will push the gate closed. The intensity of an individual's pain, therefore, is determined by a balance between noxious stimuli and Aβ fibre or descending brain activity. The wider the gate is open the more intense the pain; however, if the gate closes the pain ceases (McCaffery *et al.*, 2003).

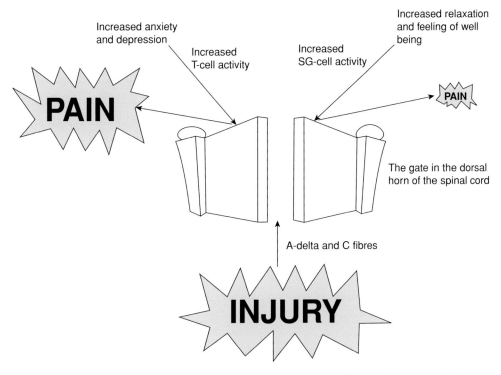

Figure 15.10 The gate control theory and the influence of T- and SG-cell activity.

Stimulation of the larger Aβ fibres with touch or heat can inhibit pain transmission via Aδ and C fibres. This explains how rubbing mild injuries, acupuncture and **transcutaneous electrical nerve stimulation (TENS)** may help reduce pain levels. Increased activity in the descending pain pathway also seeks to close the gate to pain. This helps to explain why a person's emotional state, personality and culture may determine how pain is expressed. For example, increased levels of endogenous opiates can push the gate closed. The gate control theory also proposes that pain intensity is influenced by the action of transmission cells and **substantia gelatinosa** cells, which are found within the dorsal horn of the spinal cord. Transmission, or T, cells transmit pain messages towards the brain. Substantia gelatinosa or SG cells, on the other hand, inhibit T-cell activity and thus push the gate to pain closed. The activity of both T cells and SG cells are enhanced by the descending pain pathway and therefore the individual's state of mind. In depressive and anxious states T-cell activity is enhanced, pushing the gate open and increasing pain intensity. However, in relaxed and contented states SG cell action is increased, pushing the gate closed and decreasing pain levels (Melzack and Wall, 1988; see Figure 15.10).

Pain pathophysiology and management

On completion of this section, the reader will be able to:

■ Discuss the pathophysiology of a range of pain disorders.
■ Discuss the impact of postoperative pain, neurogenic pain and oncology pain.

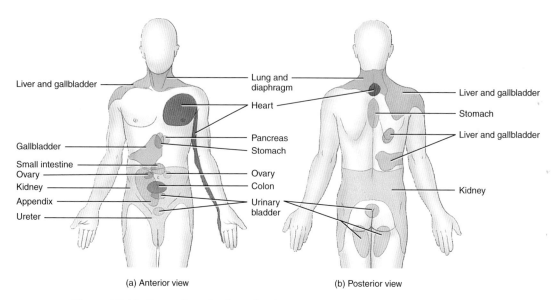

Figure 15.11 Examples of referred pain and the origin of the tissue damage.

- Identify an effective range of pain assessment strategies.
- Explain the difference between opioid and non-opioid analgesics.
- List a range of effective non-pharmacological pain control interventions.

Pathophysiology
Referred and phantom limb pain
Referred pain occurs when tissue damage in one area of the body leads to pain elsewhere, for example pain as a result of **angina**. Although the tissue damage arises in the **coronary arteries**, pain is also felt radiating down the left arm. Despite sensing intense pain, the tissue there remains healthy. Referred pain happens because the damaged or inflamed organ and the area where pain is felt are served by nerves from the same segment of the spinal cord. Other examples include pain due to liver or gallbladder inflammation being sensed in the right shoulder. Figure 15.11 highlights the main instances of referred pain (Tortora and Grabowski, 2003).

The term *phantom limb* describes the pain sensed by amputees where the removed limb once was. The pain is often described as tingling, numbness, itching or tickling and it occurs in 50–57% of all amputees (Hall, 1999). The precise pathophysiology is unknown. However, there are two possible explanations. Firstly, the brain interprets pain impulses from damaged fibres in and around the site of amputation (the stump) as pain signals for the whole (now non-existent) limb. Another possibility is that the brain contains neurones that produce an awareness of body shape and that the neurones that processed information from the removed limb are still active (Hauser, 2002).

Neuropathy
Neuropathic pain occurs when the nociceptors and neurones are damaged. There are many conditions that lead to the development of neuropathic pain (see Box 15.2). Neuropathies produce pain that is

Box 15.2 Common causes of neuropathy

- Entrapment (trapped nerve)
- Causalgia (sensory nerve damage)
- Scar tissue
- **Thoracotomy**
- **Amputation**
- Diabetes
- Herpes
- Ischaemia

described as a burning, electric or tingling pain that can be continuous or spasmodic. The nervous tissue in the ascending pain pathways is said to be plastic, meaning it can change in response to psychological and physical stimuli. This includes changes to the sensitivity of nociceptors, which can begin to generate pain impulses in response to ordinary feelings of touch. The patient may complain of pain when slight pressure is exerted on the site of injury, a phenomenon called **allodynia**. Damaged neural tissue also leads to increased sensitivity to painful stimuli and the individual will feel pain that is out of proportion to the level of tissue damage. This increase in pain sensitivity is referred to as **hyperalgesia** (Scadding, 2003).

Postoperative pain

Almost all patients undergoing surgery experience pain afterwards with up to 80% of patient reporting severe pain (Manias, 2003). A significant contributory factor to postoperative pain is anxiety, which can increase pain intensity. Anxiety and depression prior to surgery lead to high levels of anxiety postoperatively (Carr *et al.*, 2005). In order to reduce postoperative pain, nurses should invest in preoperative nursing strategies to minimise preoperative anxiety, such as patient education (Johansson *et al.*, 2005). Nurses are also ideally placed to minimise postoperative pain as they are responsible for the administration and evaluation of prescribed analgesics.

Unresolved pain leads to a complicated postsurgical recovery. Pain in the chest or abdomen, for example, can affect respiration. People in pain tend to breathe shallowly and avoid coughing. Painful movement can also render patients reluctant to mobilise. Pain also slows down gastric emptying and reduces intestinal motility, probably due to the activation of a reflex arc. Prolonged pain also increases levels of anxiety. Indeed, pain and anxiety are intertwined problems as during the postoperative period one inevitably leads to the other. The effects of unresolved anxiety can have a severe detrimental affect on the patient's postoperative recovery. Prolonged anxiety will lead to a stress response as the body attempts to maintain homeostasis. During stress the neuroendocrine system releases numerous hormones that increase blood pressure, pulse and metabolism. **Adrenaline**, for example, increases heart rate and **aldosterone** increases blood pressure. **Cortisol** and **glucagon**, on the other hand, liberate more glucose for the production of energy. Cortisol also decreases immune function (Macintyre and Ready, 2001). The combination of unresolved pain and anxiety affects many major body systems, which could lead to chest infection, impaired wound healing and deep vein thrombosis among other complications (see Table 15.2).

Respiratory system	Hypoventilation	Hypoxaemia	Gastrointestinal system	Delayed gastric emptying	Nausea and vomiting
	Decreased cough	Hypoxia		Intestinal motility	Reduced nutrition
	Tachypnoea	Retain sputum			Poor wound healing
		Chest infection			
Cardiovascular system	Tachycardia	Elevated heart workload	Renal system	Increased retention of sodium and water	ower urine output
	Hypertension	Deep vein thrombosis			
	Reduced venous return	Pulmonary embolism			
	Coronary vasoconstriction				
Musculoskeletal system	Reduced mobility	Prolonged postoperative recovery	Pancreas	Increased glucagon	Increased blood sugar levels
	Muscle atrophy	DVT		Decreased insulin	
		Pulmonary embolism			

Adapted from Cousins and Power (2003); Macintyre and Ready (2001).

Table 15.2 The effects of pain and stress on four major body systems

Cancer pain

There is a high prevalence of pain in patients with cancer. Indeed, in some studies up to 96% of patients with cancer experience pain, more than AIDS (80%), heart disease (77%), renal disease (77%) and chronic obstructive pulmonary disease (50%) (Solano *et al.*, 2006). The causes of cancer pain are wide and varied but the most common cancer pain is that caused by **bone metastases**. Cancer pain can be classified as being either nociceptive or neuropathic. Table 15.3 lists the common causes and descriptions of cancer pain.

The aim of palliative care is to minimise pain and its associated distressing symptoms (World Health Organization, 2002). Cancer pain is therefore classified according to when it occurs or if it becomes more intense and unmanageable. There are three classifications of cancer pain as follows:

- *Breakthrough pain* – pain that is more intense than normal.
- *Incident pain* – pain caused by specific activities, i.e. walking, lifting etc.
- *End of dose failure pain* – occurs if effects of analgesia subside before the next dose is due.

Type of pain	Structures affected	Causes	Patient description
Somatic nociceptor	Muscle and bone	Bone metastases Surgical incisions	Aching, sharp, gnawing or dull Easily located
Neuropathic	Nerves	Chemotherapy Tumour	Burning, itching, numbness, tingling, shooting
Visceral nociceptor	Organs of the abdomen, pelvis and thorax	Tumour	Crampy, colicky, aching, deep, squeezing, dull Less easily located

Listed in order of prevalence. Most patients have a combination of somatic and visceral nociceptor pain.

Adapted from Kochhar (2007).

Table 15.3 Types of cancer pain, their source, causes and descriptions

Breakthrough and incident pain are common even in patients whose pain is well controlled. End of dose pain, however, is an indicator that the patient's current pain control may need reviewing (Hayden, 2006).

Pain assessment

Effective pain assessment allows the practitioners to best select appropriate pharmacological and non-pharmacological interventions. However, pain is a complex multifaceted phenomenon and its assessment is very challenging. The pain experience involves four dimensions, all of which are interlinked (see Figure 15.12). Any nursing assessment must pay attention to physiological, psychological, emotional and social aspects of pain if effective holistic care is to occur (Manias *et al.*, 2002). Furthermore, pain is a subjective experience and the nurse must rely on the patient's own description of the pain. However, many patients are often unable to verbalise or describe their pain. For this reason non-verbal cues are of particular importance.

A description of pain is rarely enough to determine appropriate treatment. Further information on the location, duration and onset of pain can aid health care professionals in managing the patient's pain. Every pain assessment must also include the following:

- Location of pain – Where is the pain, does it radiate anywhere?
- Duration of pain – How long has the patient had the pain?
- Onset – When did the pain start and what was the patient doing at the time?
- Frequency – How often does the pain occur?
- Intensity – How painful is it, does the level of pain change?
- Aggravating factors – What makes the pain worse?

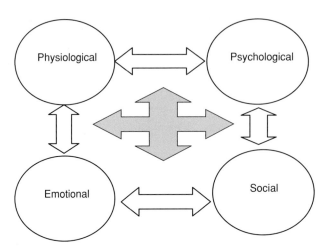

Figure 15.12 Four dimensions of the pain experience. (Adapted from Manias *et al.*, 2002.)

■ Relieving factors – What makes the pain feel better?
■ Other symptoms – Does the patient feel dizzy, nauseous, sweaty or short of breath?
■ Sleep patterns – Does the pain keep the patient awake?

(Adapted from Godfrey (2005b) and Mac Lellan (2006).)

Further information on the patient's psychological and emotional response to their pain should also be gathered. For example:

■ the patient's expectations of any potential treatments
■ the patient's concerns of the cause of their pain
■ any personal or spiritual beliefs
■ acceptable pain levels
■ pain levels that will allow the patient to return to work
■ feelings of stress and anxiety
■ any coping mechanisms
■ the patient's preferences regarding treatment options

(Mac Lellan, 2006).

Acute pain also produces an autonomic response and often patients will present with hypertension, tachycardia as well as changes in respiratory rate. Pain assessment should therefore include measurement of blood pressure, pulse, temperature and respiration rate. However, chronic pain may not have an adverse effect on these vital signs; therefore, the patient's description of the pain should remain the principal indicator of pain intensity (Lynch, 2001).

Formal structured pain assessment tools can facilitate pain assessment. There is a variety of pain assessment tools at the nurse's disposal, ranging from simple single-dimension scales to comprehensive pain questionnaires. The most common single-dimension scales are the verbal rating scale, the visual analogue rating scale and the numerical rating scale. Verbal rating scales ask the patient to select which adjective from a list best describes their pain (see Figure 15.13) and with a numerical scale the patient

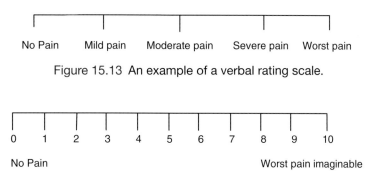

Figure 15.13 An example of a verbal rating scale.

Figure 15.14 An example of a numerical rating scale.

assigns a number to match the pain intensity (see Figure 15.14). The visual analogue scale is much simpler. The patient is shown a basic continuum which runs from no pain to worst pain possible. The patient can point or state whereabouts on the continuum their pain is (see Figure 15.15). The main advantage of simple rating scales is their ease of use. They can be utilised swiftly and do not overburden the acutely sick person. Nevertheless, they only assess one aspect of pain, its intensity, and there is an assumption that the patient will be literate (Mac Lellan, 2006).

The most common multidimensional pain assessment tool is the McGill Pain Questionnaire (see Figure 15.16). This comprehensive assessment tool contains a series of adjectives that patients can use to describe their pain. The descriptive words are divided into three classes: sensory, affective and evaluative. The questionnaire also utilises a rating scale that runs from 0–no pain to 5–excruciating. The assessment of pain is based on three measures: the pain rating index (PRI), that is based on the numerical values assigned to each number, the number of words selected and the rating scale or present pain index (PPI). The McGill Pain Questionnaire also has line drawings of the human body that can facilitate the location of the pain. The McGill Pain Questionnaire is now widely used to assess chronic pain and has been shown to be very effective when measuring pain in arthritis (Grafton *et al.*, 2005).

Pain management

Pain management or control can be either pharmacological or non-pharmacological. Pharmacological pain management involves the administration of drugs. Drugs that are used for pain control are referred to as analgesia or analgesics. There are two main types of analgesia: opioids (or opiates) and non-opioids. As the name suggests non-pharmacological pain management does not involve any drugs. As pain is a total experience, effective pain control is often achieved through a combination of both approaches (Hader and Guy, 2004).

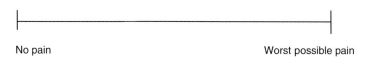

Figure 15.15 An example of a visual analogue scale.

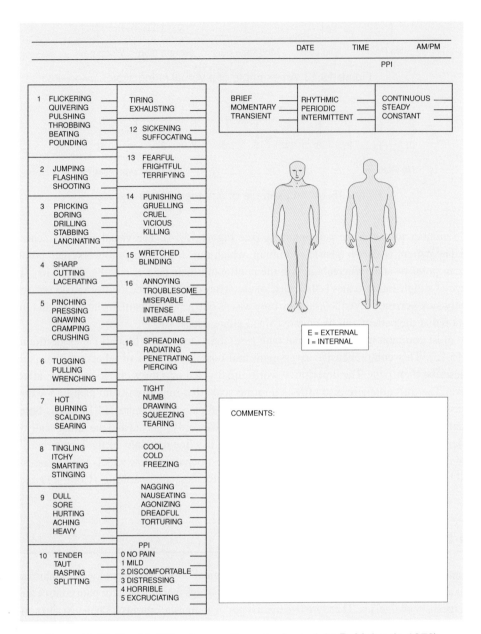

Figure 15.16 The McGill pain questionnaire (copyright R. Melzack, 1970).

Opioids

Opioid drugs are used for moderate to severe pain. They work by mimicking the body's own endogenous opiates by binding to opiate receptors in the central nervous system. Opiate receptors such as μ,κ and δ block the action of substance P when stimulated. However, unlike endogenous opiates such as endorphins, opioids are not rapidly broken down by the body (Stranc, 2002). Therefore, their analgesic

Receptor	Physiological effects
Mu (μ)	Analgesia Euphoria Respiratory depression **Bradycardia** Nausea and vomiting Inhibition of gut motility **Miosis** **Pruritus** Smooth muscle spasm Physical dependence
Kappa (κ)	Analgesia Sedation **Dysphoria** Respiratory depression Physical dependence
Delta (δ)	Analgesia Euphoria Respiratory depression Miosis Inhibition of gut motility Smooth muscle spasm Physical dependence

Table 15.4 Actions of opiate receptors

effects are powerful and long-lasting. In addition to analgesia the stimulation of opiate receptors produces many other physiological changes, which include feelings of euphoria (see Table 15.4). As a result, opioids are associated with a number of side effects which the nurse should account for (see Box 15.3). Opioids are **controlled drugs** governed by the Misuse of Drugs Act 1971 (Her Majesty's Stationery Office, 1971). Opioid drugs are classified as either weak or strong. Despite their name, weak opioids are very effective analgesics. The main weak opioids are used in combination with non-opioid analgesia such as paracetamol or aspirin. Such combinations are prescription only rather than controlled drugs (Her Majesty's Stationery Office, 1968). Tables 15.5 and 15.6 summarise the main weak and strong opioids used by the National Health Service.

In some instances patients can administer their own opioid drugs via a system known as **patient-controlled analgesia (PCA)**. The patient is attached to a small syringe driver that contains an opioid drug. The syringe is operated by a button, which when pressed by the patient delivers a set dosage. To protect against overdose, after each dose the syringe driver locks for a short time and no drug can be delivered, even if the button is pressed. The main advantage of PCA is that it fosters an individualised approach to pain management (Chumbley *et al.*, 1998).

Box 15.3 The main side effects of opiate therapies

- Respiratory depression
- Constipation
- Nausea and vomiting
- Drowsiness
- Bradycardia
- Hypotension

Non-opioid drugs

Non-opioid analgesia is used for mild to moderate pain and is rarely effective in acute or postoperative pain. However, they can enhance the effect of opioid drugs and when used in combination with opioids can reduce opioid use by 20–40% (Macintyre and Ready, 2001). The most common non-opioid drug is paracetamol (acetaminophen). The precise action of paracetamol remains controversial; however, it is widely thought to suppress the production of prostaglandins. Prostaglandins are hormone-like substances that increase inflammation and also stimulate nociceptors and promote pain (MacPherson, 2000). Paracetamol is an effective analgesia; however, it rarely acts for longer than 4 hours and therefore may not be appropriate for prolonged pain. Despite its relative safety, paracetamol can cause liver failure even in small overdoses (Heath, 1997).

Drug	Preparations	Route
Codeine	Codeine phosphate	Oral – tablet, syrup Injection (**controlled drug**)
	Co-codamol (Paracodol®) Codeine phosphate 8 mg or 30 mg with 500 mg paracetamol	Oral – capsule and dispersible tablets
	Co-codaprin® Codeine phosphate 8 mg with 400 mg aspirin	Oral – dispersible tablets
Dihydrocodeine	Dihydrocodeine (DF118®)	Oral – tablet Injection (**controlled drug**)
	Co-dyramol Dihydrocodeine 10 mg with 500 mg paracetamol	Oral – tablet
Tramadol	Tramadol (Zydol®)	Oral – capsule Injection
	Tramacet® Tramadol 37.5 mg with 325 mg paracetamol	Oral – tablet

Table 15.5 Common weak opiates and their routes of delivery

Drug	Examples	Route
Morphine	Morphine	Injection Suppository
	Oramorph®	Oral – liquid, tablet
	Sevredol®	Oral – tablet
	MST Continus®	Oral – tablet, suspension
Diamorphine	Diamorphine	Oral – tablet Injection
Oxycodone	Oxynorm®	Oral – tablet, liquid Injection
	Oxycontin®	Oral – tablet
Fentanyl	Fentanyl	Patch Injection
	Durogesic DTrans®	Patch
Pethidine	Pethidine	Oral – tablets Injection
	Pamergan P100®	Oral – tablets Injection

Table 15.6 Common strong opiates and their routes of delivery

Prostaglandins are derived from **arachidonic acid** which is released from damaged cells. The production of prostaglandins from arachidonic acid is accelerated by the presence of an **enzyme** called **cyclo-oxygenase 2** (COX-2) (see Figure 15.17). Analgesics that suppress prostaglandin production are collectively known as **non-steroidal anti-inflammatory drugs (NSAIDs)**. There are many different NSAIDs used in the United Kingdom (UK) (see Box 15.4); however, the main ones are aspirin, ibuprofen, diclofenac, indomethacin and naproxen. In addition to the suppression of COX-2, NSAIDs can also suppress another enzyme, cyclo-oxygenase-1 (COX-1), which promotes prostaglandin production in the stomach where it performs an important protective role by inhibiting gastric acid. A major side effect of NSAIDs is, therefore, the development of gastric irritation and ulcers (Gilron *et al.*, 2003). NSAIDs are also associated with hypersensitive reactions in patients with asthma (Jenkins *et al.*, 2004).

Non-opioid analgesics have other actions other than pain control, e.g. temperature control and prophylaxis of heart disease. Because prostaglandins promote fever as well as inflammation, NSAIDs

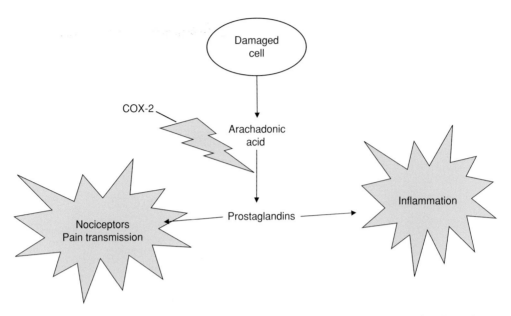

Figure 15.17 The action of cyclo-oxygenase-2 (COX-2) enhancing prostaglandin action.

and paracetamol may reduce core body temperature and are often used solely to reduce **pyrexia**. Aspirin also has **antiplatelet** properties. Used in small doses, it has been shown to reduce the risk of cardiovascular disease (Fuster *et al.*, 1993).

The analgesic ladder

The World Health Organization (WHO) produced the analgesic ladder in 1986 to help combat cancer pain. However, it is now widely used to manage many different types of pain (Godfrey, 2005b). The ladder contains three steps, each containing a recommended level of pharmacological treatment (see Figure 15.18). If pain persists the patient's treatment should be moved up to the next step. The goal is for the patient to be pain free at the lowest point on the ladder. Step one involves the use of non-opioid drugs, step two recommends adding a weak opioid whereas the final step advocates the use

---

Box 15.4 Common NSAIDs, with trade names in brackets

Aceclofenac (Preservex®)	Etoricoxib (Arcoxia®)	Mefenamic acid (Ponstan®)
Acemetacin (Emflex®)	Fenbufen (Fenbufen®)	Meloxican (Mobic®)
Aspirin (Caprin®)	Fenoprofen (Fenopron®)	Nabumetone (Relifex®)
Azapropazone (Rheumox®)	Flurbiprofen (Froben®)	Naproxen (Arthroxen®)
Celecoxib (Celebrex®)	Ibuprofen (Brufen®)	Piroxicam (Brexidol®)
Dexibuprofen (Seractil®)	Indometacin (Rimacid®)	Sulindac (Clinoril®)
Dexketoprofen (Keral®)	Ketoprofen (Orudis®)	Tenoxicam (Mobiflex®)
Diclofenac (Volterol®)		Tiaprofenic acid (Surgam®)
Etodolac		

of strong opioids. Each step also suggests the use of an adjuvant. Adjuvants are a range of drugs that have analgesic effects despite being normally prescribed for other conditions. Antidepressants, anticonvulsants, muscle relaxants, corticosteroids and local anaesthetics have all been shown to reduce pain when used in conjunction with opioid and non-opioid drugs (MacPherson, 2000).

Non-pharmacological pain management

There are many different forms of non-pharmacological pain management interventions available in the UK (see Box 15.5). However, the use of non-pharmacological pain control is controversial with many health care providers being sceptical of their effectiveness (Wigens, 2006). There is evidence for individual techniques, such as massage and cognitive behavioural therapy, for example (Furlan *et al.*, 2002; Morley *et al.*, 1999), but the overall effectiveness of non-pharmacological over pharmacological

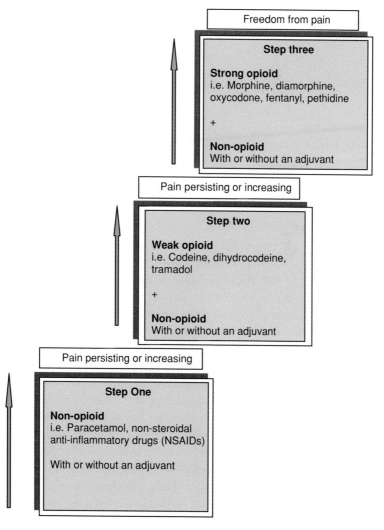

Figure 15.18 The World Health Organization analgesic ladder (WHO, 1986).

Box 15.5 Popular non-pharmacological methods of pain management

- Cognitive behavioural therapy
- Transcutaneous electric nerve stimulation (TENS)
- Application of heat and cold substances
- Acupuncture
- **Alexander technique**
- **Aromatherapy**
- Massage
- **Chiropractic**
- Hypnosis
- **Homeopathy**
- Meditation
- Osteopathy
- Reflexology
- Relaxation
- Shiatsu

Adapted from Wigens (2006).

---

methods is yet to be proven (Sindhu, 1996). Nevertheless, they remain popular with 68% of chronic pain sufferers in the USA using non-pharmacological pain control interventions regularly (Vallerand *et al.*, 2005).

Physical interventions

Many non-pharmacological pain control techniques have a physiological basis. A transcutaneous electric nerve stimulation (TENS) machine, for example, sends a constant stream of small electrical impulses through the skin (see Figure 15.19). These impulses are thought to reduce pain in two ways. Firstly, they may stimulate the large diameter Aβ fibres and interrupt the pain impulse travelling along the smaller Aδ and C fibres, the same effect as rubbing a mild injury. Secondly, the continuous electrical stimulation may increase levels of endogenous opiates such as endorphins (Sluka and Walsh, 2003). TENS machines are widely used for the treatment of postoperative pain, chronic pain and pain during labour and childbirth; however, evidence of its effectiveness remains inconclusive (Carroll *et al.*, 2000).

Acupuncture is the insertion of fine needles at strategic points around the body. It too is thought to stimulate the release of endogenous opiates (Lundeberg and Stener-Victorin, 2002). Acupuncture is widely used and is accepted as an effective analgesia in many countries; however, there is very little evidence to suggest that it is effective (Lee and Ernst, 2005).

The stimulation of large diameter Aβ fibres also helps explain the therapeutic effects of pressure- and touch-based interventions such as **osteopathy**, **reflexology** and **shiatsu**. The most widely used touch- and pressure-based intervention is massage. Massage has been shown to be potentially effective in patients with low back pain (Furlan *et al.*, 2002). As well as sensing pressure and touch Aβ fibres also respond to sensations of heat and cold. The therapeutic effects of mild heat and ice packs on injuries are well known. Heat can also be used to alleviate menstrual pain as well as joint and muscle strains.

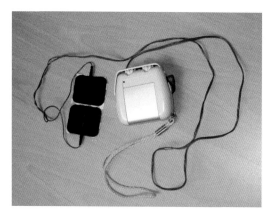

Figure 15.19 Transcutaneous electrical nerve stimulation (TENS) machine.

However, there is little evidence for the use of heat and cold substances in the clinical setting (French *et al.*, 2005).

Psychological interventions

Pain is a holistic experience and the psychological aspects of the pain experience are an integral aspect of pain sensation. The gate control theory of pain suggests that descending pain pathways from the brain influence pain intensity. Furthermore, anxiety, stress and low mood states are significant factors that can increase pain sensation. Any non-pharmacological method that can alleviate anxiety, stress or help an individual to cope with their pain could be beneficial (Williams, 1997). It is not surprising therefore that psychological-based non-pharmacological pain control methods are popular among chronic pain sufferers.

Psychological-based pain control interventions range from simplistic methods such as relaxation and distraction to more alternative therapies such as meditation, Alexandra technique and hypnotherapy. A more intense psychological approach is cognitive behavioural therapy (CBT). CBT involves a series of structured, patient-focused sessions that aim to address the individual's psychological and emotional experience of their pain. The aim is to enable to the patient to self-manage and control their anxiety and therefore their pain. CBT should complement rather than replace traditional pharmacology-based therapies. As a pain control method for those in chronic pain CBT has proved very effective (Morley *et al.*, 1999).

Conclusion

Pain is a personal experience. The brain plays a fundamental role in the interpretation of pain and therefore a patient's state of mind, personality, background and culture will all shape the way in which an individual expresses or verbalises his or her pain. Acute pain affects the function of many body systems and left unresolved can become prolonged chronic pain. Pain control therefore is essential if homeostasis is to be maintained. There are many forms of analgesia that can be used to control pain; however, as pain is an emotional as well as physiological phenomenon non-pharmacological methods should also be utilised, especially for the patient in chronic pain. Because pain is individualised the selection of appropriate pharmacological and non-pharmacological pain management strategies is reliant upon a comprehensive and holistic assessment. The nurse is therefore ideally placed to provide effective care for the patient with pain.

Multiple choice questions

1. In the ascending pain pathway, which neurones travel upwards through the spinal column towards the brain?
(a) first-order neurones
(b) second-order neurones
(c) third-order neurones
(d) interneurones

2. Which area of the brain is often referred to as the 'emotional brain'?
(a) the limbic system
(b) the reticular formation
(c) thalamus
(d) somatosensory cortex

3. Which of the following is an endogenous opiate?
(a) substance P
(b) endorphin
(c) morphine
(d) acetaminophen

4. Which of the following statements is true?
(a) superficial pain is difficult to locate
(b) somatic pain originates in structures such as bones, muscles and joints
(c) visceral pain is easily located
(d) superficial pain originates from internal organs

5. Regarding the gate control theory of pain, which of the following statements are true?
(a) pain impulses generated by nociceptors will push open the gate
(b) the wider the gate is open, the greater the pain sensation
(c) increased activity in the descending pain pathway decreases pain intensity
(d) all of the above

6. Pain that occurs in response to normal touch is called:
(a) hyperalgesia
(b) causalgia
(c) allodynia
(d) neuropathy

7. Which of the following statements is false?
(a) pain slows down gastric emptying and intestinal motility

(b) anxiety is a significant contributing factor to postoperative pain

(c) hypotension and bradycardia are likely outcomes of poor pain management

(d) unresolved pain can prolong postoperative recovery

8. Which of the following is a weak opioid drug?

(a) codeine phosphate

(b) naproxen

(c) pethidine

(d) oxycodone

9. Which of the following analgesics would inhibit the action of cyclo-oxygenase-2?

(a) paracetamol

(b) dihydrocodeine

(c) ibuprofen

(d) tramadol

10. Which non-pharmacological method of pain relief consists of structured patient-focused sessions?

(a) cognitive behavioural therapy

(b) hypnotherapy

(c) Alexander technique

(d) meditation

Answers: 1.b, 2.a, 3.b, 4.b, 5.d, 6.c, 7.c, 8.a, 9.c, 10.a.

Test your knowledge

❓ List the structures involved in the ascending pain pathway and describe their functions.

❓ Explain why two different people with the same injury may have different pain experiences.

❓ What are the main differences between acute and chronic pain?

❓ What are the major side effects of opioid analgesia and explain why they may occur?

❓ Using the gate control theory of pain, explain why a patient may find non-pharmacological methods of pain control effective.

Glossary of terms

Adrenaline: Hormone released during times of stress.

Alexander technique: A method of teaching people to improve body posture and thereby avoiding muscle tension.

Aldosterone: Hormone that increases blood pressure by increased re-absorption of water and sodium by the kidneys.

Allodynia: Pain in response to stimuli that should not cause pain.

Amputation: Surgical removal of a limb.

Analgesia: Pain killer.

Angina: Central crushing chest pain that occurs as a result of reduced blood flow through the coronary arteries.

Antiplatelet: Substance that reduces the clotting action of platelets.

Arachidonic acid: Substance found in the cell membrane, which can produce prostaglandins.

Aromatherapy: The use of odours and fragrances to alter an individual's mood.

Autonomic: Pertaining to the autonomic nervous system, associated with the maintenance of homeostasis.

Axon: The long part of a nerve cell that carries nerve impulses.

Bradycardia: Slow heart rate, less than 50 beats per minute.

Bone metastases: Cells from a tumour that have spread to bone tissue.

Central nervous system: The brain and spinal cord.

Cerebral cortex: The outer surface of the brain.

Chiropractic: The manipulation and realignment of the spine.

Controlled drugs: Therapeutic preparations governed by the Misuse of Drugs Act (1971).

Coronary arteries: Oxygenated blood supply to the heart.

Coronary vasoconstriction: Constriction of coronary blood vessels.

Cortisol: Hormone released by the adrenal glands, which increases resistance to stress.

Cyclo-oxygenase-2: Enzyme which speeds up the production of prostaglandins from arachidonic acid.

Deep vein thrombosis: Formation of a blood clot in the veins of the legs.

Diaphoresis: Excessive sweating.

Dorsal horn: The section of grey matter found on either side of a cross section of the spinal cord.

Dynorphin: Neuropeptide found in the central nervous system.

Dysphoria: Low mood, opposite of euphoria.

Endorphin: Neuropeptide found in the central nervous system. Counteracts pain sensation by inhibiting substance P.

Enkephalin: Neuropeptide found in the central nervous system. Counteracts pain sensation by inhibiting substance P.

Enzyme: A protein that speeds up chemical reactions.

Frontal lobe: Area of the cerebrum (outer part of the brain).

Glucagon: Hormone released by pancreas, which increase blood sugar levels.

Histamine: Substance released during inflammation that causes vasodilation and increased capillary permeability.

Homeopathy: Treatment based on the principle that 'like can be cured with like'.

Hyperalgesia: Increased or heightened pain sensation.

Hypertension: Abnormally high blood pressure.

Hypothalamus: Small region of the brain found in the diencephalon; important regulatory organ of the nervous and endocrine systems.

Hypoventilation: Slow and shallow breaths.

Hypoxaemia: Reduced levels of oxygen in arterial blood.

Hypoxia: Reduced levels of oxygen in the tissues.

Interneurones: Short neurones that connect nearby neurones in the brain and spinal cord.

Ischaemia: A reduction in blood supply to tissue.

Kinins: Substances released during inflammation that cause vasodilation and increased capillary permeability; also attracts phagocytes.

Limbic system: Part of the forebrain. Sometimes called the emotional brain, the limbic system controls feelings of emotion and behaviour.

Miosis: Contraction of the pupils.

Motor nerves: A nerve that travels from the brain and spinal cord out to an organ, muscle or gland.

Muscle atrophy: Muscle wasting.

Myelin: Electrically insulating phospholipid.

Myelinated: Covered by a protected sheath of myelin.

Neurone: A nerve cell.

Neuropeptide: Substance sound in the nervous system that counteracts the effects of neurotransmitters.

Neurotransmitter: Molecules that transmit messages from one nerve to another at a junction called the synapse.

Nociceptors: Special cells that detect damage and irritants that cause pain.

Non-steroidal anti-inflammatory drugs (NSAIDs): Group of non-opioid pain killers that reduce inflammation.

Opiate: Powerful analgesic agent that stimulates opiate receptors within the central nervous system.

Opiate receptors: Receptors found in the central nervous system that are stimulated by neuropeptides and opiate drugs.

Osteopathy: The manipulation of bones and joints to diagnose and treat illness.

Patient-controlled analgesia: Method of self-administration of intravenous analgesia.

Peripheral nervous system: The nervous system outside of the central nervous system.

Prostaglandins: Substances released by damaged cells. Intensify the actions of histamine and kinins.

Pruritis: Itchy sensation on the skin.

Pulmonary embolism: Reduced blood flow through the lungs due to a blood clot.

Pyrexia: Raised body temperature or fever.

Reflex arc: Nervous pathway from sensory nerve to motor nerve via spinal cord.

Reflexology: The manipulation of various area of the feet and hands in order to promote well-being.

Reticular formation: A network of neurones found in the central part of the brain stem.

Sensory fibres: Special nerve fibres that transmit sensations of pain, heat, cold and touch.

Serotonin: Neurotransmitter found in central nervous system; associated with pain sensation.

Shiatsu: Finger pressure applied to various areas of the body in order to stimulate the internal energy of the body and thus promote healing.

Somatosensory cortex: Region of the cerebral cortex that processes feelings of touch, pain, heat, cold and muscle and joint position.

Spinothalamic tract: Sensory pathway which transmits messages of pain, temperature, touch and pressure upwards along the spinal cord.

Substance P: Neurotransmitter found in sensory nerves, spinal cord and brain associated with the sensation of pain.

Substantia gelatinosa: Part of the spinal cord's grey matter; it is composed of large amounts of small nerve cells.

Synapse: The junction where two neurones meet, or where a neuron meets tissue.

Syndrome: A collection of symptoms that characterise a specific disorder.

Tachycardia: Pulse rate greater than 100 beats per minute.

Tachypnoea: Rapid and usually shallow respiration rate, greater than 20 breaths per minute.

Thalamus: A pair of oval masses of grey matter which accounts for 80% of the diencephalon area of the brain.

Thoracotomy: Incision in the chest.

Transcutaneous electrical nerve stimulation (TENS): Method of pain control which stimulates Aβ, Aδ and C fibres with small electrical currents.

Ulceration: The erosion of skin or internal surface.

Venous return: The volume of blood entering the right atrium.

White matter: Tissue of spinal cord that surrounds the grey matter.

References

Adams, N. and Field, L. (2001). Pain management 1: Psychological and social aspects of pain. *British Journal of Nursing, 10*(14), 903–911.

Carr, E.C.J., Thomas, V.N. and Wilson-Barnet, J. (2005). Patient experiences of anxiety, depression and acute pain after surgery: A longitudinal perspective. *International Journal of Nursing Studies, 42*, 521–530.

Carroll, D., Moore, R.A., McQuay, H.J., Fairman, F., Tramer, M. and Leijon, G. (2000). Transcutaneous electrical nerve stimulation (TENS) for chronic pain. *The Cochrane Database of Systematic Reviews, 2002*, Issue 4.

Chumbley, G.M., Hall, G.M. and Salmon, P. (1998). Patient controlled analgesia: An assessment of 200 patients. *Anaesthesia, 53*, 216–221.

Cousins, M. and Power, I. (2003). Acute and postoperative pain. In: Melsack, R. and Wall, P.D. (eds) *Handbook of Pain Management: A Clinical Companion to Wall and Melzack's Textbook of Pain*. Edinburgh: Churchill Livingstone.

French, S.D., Cameron, M., Walker, B.F., Reggars, J.W. and Esterman, A.J. (2005). Superficial heat or cold for low back pain. *The Cochrane Database of Systematic Reviews, 2006*, Issue 1.

Furlan, A.D., Brosseau, L., Imamura, M. and Irvin, E. (2002). Massage for low back pain. *The Cochrane Database of Systematic Reviews, 2002*, Issue 2.

Fuster, V., Dyken, M.L., Vokonas, P.S. and Hennekens, C. (1993). Aspirin as a therapeutic agent in cardiovascular disease. *Circulation, 87*(2), 659–675.

Gilron, I., Milne, B. and Hong, M. (2003). Cyclooxygenase-2 inhibitors in postoperative pain management. *Anaesthesiology, 99*(5), 1198–1208.

Godfrey, H. (2005a). Understanding pain, part 1: Physiology of pain. *British Journal of Nursing, 14*(16), 846–852.

Godfrey, H. (2005b). Understanding pain, part 2: Pain management. *British Journal of Nursing, 14*(17), 904–909.

Gould, D. and Thomas, V.N. (1997). Pain mechanisms: The neurophysiology and neuropsychology of pain perception. In: Thomas, V.N. (ed) *Pain: Its Nature and Management*. London: Bailliere Tindall.

Grafton, K.V., Foster, N.E. and Wright, C.C. (2005). Test-retest reliability of the short-form McGill pain questionnaire. *Clinical Journal of Pain, 21*(1), 73–82.

Hader, C.F. and Guy, J. (2004). Your hand in pain management. *Nursing Management, 35*(11), 21–28.

Hall, A. (1999). Phantom limb pain: A review of the literature on attributes and potential mechanisms. *Journal of Pain and Symptom Management, 17*(2), 125–142.

Hauser, S.A. (2002). Phantom limb pain. In: Warfield C.A. and Fausett, H.J. (eds) *Manual of Pain Management*, 2nd edn. Philadelphia: Lippincott Williams & Wilkins.

Hayden, D. (2006). Pain management in palliative care. In: Mac Lellan, K. (ed) *Expanding Nursing and Health Care Practice: Management of Pain*. Cheltenham: Nelson Thornes.

Heath, M.L. (1997). The use of pharmacology in pain management. In: Thomas, V.N. (ed) *Pain: Its Nature and Management*. London: Bailliere Tindall.

Her Majesty's Stationery Office (1968). *The Medicine's Act*. London: HMSO.

Her Majesty's Stationery Office (1971). *The Misuse of Drugs Act*. London: HSMO.

Jenkins, C., Costello, J. and Hodge, L. (2004). Systematic review of prevalence of aspirin induced asthma and its implications for clinical practice. *BMJ, 328*, 434–440.

Johansson, K., Nuutila, L., Virtanen, H., Katajisto, J. and Salantera, S. (2005). Preoperative education for orthopaedic patients: Systematic review. *Journal of Advanced Nursing, 50*(2), 212–223.

Johnson, M. (2005). Physiology of chronic pain. In: Banks, C. and Mackrodt, K. (eds) *Chronic Pain Management*. London: Whurr Publishers.

Julius, D. and Basbaum, A.I. (2001). Molecular mechanisms of nociception. *Nature, 413*, 203–210.

Kochhar, S.C. (2002). Cancer pain. In: Warfield, C.A. and Fausett, H.J. (eds) *Manual of Pain Management*, 2nd edn. Philadelphia: Lippincott Williams & Wilkins.

Large, R.G., New, F., Strong, J. and Unruh, A.M. (2002). Chronic pain and psychiatric problems. In: Strong, J., Unruh, A.M., Wright, A. and Baxter, G.D. (eds) *Pain: A Textbook for Therapists*. Edinburgh: Churchill Livingstone.

Lee, H. and Ernst, E. (2005). Acupuncture analgesia during surgery: A systematic review. *Pain, 114*(3), 511–517.

Lin, L. and Wang, R. (2005). Abdominal surgery, pain and anxiety: Preoperative nursing intervention. *Journal of Advanced Nursing, 51*(3), 252–260.

Lundeberg, T. and Stener-Victorin, E. (2002). Is there a physiological basis for the use of acupuncture in pain? *International Congress Series, 1238*, 3–10.

Lynch, M. (2001). Pain as the fifth vital sign. *Journal of Intravenous Nursing, 24*(2), 85–94.

MacIntyre, P.E. and Ready, L.B. (2001). *Acute Pain Management: A Practical Guide*, 2nd edn. London: W.B. Saunders.

Mac Lellan, K. (2006). *Expanding Nursing and Health Care Practice: Management of Pain*. Cheltenham: Nelson Thornes.

MacPherson, R.D. (2000). The pharmacological basis of contemporary pain management. *Pharmacology and Therapeutics, 88*, 163–185.

Main, C.J. and Spanswick, C.C. (2000). *Pain Management: An Interdisciplinary Approach*. Edinburgh: Churchill Livingstone.

Manias, E. (2003). Pain and anxiety management in the postoperative gastro-surgical setting. *Journal of Advanced Nursing, 41*(6), 585–504.

Manias, E., Botti, M. and Bucknall, T. (2002). Observation of pain assessment and management – the complexities of clinical practice. *Journal of Clinical Nursing, 11*, 724–733.

Marieb, E. and Hoehn, K. (2007). *Human Anatomy and Physiology*, 7th edn. San Fransisco: Pearson Benjamin Cummings.

McCaffery, M. (1979). *Nursing Management of the Patient with Pain*, 2nd edn. New York: J.B. Lippincott Company.

McCaffery, M. and Beebe, A. (1994). *Pain: Clinical Manual for Nursing Practice*. Aylesbury: Mosby.

McCaffery, R., Frock, T.L. and Garguilo, H. (2003). Understanding chronic pain and the mind–body connection. *Holistic Nursing Practice, 17*(6), 281–287.

Melzack, R. and Wall, P. (1988). *The Challenge of Pain*, 2nd edn. London: Penguin.

Morley, S., Eccleston, C. and Williams, A. (1999). Systematic review and meta-analysis of randomized controlled trials of cognitive behaviour therapy and behaviour therapy for chronic pain in adults, excluding headache. *Pain, 80*, 1–13.

Scadding, J.W. (2003). Peripheral neuropathies. In: Melzack, R. and Wall, P.D. (eds) *Handbook of Pain Management: A Clinical Companion to Wall and Melzack's Textbook of Pain*. Edinburgh: Churchill Livingstone.

Sindhu, F. (1996). Are non-pharmacological nursing interventions for the management of pain effective? A meta-analysis. *Journal of Advanced Nursing, 24*(6), 1152–1159.

Skevington, S. (1995). *Psychology of Pain*. Chichester: John Wiley and Sons.

Sluka, K.A. and Walsh, D. (2003). Transcutaneous electrical nerve stimulation: Basic science mechanisms and clinical effectiveness. *The Journal of Pain, 4*(3), 109–121.

Solano, J.P., Games, B. and Higginson, I.J. (2006). A comparison of symptom prevalence in far advanced cancer, AIDS, heart disease, chronic obstructive pulmonary disease (COPD) and renal disease. *Journal of Pain and Symptom Management, 31*(1), 58–69.

Stranc, D.S. (2002). Endogenous opioids. In: Warfield, C.A. and Fausett, H.J. (eds) *Manual of Pain Management*, 2nd edn. Philadelphia: Lippincott Williams & Wilkins.

Tortora, G.J. and Grabowski, S.R. (2003). *Principles of Anatomy and Physiology*, 10th edn. New York: John Wiley and Sons.

Vallerand, A.H., Fouladbakhsh, J. and Templin, T. (2005). Patients' choices for the self-treatment of pain. *Applied Nursing Research, 18*, 90–96.

Wigens, L. (2006). The role of complimentary and alternative therapies in pain management. In: Mac Lellan, K. (ed) *Expanding Nursing and Health Care Practice: Management of Pain*. Cheltenham: Nelson Thornes.

Williams, A. (1997). Psychological techniques in the management of pain. In: Thomas, V.N. (ed) *Pain: Its Nature and Management*. London: Bailliere Tindall.

World Health Organization (1986). *Cancer Pain Relief*. Geneva: WHO.

World Health Organization (2002). *National Cancer Control Programmes: Policies and Management Guidelines*, 2nd edn. Geneva: WHO.

Chapter 16

The musculoskeletal system and associated disorders

Ian Peate

Test your prior knowledge

- ❓ How many bones are there in the human body?
- ❓ Discuss a range of factors that can impinge on a person's ability to mobilise independently.
- ❓ What are the key functions of the skeleton?

Learning outcomes

On completion of this section, the reader will be able to:

■ Discuss the development and growth of healthy bone.

■ Describe the function of the musculoskeletal system.

■ Describe some of the pathophysiological changes that may occur to the skeleton.

■ Highlight the role and function of the nurse when caring for those who may suffer with a musculoskeletal condition.

■ Describe some of the complications that may occur as a result of immobility.

■ Outline the activities the nurse must take to reduce complications and promote healing.

Introduction

Every activity that an individual performs is associated with movement, for example non-verbal communication in the form of facial expression, which allows another person to interpret or begin to interpret what we are attempting to communicate. In order to function in an optimal manner a fully functioning musculoskeletal system is required. When breathing occurs and gases are exchanged, mobility is needed for this life-sustaining activity to take place. It is the musculoskeletal system that allows these activities to occur. Mobility is an intrinsic aspect of living.

When injury or disease occurs and this affects the musculoskeletal system, it can result in the person becoming dependent on another person (nurse/carer), the independence usually enjoyed by the person becomes a dependency. Davis (2006) states that diseases of the musculoskeletal system are a major cause of health problems and for the older population they are the biggest, non-neurological threat to health and well-being.

The protection of internal structures is also the responsibility of the musculoskeletal system. Support is provided to the various internal structures, for example the ribs and the protection and support they offer to the lungs and the heart and the kidneys.

In order to provide safe and effective care (for both the patient and the nurse) the nurse needs to understand the fundamental issues related to the musculoskeletal system and how this works. This chapter outlines how the musculoskeletal system operates in order to enable an individual to mobilise. The reader is provided with an overview of the musculoskeletal system and a number of musculoskeletal-related conditions are outlined alongside their associated nursing care.

The nurse's role is to prevent or reduce further injury, identify and reduce the risk of complications, assist in the promotion of healing and promote and maximise independence. If there is a need, then the nurse will also be involved in the rehabilitation process.

The musculoskeletal system

Sometimes the musculoskeletal system is also known as the locomotor system. There are 206 bones in the adult human, of various shapes and sizes; babies are born with 300 bones, but as humans age a number of bones fuse to become bigger bones. Baby's bones are primarily made up of **cartilage** and over time most of this cartilage turns into bone thorough a process called **ossification**. Half of the bones in the adult are in the feet and hands. See Figure 16.1 for the skeleton.

The presence of joints in the limbs (i.e. the elbow and knee joints) allows movement; if there were no joints then there could be no movement, and the skeleton would be rigid. Cartilage, a type of cushion, provides protection for those joints that are exposed to force that is generated during movement. **Ligaments** help to provide joint strength and are either incorporated into the joint capsule or they may be independent of it. Movement at the joint is achieved by contraction of muscles that pass across it.

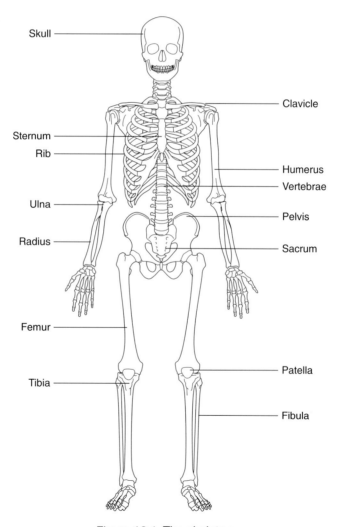

Figure 16.1 The skeleton.

The skeleton, the joints and skeletal muscle work together to provide basic functions that are essential to life:

■ protection for internal organs and to provide support to soft tissue
■ support – maintains an upright posture
■ blood formation – in red bone marrow, **haemopoiesis**
■ mineral homeostasis, storage and release of minerals as the body requires them. The bones store most of the bodies' calcium requirement
■ storage – fat and minerals in the yellow bone marrow
■ leverage, working with the muscles and the bones in the upper and lower limbs pull and push allowing for movement

Bone structure

Bone is a collagen-based matrix with minerals laid upon it; its strength depends on both components. The mineral aspect is composed primarily of calcium, magnesium and phosphorus, and the collagen fibres help with the tension and compression the bone is being subjected to. The collagen fibres and the minerals are densely packed together resulting in a hardening of bone. Vitamin D, parathyroid hormone and calcitonin are important factors in bone mineralisation (Forbes and Jackson, 2003). Bone formation is controlled by osteoblastic and osteoclastic activity. **Osteoblasts** control bone formation and **osetoclasts** are responsible for bone destruction. Throughout life, bone will continue to reform and remodel itself – it is firm, rigid and elastic and dynamic. Bone is more than a rigid structure, and it constantly changes and remodels itself.

The way an individual moves, the amount and type of exercise taken and the diet a person eats and drinks will all influence bone structure (see Figure 16.2).

The skeleton is the body's supporting framework and there are four types of bone:

■ long, i.e. the femur
■ short, i.e. tarsal bones
■ flat, i.e. ribs
■ irregular, i.e. the mandible

Bone structure can be seen in Figure 16.3.

Joints

At the end of where one bone meets another are the joints. Joints are classified threefold:

■ those that allow free movement (i.e. diarthrosis)
■ those that are fixed (i.e. synarthrosis)
■ those that permit limited movement (amphiarthroses)

Heath (2000) considers four classifications of joints:

■ synostotic
■ cartilaginous
■ fibrous
■ synovial

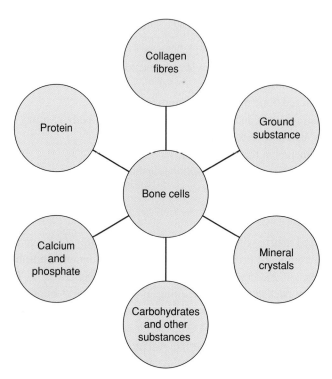

Figure 16.2 Bone production. (Adapted from Davis, 2006.)

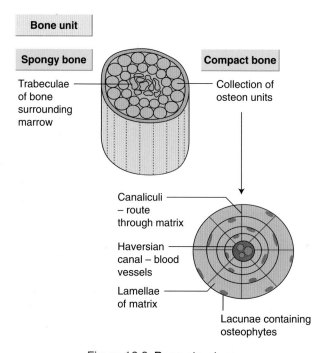

Figure 16.3 Bone structure.

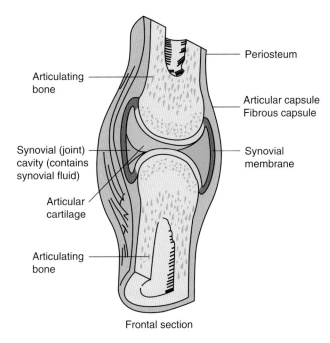

Figure 16.4 A synovial joint.

The synovial joint allows free movement. Bony surfaces (the ends of the bones) are covered by articular cartilage and are connected by ligaments; the types of synovial joints include:

- pivotal joints (i.e. the joint between the humeral radius and the ulna)
- ball and socket joints (i.e. the hip joint)
- hinge joints (i.e. the interphalangeal joints of the fingers)

In synovial joints, a space exists between the bone surface which allows movement of one bone against the other. Synovial fluid present in the synovial joint provides nutrition for the articular cartilage and lubrication for the joint surfaces (Epstein *et al.*, 2003). Throughout life, synovial joints are subjected to a lifetime of wear and tear as a result of the stress placed upon them. The wear and tear is usually seen in the cartilage at the end of the bone where the end of another bone rubs against it; when this occurs it can cause an inflammatory process to occur and can bring with it pain and loss of movement. Figure 16.4 demonstrates a synovial joint.

Muscle

Skeletal muscle has the ability to contract and relax. A motor neuron innervates 100–1000 skeletal muscle fibres and when contraction of the muscle occurs, the impulse that travels from the nerve to the muscle does so across the neuromuscular junction. The electrical activity causes thin **actin** containing filaments to shorten, resulting in contraction of muscle. Removal of this actin-rich stimulus results in relaxation of the muscle (see Figure 16.5). Electrical activity and the relationship between skeletal muscle is discussed later on in this chapter.

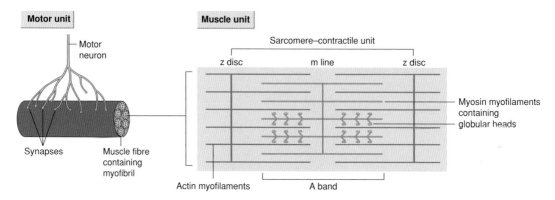

Figure 16.5 Muscle.

Muscles are often arranged in pairs associated with two or more bones and a joint. Those muscles that are associated with movement are to be found within the skeletal region where movement is caused by leverage. The pair of muscles have opposing functions: one muscle acts as the flexor (contracting and flexing) and the other as the extensor (relaxing and extending). The muscles that are attached to the bones provide the necessary force to move an object.

Body mechanics is a term used to incorporate the following coordinated efforts of the musculoskeletal and nervous systems (Heath, 2000):

- to maintain balance
- to provide posture
- to ensure body alignment

There are certain muscles that are associated with posture; these muscles are primarily the muscles of the trunk, neck and back. They converge obliquely at a common tendon, are short and featherlike in appearance. Working together they provide stability and support body weight, thus allowing a sitting or standing posture to be maintained.

The nervous system

Movement and posture are both regulated by the nervous system. There is an area in the brain (the cerebral cortex) that houses the voluntary motor area. The specific area in the cerebral cortex – the precentral gyrus or motor strip – sends impulses down the motor strip to the spinal cord during voluntary movement. Muscles are stimulated after a variety of very complex neural and chemical activities have taken place and movement occurs.

Movement can be impaired by a number of disorders that impede neural and chemical activity to take place; if the muscles will not be stimulated movement will not occur. The concept – mobility – is complex, and there are various texts available that will explain in more detail this multifaceted activity. This aspect of the chapter has merely touched on the complexities associated with the activity – mobility. Suffice it to say that in order to care for a patient with problems related to mobility, the nurse needs to have a sound understanding of the many principles underpinning it.

Assessing the patient with a musculoskeletal disorder

In order to help people who present with altered pathophysiology of the musculoskeletal system, the nurse needs to take an in-depth nursing and medical history; this combined with a physical examination can help the nurse help the patient. There may be further diagnostic tests that are needed to confirm diagnosis and aid in the management of care.

Taking a history requires the nurse to have excellent effective communication skills. The competent nurse will be able to identify serious conditions that need urgent attention quickly, many patients will communicate to the nurse that they are in pain (verbally or non-verbally). The type of pain will determine if the patient has an inflammatory or mechanical condition (Wakley *et al.*, 2001); a physical examination provides information about what aspect of the anatomy has been injured.

Finding out as much as possible about the pain the person is experiencing can be done by asking three questions:

- Where is the pain?
- What type of pain?
- What makes it better or worse?

Table 16.1 highlights some important issues associated with pain in relation to the musculoskeletal system.

Examining the patient provides the nurse with information in relation to the anatomical site. When examining the person with a musculoskeletal problem the nurse is generally able to make a comparison with the unaffected side of the body; usually it is advised that the unaffected side be examined first to determine what is normal for the patient. See Table 16.2 for some issues associated with physical examination and the musculoskeletal system.

When the history has been taken and a physical examination performed there may be a need for further investigations such as blood tests, X-rays and various other imaging procedures, for example, magnetic resonance imaging (MRI) and computer tomography (CT).

Disorders of the musculoskeletal system

There are many issues that may result in a disorder of the musculoskeletal system:

- congenital anomalies
- infection
- inflammation
- degenerative processes
- trauma
- cancer
- vascular disease
- metabolic disorders

Characteristic	Possible meaning
Numb, burning shooting, 'pins and needles'	May be neurological in nature
Pain that is relieved by rest is known as **claudication** pain	This type of pain can mean that there is arterial insufficiency
Pain that is worse on movement or when weight bearing and is relieved by rest	It is likely to be associated with damage to articular structures
Some types of pain that are associated with a joint but in a vague way, when examined the joint seems normal, pain that is unceasing even at night	This pain may be due to referred pain or a bone **lesion**
Multiple painful joints, morning stiffness that improves with exercise. The patient may also be feeling unwell, has a pyrexia and experienced weight loss	These may be signs of inflammation. Could be the result of rheumatoid arthritis
Short duration of morning stiffness, with little or no pain at rest. The pain may become worse during or after sustained exercise and particularly if there is no evidence of systemic disease (for example, the patient feels unwell, has a pyrexia and has lost weight loss)	This can suggest local mechanical problems, for example osteoarthritis, a sprain or strain

Table 16.1 Pain and its possible causes in association with musculoskeletal system

Characteristic	Possible meaning
Warmth over the joint, for example the elbow	Can indicate an inflammatory process
Swelling of the joint, for example the knee	There may be joint **effusion**, enlargement of the bone or synovial thickening
Reduced range of movement with tenderness	Soft tissue injury or muscle injury
Unable to move the limb independently or with help	Structurally abnormal joint
Crepitus with pain	Could suggest damage to articular surfaces
Knee or ankle muscle weakness (unstable)	Ligament tear

Table 16.2 Issues associated with examination of the musculoskeletal system

Musculoskeletal conditions can usually be divided into acute or chronic (long-term) conditions and the care and treatment required will reflect this. Acute conditions are often the result of injury or over-use and are treated according to the acronym **RICE**:

Rest until the swelling and the worse of the pain has settled down.
Ice packs can reduce the swelling, but be careful that the patient does not suffer with ice burns to the skin.
Compression and compassion, support in the form of Tubigrip may be required and the nurse must take care when applying it so as not to cause the person any more pain.
Elevation, swelling can be reduced by elevating the limb.

Pain relief may be required and this can be prescribed; however, some patients will buy over-the-counter medications such as ibuprofen or paracetamol. The person should be encouraged to mobilise as soon as possible; this may be gradual and in the form of non-weight bearing. Referral to a physiotherapist or sports physiotherapist can be arranged as they can provide expert advice on how to return to normal functioning in a safe way.

Chronic musculoskeletal pain is, according to Woolf (2002), reported in surveys by one in four people – musculoskeletalconditions have an enormous and growing impact worldwide. Chronic diseases can be defined as illnesses that are long-lasting, do not resolve of their own accord and are rarely cured completely. Osteoarthritis is an example of a chronic musculoskeletal condition.

Fractures and bone healing

Many patients refer to fractures as 'broken bones': fractures are defined as a break in the continuity of bone and this can be the result of direct or indirect trauma, underlying disease or repeated stress on a bone. Those fractures that are caused by underlying disease are known as pathological fractures and those by repeated stress are called stress fractures (Langstaff, 2000).

It has already been stated that one of the unique functions of bone is its ability to regenerate; it is able to produce new cells and remove those cells that have died. Tortora and Grabowski (2003) suggest that the balance of calcium is a critical element in bone growth and repair; this is affected by the level of vitamin D in the body as well as renal and intestinal functioning, parathyroid gland functioning and the ability of the adrenal glands to work effectively.

Osteology is the scientific study of bones. Bone has the ability to heal by itself; however, it can be aided by making the broken bone immobile, restricting movement or by surgical intervention. A well-balanced diet will also aid bone healing. A well-balanced diet includes foods from the five main food groups, they are:

- bread cereal and potatoes
- fruit and vegetables
- meat and fish
- milk and diary foods
- fat and sugar

Fibroblasts (cells that take part in bone healing) originate within the connective tissue of the periosteum; therefore, the more damage that occurs to the periosteum, the more difficult it will be for the bone to

Time scale	Bone activity
Within the first 6 hours	As result of the blood vessels in the bone becoming ruptured, **haematoma** formation occurs
6–48 hours	The inflammatory process begins and **cytokines** are released, this causes fibroblasts to migrate to the haematoma and tissue granulation begins
2–7 days	As granulation tissue begins to form, it becomes denser and more stable and joins with infiltrating cartilage tissue. **Macrophages** begin to work on the haematoma and osteoclasts resorb the damaged bone
Weeks	Callus formation occurs, this is where the structure surrounding the fracture area becomes hard. This harder woven bone is eventually remodelled and becomes lamellar bone
Months	The callus, within time, becomes smaller as the bone is reconstructed

Source: Adapted from McRae (2006).

Table 16.3 Osteology

heal (Tortora and Grabowski, 2003). McRae (2006) describes the bone-healing process and states that it can take months for full bone healing to take place. There are several stages involved in the bone healing process. Table 16.3 provides information about the bone-healing process and the approximate time scales involved.

Fracture of the bone can occur for a variety of reasons; however, the most common type of fractures are those sustained by the older population as result of osteoporosis, with most fractures occurring near the **proximal** aspect of the head of the humerus (Docherty, 2007). There are five ways of classifying the type of fracture sustained:

- hairline – usually this type of fracture only affects the outer bone
- simple – bone damage but little or no soft tissue injury
- incomplete (also known as greenstick) – commonly seen (but not exclusively) in children, only one side of the bone is fractured
- comminuted – more than two fragments of bone have been broken, the bone has broken off
- compound – a very complicated type of fracture where the bone breaks through the skin. There is high risk of haemorrhage and infection when this type of fracture is sustained

Figures 16.6(a)–16.6(d) demonstrate four types of fractures.

The aim of bone healing is to restore the normal anatomy and function of the fractured bone. The nurse also has a responsibility to reduce the complications that can occur as a result of immobility. Some of the complications associated with immobility are found in Box 16.1.

Spray (2003) suggests that adult patients who were confined to bed rest for approximately 27 days, average a 0.9% loss in mineral content, such as calcium per week. It can be seen that bed rest is not

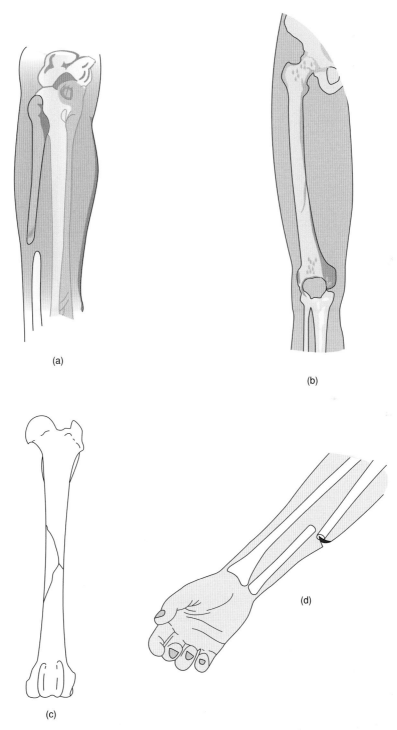

Figure 16.6 The four types of fractures: (a) simple, (b) incomplete (greenstick), (c) comminuted and (d) compound.

Box 16.1 Some potential complications associated with immobility

Deep vein thrombosis
Pulmonary embolism
Increased cardiac work load
Orthostatic hypotension
Decreased cardiac output and reduced tissue perfusion
Chest infection
Renal stones
Incontinence
Muscle wasting
Joint contractures
Loss of self-esteem
Frustration
Boredom
Isolation

Source: Peate (2005).

without serious complications. The nurse must be aware of these actual and potential complications such as constipation and chest infection and be proactive when planning nursing interventions to prevent or reduce the harmful consequences of bed rest. Bed rest can be considered as therapeutic interventions that will help achieve several objectives (Day, 2004) such as:

■ the provision of rest for those patients who are exhausted
■ decrease the body's oxygen consumption
■ reduce pain and discomfort

These objectives also link with the key role of the nurse:

■ to act as a preventative agent
■ to educate
■ to provide comfort

Although there are good reasons for bed rest it can be counterproductive to the patient's recovery. The nurse has a key role to play in helping to promote independence and provide the patient with a sense of well-being (Courtenay, 2002). In some instances, the nurse may need to move the patient when he/she is unable to do so. Jamieson *et al.* (1997) suggest that it may be necessary for one, two or more staff using mechanical aids to move a patient, and the nurse must ensure that safe moving and handling techniques are being used to prevent injury to themselves as well as the patient.

Osteoarthritis

Osteoarthritis is the most common disorder to affect joints (Doherty and Lohmander, 2002); as a person ages its frequency increases, causing pain and disability. Osteoarthritis is the single most important cause of locomotor disability. The following joints can be affected:

Box 16.2 Risk factors associated with osteoarthritis

- ■ Those aged 45 years and over (uncommon in younger people)
- ■ Women are more at risk than men
- ■ A higher incidence in Black and Asian populations
- ■ Those who have a genetic predisposition
- ■ Those who are overweight and obese
- ■ Those with poor muscle function
- ■ Some occupations, for example farming
- ■ Those who have experienced a previous fracture
- ■ Those people who have experienced **menisectomy**

Source: Adapted from Davies *et al*. (2006).

- ■ the small joints of the hands
- ■ the neck
- ■ the lower back
- ■ the big toe
- ■ the knee
- ■ the hip

Osteoarthritis can be said to be a degenerative disease (due to wear and tear) of articular cartilage; it is now suggested that the cause of osteoarthritis is also as a result of metabolic disease. The disease causes damage to the cartilage surfaces of synovial joints. In more severe cases the joint space becomes narrow and **osteophytes** form. The patient tends to seek help because of the pain caused by osteoarthritis and the way it infers with their ability to mobilise. There are known risk factors associated with the disease (see Box 16.2).

Signs and symptoms

The patient presents with joint pain and there is a history of joint stiffness. On examination there may be evidence of **creptius**, swelling and muscle weakness and wasting; often the person becomes increasingly immobile – loss of function can occur. Most commonly the patient usually complains of pain in the hands, hip or knee.

Diagnosis

History and examination are vital. Analysis of X-ray may demonstrate a reduced joint space, osteophyte formation and other abnormalities (see Figure 16.7). Other investigations will also need to be carried out to exclude other causes of pain, for example blood tests to rule out inflammatory disease such as inflammatory arthritis.

Nursing care and management

The role of the nurse is to reduce pain, increase mobility and independence and to minimise progression of the disease. Pain control can be managed by some patients with the use of paracetamol, and there may

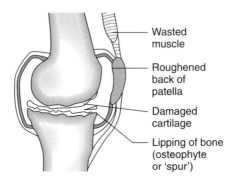

Wasted muscle

Roughened back of patella

Damaged cartilage

Lipping of bone (osteophyte or 'spur')

Figure 16.7 A knee joint with osteoarthritis.

be some patients who will benefit from the use of non-steroidal anti-inflammatory drugs (NSAIDs) either orally or topically applied. Local heat or cold applied to the affected region may help to ease the pain.

The patient may need to be referred to a physiotherapist who can advise about exercise regimens and the occupational therapist who can help with adaptations to the home if they are needed. Referral to an orthopaedic surgeon may be required if joint replacement is an issue. If the patient is overweight or obese, weight reduction is recommended as this can reduce weight on the joint, decrease other symptoms and prevent progression of osteoarthritis in the affected joint.

Osteoporosis

In the elderly, osteoporosis is a major cause of death. The impact of fractures as a result of osteoporosis can have an overwhelming effect on the quality of an individual's life. Osteoporosis is a metabolic disease resulting in loss of bone mass, particularly in postmenopausal women (Proctor, 2004). Khot and Polmear (2006) suggest that osteoporosis is a disorder of diminished bone density and degenerate microarchitecture leading to increased fragility and threat of fracture. The skeleton is affected, the bones become weak and break, bone breakdown occurs faster than bone is being built.

Osteoporosis means porous bones and is defined as a reduction in bone density, along with skeletal fragility and an increase in the risk of fracture after minimal trauma. Everyone loses bone as they age, and the amount varies from person to person. Some people lose much more bone than others and their bones become fragile and break more easily.

Risk factors

Everyone is at risk of developing osteoporosis as they age, there are some factors that make some people more at risk. Risk factors that are associated with the development of osteoporosis are associated with an interaction of multiple factors in a genetically susceptible person:

- advancing age – risk of osteoporosis and fractures increases with age
- sex hormone deficiency
- low body mass index (underweight)
- medications (such as steroid use)
- chronic disease, for example chronic liver disease, inflammatory bowel or coeliac disease
- previous fracture
- early menopause

- family history of maternal hip fracture
- immobility
- environmental hazards such as an unsafe carpets and rugs in the home
- smoking
- alcohol abuse

The person who suffers with osteoporosis may experience immobility and this can bring with it an increase in dependence on others; for some people the result may be death. There is personal distress as a result and this is also accompanied with financial expense.

Diagnosis

Diagnosis is usually made after the patient has suffered a fracture, and sometimes diagnosis of osteoporosis can be overlooked. Diagnosis can also be made by carrying out a number of investigations as well as taking an in-depth nursing and medical history, coupled with physical examination. X-ray cannot diagnose osteoporosis; it can, however, reveal fractures of the vertebra that have occurred as a result of osteoporosis. Special scans called dual energy X-ray absorptionmetry (DEXA) can be used to measure the density of the bone (bone mineral density); this can confirm diagnosis as well as quantifying the risk of fracture that may be due to osteoporotic changes. Blood tests are required to assess a variety of biochemical substances, for example:

- serum calcium, albumin, phosphate
- serum creatinine
- serum thyroid-stimulating hormone
- alkaline phosphatase and liver transaminases

Nursing care and management

Increasing awareness and encouraging activities to reduce risk can prevent the personal and financial hardships from occurring. Pain is a key feature of osteoporosis immediately when a bone fractures or in the long-term in association with hip, wrist or vertebral fractures; the pain of osteoporotic fractures can be both acute and chronic. There are some over-the-counter analgesics that may help some patients and the pharmacist may be able to provide advice; there are some patients who may, however, need stronger analgesia. Acute pain can be incapacitating and the nurse may need to engage the help of other health care professionals, for example, those working in pain services; strong analgesics may be required for **opiates**.

Lifestyle advice is also a part of the care and management of the person with osteoporosis and the person requires advice concerning:

- regular weight-bearing exercise
- adequate nutrition (eating foods that are rich in calcium and vitamin D)
- avoidance of smoking
- avoidance of excessive alcohol intake

There is a range of pharmacological interventions that can be used to improve bone mass (see Table 16.4). Alternative methods of pain relief include:

Drug	Action
Bishosphonates	Decreases bone loss and fracture rate
Strontium ranelate	Increases bone formation and decreases resorption of bone
Selective oestrogen receptor modulator (SERM)	These inhibit bone resorption
Hormone replacement therapy (HRT)	Postpones postmenopausal bone loss and decreases fractures

Source: Adapted from Davies *et al*. (2006).

Table 16.4 Some of the pharmacological agents that may be used in the treatment for osteoporosis

■ Transcutaneous electrical nerve stimulation (TENS) – electrical signals are used to block or reduce pain impulses from getting to the brain.
■ Complementary therapies, for example aromatherapy, homeopathy and acupuncture, may help to relieve pain as well as increasing well-being.

As well as the physical issues the nurse must also consider the psychological aspects associated with osteoporosis. Being in pain can result in lack of sleep, as well as having the potential to make the patient depressed. Psychological assessment and interventions may be required, as well as considering the use of antidepressants.

Measures must be taken to reduce the risk of falls and the damage that can be caused by falls (i.e. fractures). Falls are one of the biggest risk factors for fractures and there is an increase in the tendency to fall as the patient ages.

Gout

Gout also known as crystal-induced arthritis is an inflammatory disease (Davies *et al*., 2006; Wakley *et al*., 2001) of the joints as the result of the deposition of crystals of the sodium salt of **uric acid**; it is the most common cause of inflammatory joint disease in men aged 40 years and over. The patient experiences intermittent episodes of joint pain due to the uric crystals. Uric acid is the waste product formed from the breakdown of food and protein in the blood and tissues; the crystals, formed after supersaturation of the tissues are needle-like and can cause inflammation and painful swelling of the joints. There are three joints that are commonly (but not exclusively) affected:

■ the first metatarso-phalangeal joint
■ the midtarsal joints
■ the knee

Gout is more common in men than women and has prevalence of 1% of the population (Perkins and Jones, 1999), affecting those aged between 40 and 50 years. Gout is rare in those men under 25 years

Box 16.3 Some predisposing factors associated with gout

Family history
Obesity
Excess alcohol intake
High purine diet (purines are found in many foods, for example meat, game and seafood)
Use of diuretics
Acute infection
Ketosis
Surgery
Leukaemia
Cytotoxic drugs
Hypertension
Renal failure

and in those women who are premenopausal. There are a number of predisposing factors that puts a person more at risk of contracting gout (see Box 16.3).

Diagnosis

The person may experience intermittent episodes of acute joint pain; this is a characteristic sign, often beginning during the night and can be brought about by trauma or another illness and reaches a peak within a few hours. The pain may be so great that the patient is unable to tolerate the weight of bed clothes. As well as painful swollen joints the skin over the affected area may be red and shinny, it may also peel, there may be pyrexia and fever and the patient may have loss of appetite and malaise. More than one joint can be affected (this is termed polyarticular) particularly in the elderly person, and the joint may feel hot to touch.

Diagnosis is confirmed by in-depth history taking, examination and investigation; investigations are not carried out until the acute phase is over. Blood tests are required that may show an elevated white blood cell count and an increase in blood urate. In some instances the fluid in the joint (the synovial fluid) may be aspirated (fluid removed through a needle and syringe) and analysed; analysis of the synovial fluid will exclude the possibility of **septic arthritis**. Renal function tests may also be needed to rule out renal disease. X-rays will be unhelpful as they will usually only reveal soft tissue swelling.

Nursing care and management

Treatment is threefold:

1. pain management
2. lifestyle modification
3. lowering of urate levels

Pain relief is a central aspect of the care and management of the person with gout. NSAIDs such as diclofenac or indomethacin may help, but the nurse must be aware that such medications may cause gastrointestinal disturbances (for example, gastric haemorrhage); if this is the case alternative medications must be given. The patient should rest and the affected limb should be elevated and the application of an ice pack may help; a bed cradle should be used to take the weight of the bed clothes off the patient's joints. The injection of steroid preparations into the joint is also effective.

The nurse as health educator should encourage the patient to reduce weight if overweight or obese, and alcohol should be reduced as well as those foods that are high in purine (for example sardines, liver and red meats) – lifestyle modification is needed. If the patient is receiving aspirin (salicylate) or diuretic medications these should be reviewed with a view to stopping them if possible.

There are some medications, for example allopurinol, that act in order to lower the level of uric acid. Wakley *et al.* (2001) point out that once this drug is started it has to be taken for a lifetime; therefore, the decision to commence this type of medication must be carefully explained to the patient using a language that they understand in order for them to arrive at an informed decision.

Myasthenia gravis

This condition is known as an autoimmune disease (Henry and Kilpatrick, 2006); it is a chronic autoimmune disease and is cited as a neurological disease by Clarke (2005). According to the Myasthenia Gravis Association (2004), myasthenia gravis is a complicated condition that is not fully understood, the condition fluctuates in severity as well its distribution throughout the body and the person can experience relapses and remissions. In some patients, the condition resolves spontaneously but in others it persists for life. There are three myasthenias:

1. myasthenia gravis
2. congenital myasthenias
3. the Lambert–Eaton myasthenic syndrome

This aspect of the chapter will briefly consider myasthenia gravis.

The disease is a progressive neuromuscular disease of the lower motor neurones characterised by muscle weakness and fatigue. Chapter 10 of this book discusses the central nervous system and associated disorders in more detail. Clarke (2005) notes that the condition is twice as common in women as it is in men, with a peak age incidence of approximately 30 years of age.

Electrical activity in the muscles

For skeletal muscles to contract, it needs to receive electrical nerve impulses from the fibres of motor neurones – these are nerve cells. In the central nervous system (the brain or spinal cord), the electrical impulses originate (Davis, 2006). The electrical impulses travel to a nerve cell close to the muscle via the nervous system where chemical messengers (also called neurotransmitters) are released into the gap between the nerve cell and muscle cell. A neuromuscular junction is formed when the end of the nerve cell is in close contact with the muscle cell membrane; this structure is similar to a **synapse**. Acetylcholine is the neurotransmitter that is released into the neuromuscular junction (Marieb, 2006).

Acetylcholine has short distance to travel across the nerve cell to the muscle membrane, when it reaches the muscle membrane it attaches itself to receptors generating electrical impulses in the muscle. Calcium is released into the muscle cell when the impulses occur and this usually results in muscle contraction.

In myasthenia gravis, the action of acetylcholine is not fully effective. The body's immune system produces autoantibodies that attack the muscle cells (receptors) at the neuromuscular junction and neurones are unable to stimulate the muscle cells adequately (Richardson, 2006). The result of this ineffective activity is that muscular contraction becomes weak and ineffective. Muscle weakness particularly in the face, throat and eyes progressing to all four limbs and the muscles of the respiratory tract occurs.

There are some patients who may be more at risk of developing myasthenia gravis than others, it can affect all races. Those who have a tendency to inherit autoimmune diseases, such as diabetes mellitus and thyroid disease, are at an increased risk. Risk also increases if the person has a relative with an autoimmune disease. Myasthenia gravis is not an inherited disease and does not occur in families.

Diagnosis

Patient history and examination will help to reveal a diagnosis. The patient may experience abnormal muscle fatigability and muscle weakness. The most common manifestations are **ptosis** and **diplopia**. There may also be an accompanying **dysarthria**, **dysphagia**, ocular palsy, facial and limb weaknesses. Respiratory involvement will lead to breathlessness, in the acute stage respiratory distress can occur and this may lead to respiratory arrest followed by cardiac arrest.

There are a number of tests that can be used to confirm or refute the diagnosis. The most common test used to confirm diagnosis is the Tensilon test (Cunning, 2000). Tensilon (edrophonium) is an **anticholinesterase** and is injected intravenously; those patients who show an improvement in muscular strength after the test have tested positive for the disease. This anticholinesterase increases the effective amount of acetylcholine at the neuromuscular junction in those patients with myasthenia gravis. The response is measured over 1 minute and lasts no longer than 5 minutes; it is vital that resuscitation an equipment is at hand when performing this test.

Blood tests may also be needed, for example, testing for the antibodies to acetylcholine receptors. These antibodies according to Clarke (2005) are found in no other condition. An electro-myogram (EMG) is a test that involves measuring the electrical activity within the muscle after a fine needle is inserted into the muscle; however, not all centres offer such a facility. There are some patients with myasthenia gravis who also have an enlarged thymus gland (this may be due to a tumour) and a scan of the chest or a chest X-ray may need to be performed.

Nursing care and management

No single treatment works for all patients; it advocated that an individualised care package be produced once a diagnosis has been made. The condition can be life-threatening, but with appropriate treatment, advice and support the majority of patients can become symptom free. Careful explanation regarding the condition must be provided and the patient should be advised to avoid activities that may put them in danger if they suddenly become weak, for example swimming alone. The nurse should communicate clearly with the patient, encouraging concordance with medications and to avoid activities such as stress inducing activities that may exacerbate the condition. As some patients with myasthenia gravis suffer with respiratory difficulties the patient should be advised to have annual influenza immunisations. A coordinated, multidisciplinary approach to care should be adopted as there are several health care professionals that may be needed to intervene and provide care for the patient, for example physiotherapist, occupational therapist and dietician. The diagnosis of a long-term potentially life-threatening disease can instil fear and anxiety in patients and they may as a result experience depression, careful assessment of the patient's psychological state is required and where appropriate referral to the most suitable health care professional, for example, a psychologist and/or counsellor.

Medications such as oral anticholinesterase can be prescribed, for example, pyridostigmine, this medication prolongs the action of acetylcholine by inhibiting the production of cholinesterases.

Immunosuppressive medications, for example corticosteroids, may be of value as these medicines have an **immunosuppressive** effect. If there is thymus involvement then thymectomy may improve prognosis. Special procedures, for example **plasmapheresis**, can also have some impact for some patients as this procedure attempts to remove the destructive antibodies. One other option is the injection of intravenous immune globulin; this, it is thought, reduces the function or production of antibodies (Clarke, 2005). **Plasmapheresis** intravenous immunoglobulins produce a rapid improvement in symptoms but only last for approximately 6 weeks.

Conclusion

Every activity of living is associated with mobility and the degree of mobility/immobility will alter as the patient traverses the lifespan. The ability to move about freely allows us to meet our basic needs, for example eating, drinking and elimination as well as being able to carry out leisure and work-related activities that will enable us to maintain our social contact and enhance our self-esteem.

Some patients may become totally dependent on others for their care; some may become transiently dependent on others and will then return to carrying out their activities of living in an independent manner. All body systems can be affected by the hazardous effects of immobility; the longer the patient is immobilised the greater the consequences (McCance and Huether, 2006). There are many potential complications associated with bed rest that can cause discomfort (physically and psychosocially); the nurse, therefore, has to assume an active role in the prevention or minimisation of the potential problems. The role of the nurse is predominantly threefold – to comfort, educate and prevent.

It is not possible in a chapter of this size to address in depth all concerns associated with the musculoskeletal system and the reader is advised to read more detailed texts in order to inform clinical practice with the aim of improving their clinical nursing skills.

Multiple choice questions

1. Babies are born with 300 bones in their bodies, when they reach adulthood this number is:
(a) 320
(b) 299
(c) 196
(d) 206

2. The largest bone in the human body is the:
(a) clavicle
(b) ulna
(c) femur
(d) tibia

3. What is the smallest bone in the human body?
(a) mandible
(b) radius
(c) sternum
(d) stirrup

4. A joint that allows free movement is known as:
(a) diarthrosis
(b) haemarthrosis
(c) synarthrosis
(d) amphiarthroses

5. When electrical activity occurs in the muscle this causes thin actin-containing filaments to:
(a) lengthen
(b) shorten
(c) stay the same
(d) rupture

6. When the actin-rich stimulus is removed, this results in:
(a) relaxation of the muscle
(b) contraction of the muscle
(c) no change in the muscle
(d) rupture of the muscle

7. The area in the brain that houses the major voluntary motor area is called the:
(a) precentral gyrus

(b) the medulla oblongata

(c) the midbrain

(d) the cerebral cortex

8. Opiates are:

(a) antibiotics

(b) antifungals

(c) strong analgesics

(d) antiplatelets

9. How long can the effects of plasmapheresis be expected to last in patients with myasthenia gravis?

(a) 2 days

(b) 6 months

(c) 2 years

(d) 6 weeks

10. The most common test used to confirm diagnosis in myasthenia gravis is:

(a) the Tensilon test

(b) electromyography

(c) gelectrocardiography

(d) blood tests

Answers: 1.d, 2.c, 3.d, 4.a, 5.b, 6.a, 7.d, 8.c, 9.d, 10.a.

Test your knowledge

❓ Describe the role and function of the nurse in relation to the care of the person who has a musculoskeletal problem.

❓ Discuss the environmental, physical, psychological, politicoeconomic and sociocultural factors that need to be taken into account when caring for a person with a musculoskeletal problem.

❓ Describe the ways in which the musculoskeletal system is able to perform and fulfil several different roles.

Glossary of terms

Actin: This is a contractile protein of muscle.

Anticholinesterase: An agent that blocks nerve impulses by inhibiting the activity of an enzyme called cholinesterase.

Cartilage: Strong tough material on the bone ends that helps to distribute the load within the joint, the slippery surface allows smooth movement between the bones.

Cholinesterase: An enzyme that breaks down acetylcholine to stop its action.

Claudication: Ischaemia of the muscles, causing lameness and pain brought on by walking particularly in the calf muscles.

Crepitus: A crinkling, cracking or grating feeling or sound in the joints.

Cytokines: A hormone-like protein that regulates the intensity and duration of immune responses.

Diplopia: A condition where a single object is perceived as two objects.

Dyarthria: A disturbance of speech and language.

Dysphagia: Difficulty on swallowing.

Effusion: A collection of fluid.

Haematoma: A localised collection of blood that is often clotted due to a break in the wall of a blood vessel.

Haemopoiesis: The formation and development of blood cells.

Immunosuppressive: Pertaining to immunosuppression – prevention or interference with the development of immunologic response.

Lesion: Wound or injury, refers to a change in the tissues.

Ligaments: Tough fibrous bands that hold two bones together in a joint.

Macrophage: Cells that engulf and digest cellular debris and pathogens.

Menisectomy: Removal of the meniscus (ligament within the knee).

Opiates: A preparation that is derived from opium, narcotic substances, a powerful analgesic.

Ossification: The formation of bone.

Osteoblasts: Cells that arise from fibroblasts, a bone-forming cell.

Osteoclasts: Cells associated with absorption and removal of bone.

Osteophytes: Overgrowth of new bone around the side of osteoarthritic joints, also known as spurs growth.

Plasmapheresis: Removal of whole blood from the body, separation of cellular elements.

Proximal: Nearest to the trunk or point of origin.

Ptosis: Drooping of the upper eye lid.

Resorption: To absorb what has been excreted.

Septic arthritis: A pus forming bacterial infection of a joint space.

Synapse: A connection between excitable cells.

Uric acid: The end product of purine nucleotide (nucleoprotein).

References

Clarke, C.R.A. (2005). Neurological disease. In: Kumar, P. and Clark, M. (eds) *Clinical Medicine*, 6th edn. Edinburgh: Saunders, pp. 1173–1271.

Courtenay, M. (2002). Movement and mobility. In: Hogston, R. and Simpson, P.M. (eds) *Foundations of Nursing Practice: Making the Difference*, 2nd edn. London: Palgrave, pp. 262–285.

Cunning, S. (2000). When the Dx is myasthenia gravis. *RN*, *63*(4), 26–30.

Davies, R., Everitt, H. and Simon, C. (2006). *Musculoskeletal Problems*. Oxford: Oxford University Press.

Davis, G. (2006). The musculoskeletal system: Physiology, conditions and common drug therapies. *Nurse Prescribing*, *4*(10), 406–411.

Day, A. (2004). Mobility and biomechanics. In: Daniels, R. (ed) *Nursing Fundamentals: Caring and Clinical Decision Making*. New York: Thompson, pp. 1162–1236.

Docherty, B. (2007). Skeletal system. Part two – Bone growth and healing. *Nursing Times*, *103*(6), 28–29.

Doherty, M. and Lohmander, S. (2002). The future diagnosis and management of osteoarthritis. In: Woolf, A.D. (ed) *Bone and Joint Futures*. London: British Medical Journal Books, pp. 62–78.

Epstein, O., Perkin, G.D., Cookson, J. and de Bono, D.P. (2003). *Clinical Examination*. London: Mosby.

Forbes, C.D. and Jackson, W.F. (2003). *Clinical Medicine*, 3rd edn. London: Mosby.

Heath, H.B.M. (ed) (2000). *Foundations in Nursing Theory and Practice*. London: Mosby.

Henry, M. and Kilpatrick, C. (2006). Disorders of the immune system, infection control and infectious diseases. In: Alexander, M.F., Fawcett, J.N. and Runciman, P.J. (eds) *Nursing Practice, Hospital and Home: The Adult*, 3rd edn. Edinburgh: Churchill Livingstone, pp. 653–689.

Jamieson, E.M., McCall, J.M., Blythe, R. and Whyte, L.A. (1997). *Clinical Nursing Practices*, 3rd edn. Edinburgh: Churchill Livingstone.

Khot, A. and Polmear, A. (2006). *Practical General Practice: Guidelines for Effective Clinical Management*. Edinburgh: Butterworth Heinemann.

Langstaff, D. (2000). Fracture healing and principles of fracture management. In: Langstaff, D. and Christie, J. (eds) *Trauma Care: A Team Approach*. Oxford: Heinemann.

Marieb, E.N. (2006). *Essentials of Human Anatomy and Physiology*, 8th edn. San Francisco: Pearson.

McCance, K.L. and Huether, S.E. (2006). *Pathophysiology: The Biologic Basis for Disease in Adults and Children*, 5th edn. St. Louis: Mosby.

McRae, R. (2006). *Pocket Book of Orthopaedics and Fractures*, 2nd edn. Edinburgh: Churchill Livingstone.

Myasthenia Gravis Association (2004). *Information Pack. Vol. 5: Medical Information (Medical professions)*. Derby: MGA.

Peate, I. (2005). Mobility and movement. In: Peate, I. (ed) *Compendium of Clinical Skills for Student Nurses*. London: Whurr, pp. 194–206.

Perkins, P. and Jones, A.C. (1999). Gout. *Annals of Rheumatic Disease*, *58*, 611–616.

Proctor, J. (2004). Arthritis. In: Martin, J. and Lucas, J. (eds) *Handbook of Practice Nursing*, 3rd edn. Edinburgh: Churchill Livingstone, pp. 233–249.

Richardson, M. (2006). Muscle physiology. Part 4: Movement and muscle problems. *Nursing Times*, *102*(50), 26–27.

Spray, M.E. (2003). Care of the patient with a musculoskeletal disorder. In: Kockrow, V. (ed) *Adult Health Nursing*, 4th edn. St. Louis: Mosby, pp 102–169.

Tortora, G.J. and Grabowski, S.R. (2003). *Principles of Anatomy and Physiology*, 10th edn. New Jersey: Wiley.

Wakley, G., Chambers, R. and Dieppe, P. (2001). *Musculoskeletal Matters in Primary Care*. Oxford: Radcliffe Medical Press.

Woolf, A.D. (2002). The future provision of care for musculoskeletal conditions. In: Woolf, A.D. (ed) *Bone and Joint Futures*. London: British Medical Journal Books, pp. 1–18.

amazon.co.uk

Thank you for shopping at Amazon.co.uk!

Invoice for

Invoice for	Billing Address
Your order of 9 November 2010	Joanna mayo
Order ID 202-2348141-1675561	148 Snack Wc
Invoice number Dc20r8qsk	Lea
Invoice date 10 November 2010	Preston Lanca
	United Kingdo

Qty.	Item	
1	**Fundamentals of Applied Pathophysiology: An Essential Guide for Nursing Students** Paperback, Nair, Muralitharan 04/10 1/9/56 (** P-1-A148E132 **)	Shipping Add...

Shipping charges
Subtotal (excl. VAT) 0%
Total VAT
Total

Conversion rate - £1.00 EUR 1.14

This shipment completes your order.

You can always check the status of your orders...

Thinking of returning an item? PLEASE USE OUR ON LINE RETURNS SUPPORT CENTRE

Our Returns Support Centre (www.amazon...
return label. Please have your order...

Please note - this is not...

49/DVZbrDqsKV-1 of 1/19/cca/dk/5...

Chapter 17

Fluid and electrolyte balance and associated disorders

Muralitharan Nair and Ian Peate

KEY WORDS

- Diffusion
- Hypovolaemia
- Intracellular
- Oedema
- Electrolytes
- Hypervolaemia
- Osmosis
- Extracellular
- Interstitial fluid
- Osmotic pressure

Test your prior knowledge

- In the human body, where are the extracellular compartments?
- Where is most of the fluid volume found, intracellular or extracellular compartments?
- Define the function of body fluids and electrolytes.
- Define the terms *hypotonic*, *hypertonic* and *isotonic* solutions.

> ## Learning outcomes
>
> On completion of this section, the reader will be able to:
> - Identify the fluid compartments of the body.
> - List the major electrolytes of the extracellular and intracellular compartments of the body.
> - Define the term *osmosis*.
> - Define the term *diffusion*.

Introduction

Fluid and **electrolytes** are essential for body function and to maintain homeostasis. Fluid and electrolytes are not stationary in the body. There is constant movement of fluid and electrolytes between the **intracellular** and **extracellular compartments**. The movement of fluid and electrolytes ensures that the cells are in constant supply of electrolytes such as sodium, chloride, potassium, magnesium, phosphates, bicarbonate and calcium for cellular function. See Chapter 1 for cellular functions. Changes in the movement of fluid and electrolytes between compartments occur as a result of disease. This chapter considers fluid and electrolyte balance and some diseases resulting from fluid and electrolyte imbalance.

Body fluid compartments

The fluid in the body forms approximately 60% of the body weight in an adult male, 50% in an adult female and 70% in an infant (McCance and Huether, 2006). The percentage of fluid distribution varies with age and gender. Women have less body fluid compared to men as women have more body fat and men have more muscle mass (McCance and Huether, 2006). Fat cells contain less water compared to muscle cells.

The two principal body fluid compartments are intracellular and extracellular. The intracellular compartment is the space inside a cell and the fluid inside the cell is called intracellular fluid (ICF). The extracellular compartment is found outside the cell and the fluid outside the cell is called extracellular fluid (ECF). However, the extracellular compartment is further divided into the interstitial compartment and the intravascular compartment (see Figure 17.1). Two-thirds of body fluid is found inside the cell and one-third of the fluid outside the cell. Eighty per cent of the ECF is found in the **interstitial** compartment and 20% in the intravascular compartment as **plasma** (see Figure 17.2).

Composition of body fluid

The body fluid is composed of water and dissolved substances such as electrolytes (sodium, potassium and chloride), gases (oxygen and carbon dioxide), nutrients, enzymes and hormones. The total body

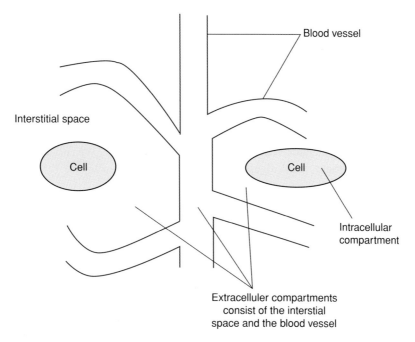

Figure 17.1 Fluid compartments.

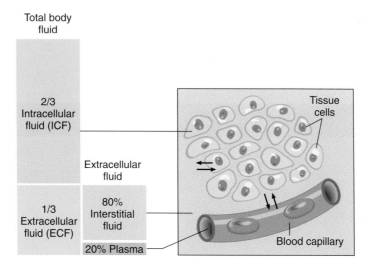

Figure 17.2 Fluid distribution.

water constitutes 60% of the total body weight (Lemon and Burke, 2004) and water plays an important part in cellular function. Water is essential for the body as it:

■ acts as a lubricant
■ transports nutrients, gases such as oxygen, hormones and enzymes to the cells and waste products of metabolism, for example, carbon dioxide, urea and uric acid from the cells for excretion
■ helps in the regulation of body temperature
■ provides an optimum medium for the cells to function
■ provides a medium for chemical reactions
■ breaks down food particles in the digestive system
   (Lemon and Burke, 2004).

Body fluid balance

The term *fluid balance* indicates the body's required amount of water is present and distributed proportionally among the compartments. Generally, water intake equals water loss and the body fluid remains constant. However, fluid intake varies with individuals; but the body regulates fluid volume within a narrow range. Most of the water essential for body function is obtained from drinking water, some from the food consumed and some from cellular **metabolism**. The kidneys play a vital role in fluid balance as water is excreted in the urine, some water is lost in respiration, skin and in faeces. See Table 17.1 for fluid intake and output.

The body regulates body fluid volume via the thirst receptors. When there is an excess of water loss through excessive sweating or by not drinking then the body fluid balance is disrupted which could result in **dehydration**. Dehydration stimulates the thirst reflex in three ways:

■ the blood osmotic pressure increases resulting in the stimulation of the osmoreceptors of the hypothalamus

Intake		Output	
Drinking	1500–2000 mL	Urine	1500–2000 mL
Water from food	700–1000 mL	Faeces	100 mL
Cellular metabolism	300–400 mL	Expiration	600–800 mL
		Skin	300–600 mL
Total balance	2500–3400 mL		2500–3400 mL
Adapted from McCance and Huether (2006).			

Table 17.1 Fluid intake and output

■ circulating blood volume decreases which initiates the renin–angiotensin system resulting in the stimulation of the thirst centre in the hypothalamus

■ as a result of dehydration, the mucosal lining of the mouth is dry and the production of saliva decreases which stimulates the thirst centre in the hypothalamus

Osmosis

Osmosis is a process by which water moves from an area of high volume to an area of low volume through a selective permeable membrane. The movement of water depends on the number of solutes dissolved in the solution and not their weights (Metheny, 1996). Therefore, the number of dissolved particles determines the concentration of the solution which is expressed as the **osmolality** of the solution. The selective permeable membrane will allow water molecules to move across but is not permeable to solutes such as sodium, potassium and other substances. Water accounts for the **osmotic pressure** in tissues and cells of the body. Water movement between the intracellular and the extracellular compartments occur through osmosis.

At times the term **tonicity** is used instead of osmolality. Thus, solutions could be regarded as **hypertonic**, **hypotonic** or **isotonic**. The term *hypertonic* solution indicates that the solution has high amount of solutes dissolved in the solution. An example of a hypertonic solution is 5% dextrose. *Hypotonic* solution is one that has a low concentration of solutes dissolved in the solution. An example of a hypotonic solution is 0.45% normal saline. An *isotonic* solution has the same osmolality as body fluids and an example is 0.9% normal saline (Metheny, 1996).

Electrolytes

Fluid balance is linked to electrolyte balance. Electrolytes are chemical compounds that dissociate in water to form charged particles called ions (Lemon and Burke, 2004). They include potassium (K), sodium (Na), chloride (Cl), magnesium (Mg) and phosphate (HPO_4). Electrolytes are either positively or negatively charged. Positively charged ions are called **cations** (for example, Na^+ and K^+) and negatively charged ions are called **anions** (for example, Cl^- and HCO_3^-). Remember that an anion and a cation will combine to form a compound, for example, potassium (K^+) and chloride (Cl^-) will combine to form potassium chloride (KCl). The composition of electrolytes differs between the intracellular and the extracellular compartments (see Figure 17.3).

Functions of the electrolytes

Electrolytes have numerous functions in the body. They:

■ regulate fluid balance
■ regulate acid–base balance
■ are essential in neuromuscular excitability
■ are essential for neuronal function
■ are essential for enzyme reaction

See Table 17.2 for a summary of the principal electrolytes and their functions.

Diffusion

Diffusion is a process by which solutes move from an area of high concentration to an area of low concentration. Diffusion is further subdivided into simple and facilitated diffusion. Liquid-soluble

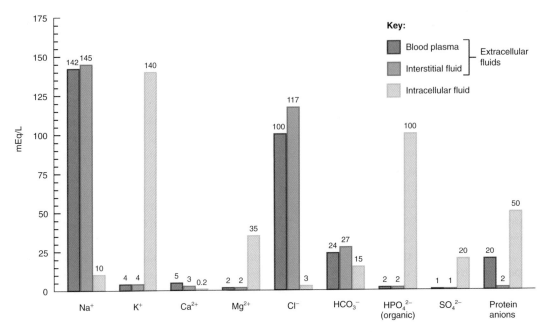

Figure 17.3 Electrolytes of intracellular and extracellular compartments.

molecules and gases move by a process of simple diffusion through a concentration gradient (see Figure 17.4). Larger molecules such as glucose and amino acids are transported across cell membrane by a carrier protein and concentration gradient (see Figure 17.5).

Hormones that regulate fluid and electrolytes

The two principal hormones that regulate fluid and electrolyte balance are antidiuretic hormone (ADH) and aldosterone (Thibodeau and Patton, 2007). Antidiuretic hormone regulates fluid balance in the body. This hormone is produced in the hypothalamus by neurons called osmoreceptors and the hormone is stored by the posterior pituitary gland. Osmoreceptors are sensitive to plasma **osmolality** and a decrease in blood volume. The target organs for ADH are the kidneys. ADH acts on the distal convoluted tubule and the collecting ducts (see Chapter 6) which make the tubules more permeable to water thus increasing reabsorption of water.

Aldosterone is a steroid hormone produced by the adrenal glands which are situated on top of each kidney (see Figure 17.6). The adrenal gland is divided into cortex and the medulla (see Figure 17.7). The cortex produces the steroid hormone aldosterone. Aldosterone regulates electrolyte and fluid balance by sodium and water retention.

Oedema

Oedema is the abnormal accumulation of fluid, mainly water in the body (Kumar and Clark, 2005) in the interstitial space. It is a problem of fluid distribution and does not indicate fluid excess (McCance and Huether, 2006). The term is derived from the Greek word meaning swollen condition. The accumulation of fluid may be localised as in thrombophlebitis or generalised as in heart failure affecting all tissues.

Electrolytes	Normal values in extracellular fluid	Function	Main distribution
Sodium (Na$^+$)	135–145 mmol/L	Important cation in generation of action potentials. Plays an important role in fluid and electrolyte balance	Main cation of the extracellular fluid
Potassium (K$^+$)	3.5–5 mmol/L	Important cation in establishing resting membrane potential. Regulates pH balance. Maintains intracellular fluid volume	Main cation of the intracellular fluid
Calcium (Ca^{2+})	2.1–2.6 mmol/L	Important clotting factor. Plays a part in neurotransmitter release in neurons. Maintains muscle tone and excitability of nervous and muscle tissue	Mainly found in the extracellular fluid
Magnesium (Mg^{2+})	0.5–1.0 mmol/L	Help to maintain normal nerve and muscle function; maintain regular heart rate, regulate blood glucose and blood pressure. Essential for protein synthesis	Mainly distributed in the intracellular fluid
Chloride (Cl$^-$)	98–117 mmol/L	Maintains a balance of anions in different fluid compartments	Main anion of the extracellular fluid
Hydro carbons (HCO$_3^-$)	24–31 mmol/L	Main buffer of hydrogen ions in plasma. Maintains a balance between cations and anions of intracellular and extracellular fluids	Mainly distributed in the extracellular fluid
Phosphate – organic (HPO$_4^{2-}$)	0.8–1.1 mmol/L	Essential for the digestion of proteins, carbohydrates and fats and absorption of calcium. Essential for bone formation	Mainly found in the intracellular fluid
Sulphate (SO$_4^{2-}$)	0.5 mmol/L	Involved in **detoxification** of phenols, alcohols and **amines**	Mainly found in the intracellular fluid

Table 17.2 Principal electrolytes and their functions

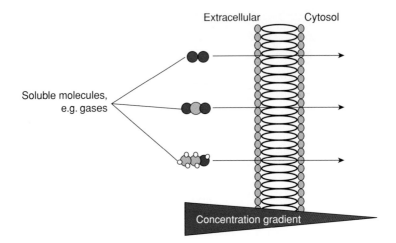

Figure 17.4 Simple diffusion.

Localised oedema is normally temporary and would resolve without intervention. Generalised oedema is regarded as abnormal condition which will require treatment.

Oedema can either be pitting or non-pitting. If an indentation develops after gently pressing the swollen lower limb, with a finger, of a patient it is termed *pitting oedema*. The causes of oedema include:

- heart failure
- obesity resulting in increased fluid pressure and salt retention
- drugs such as calcium antagonists, for example verapamil and nifedipine and prolonged steroid therapy
- renal condition such as nephrotic syndrome
- venous stasis resulting from immobility
- varicose veins
- liver cirrhosis causing hypoalbuminaemia

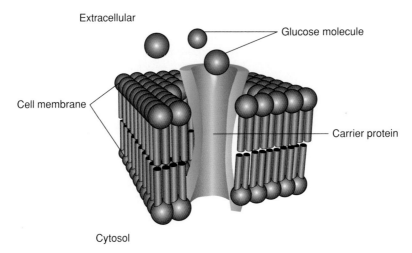

Figure 17.5 Carrier protein (facilitated diffusion).

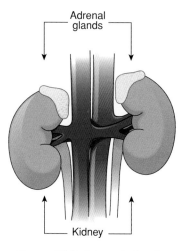

Figure 17.6 Adrenal glands.

Pulmonary oedema

Pulmonary oedema is a condition where there is accumulation of fluid in the lungs resulting in impaired gas (oxygen and carbon dioxide) exchange and pulmonary function. Pulmonary oedema could result from:

- congestive heart failure (see Chapter 5)
- fluid overload as a result of renal failure

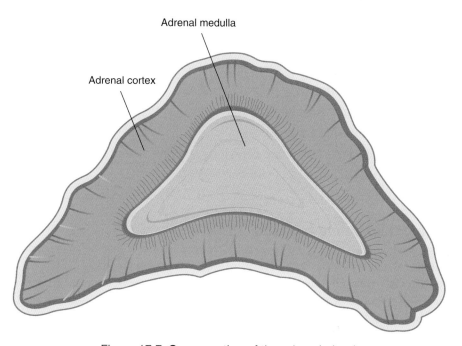

Figure 17.7 Cross section of the adrenal gland.

- myocardial infarction with left ventricular failure
- chest injury as a result of road traffic accident
- upper airway obstruction
- severe chest infection

Peripheral oedema

Peripheral oedema is a condition where there is localised soft tissue swelling as a result fluid accumulation in the interstitial space. Fluid accumulates in parts of the body affected by gravity, for example the lower limbs in a mobile patient or around the sacral region in a patient who is immobile and on bed rest. Peripheral oedema could result from:

- immobility
- obesity
- heart failure
- pregnancy as a result of fluid retention and venous stasis
- liver diseases such as cirrhosis of the liver
- prolonged steroid therapy

Disorders associated with fluid and electrolyte imbalance

Learning outcomes

On completion of this section, the reader will be able to:

- Describe the importance of maintaining a fluid balance chart.
- Discuss the significance of adequate hydration and the benefits of this for the health and well-being of the patient.
- Outline the nursing management and interventions related to the patient who is nauseous and maybe vomiting.
- Outline the nursing management and interventions related to the patient who has pulmonary and/or peripheral oedema.

Maintaining fluid balance charts

Fluid balance according to Carter (2007) is a state where the amount of fluid taken into the body equals the amount of fluid that leaves the body. Sometimes these charts are known as fluid intake and output charts or intake and output flow charts. Maintenance of fluid balance is an important nursing activity and is essential for optimal health. If a patient has too much fluid and there is an imbalance this can cause health problems; likewise if the patient has too little fluid this too can cause problems. There are some pathophysiological conditions that can result in fluid overloading, for example kidney disease and

	Fluid intake			Fluid output		
Ward:				Date:		
Surname:				Hospital Number:		
Forename:						
Date of Birth:						

	Fluid intake			**Fluid output**		
Time	**Oral**	**Intravenous**	**Other (specify)**	**Urine**	**Vomit**	**Other (specify)**
01.00						
02.00						
03.00						
04.00						
05.00						
06.00						
07.00						
08.00						
09.00						
10.00						
11.00						
12.00						
13.00						
14.00						
15.00						
16.00						
17.00						
18.00						
19.00						
20.00						
21.00						
22.00						
23.00						
24.00						
Total						

Figure 17.8 A fluid balance chart.

some types of heart disease; when this occurs the person finds it difficult to rid the body of excess water. When this occurs the person can experience oedema, this is where there is too much fluid in the tissues of the body (care of the patient with oedema is discussed later).

For those patients who are experiencing problems associated with fluid balance the monitoring of fluid balance becomes important. The nurse uses a chart called a fluid balance chart in order to monitor the patient's input and output (see Figure 17.8). Each time the patient takes in fluids or fluids leave the body, the nurse has a responsibility to record this on the fluid balance chart. The amounts are calculated at the end of a 24-hour period – usually this is from 12 midnight to 12 midnight the next night. A comparison is made between the amounts of fluid taken in and the amount of fluid the patient passes out; this is the patient's fluid balance.

Reid *et al.* (2004) suggest that fluid balance charts that are family-friendly should be provided. Family-friendly (user-friendly) fluid balance charts encourage patients and their families to fill them in themselves; this can help to promote independence.

Measuring fluid balance
Intake
All of the fluid that a patient drinks and also those foods that are liquid, milk on cereals and ice cream are deemed fluid intake. There are other fluids that are considered a part of fluid intake, for example enteral feeds and intravenous fluids. All fluid intake must be measured and documented on the patient's fluid balance chart. The nurse needs to know how much various receptacles, such as cups and glasses, hold in order to chart intake effectively.

The amount of enteral feed, gastrostomy and nasogastric feeding and intravenous fluid (including the infusion of blood and or blood products) being infused must also be monitored, measured and documented. There are some patients who require fluid via the subcutaneous or rectal route and the same is required here; the fluid intake must be recorded.

Output
The following are deemed fluid output, and these (just like intake) must be monitored, measured and documented on the fluid balance chart:

- urine (in seriously ill patients with a urinary catheter in situ this may need to be measured and recorded hourly)
- vomit
- aspirate from a nasogastric tube
- diarrhoea
- effluent from a stoma
- exudate from a wound and wound drain

There may be some instances when it is impossible to measure output accurately, for example where the patient has diarrhoea or a wound has excessive exudate, in these instances the nurse may need to weigh incontinence pads or dressings to determine the amount of fluid being lost via this route.

A positive fluid balance exists when the patient's intake exceeds their output and a negative balance occurs when output exceeds intake. Brooker (2007) points out that a record of the daily balance over several days should be carried out so that an assessment of trend can occur.

Maintaining hydration
Florence Nightingale stated that the very first requirement in a hospital is that it should do the sick no harm; this statement was made back in 1854. Having enough to eat and drink is one of the most basic of human needs (DH, 2007). Most people are able to maintain an adequate level of hydration – they are prompted by thirst or hunger to seek fluids or food; however, those who are ill and dependent are unable to do this and they may be at risk of becoming dehydrated. Hodgkinson *et al.* (2003) point out that dehydration is the most common fluid and electrolyte imbalance in older people.

This aspect of the chapter considers the nursing responses that need to be made to ensure that patients are adequately hydrated. It draws on previous aspects of the chapter in respect to fluid and electrolyte balance. Green and Simpson (2007) define hydration as the state of fluid balance of the body. Rapid weight loss as a result of dehydration could be the consequence of a lack of fluid intake or hyponatraemia (sodium depletion) with an accompanying loss of water.

Benefits of good hydration

Water is vital to health and should be seen as an essential nutrient, as people age their body's needs and health concerns change as a result of an increasing susceptibility to pathophysiological disease (Water UK, 2005). There are many benefits associated with good hydration. The implications of poor hydration from a pathophysiological perspective can have many ramifications and some of these are discussed below.

Casimiro *et al.* (2002) describe how those patients who are poorly hydrated have the potential to develop pressure sores (decubitus ulcers); the more an individual becomes dehydrated, the more at risk they become. Dehydration results in a reduction in padding over bony prominences. Fluid intake taken to correct poor hydration can increase oxygen levels with the possibility of enhancing ulcer healing (Stotts and Hopf, 2003).

One of the most frequent causes of chronic constipation is inadequate fluid intake. Those patients who are inadequately hydrated can, by drinking more water, increase stool frequency and enhance the beneficial effects of daily dietary fibre intake (Registered Nurse Association of Ontario, 2005).

It is important in the prevention of urinary tract infection to ensure that the patient maintains adequate hydration. Gray and Krissovich (2003) note that water helps to maintain a healthy urinary tract and promotes renal function. Consumption of water at regular intervals can help by diluting bile and stimulating gall bladder emptying, which in turn has the potential to reduce and prevent gall stone formation.

Chan *et al.* (2002) in relation to heart disease, point out that hydration reduces the risk of coronary heart disease by 46% in men and in women this is 59%. Adequate hydration acts by decreasing blood viscosity, thereby protecting against clot formation.

Dehydration can worsen diabetic control, and water is an essential aspect of dietary management of diabetes mellitus. In those patients who have poorly controlled diabetes they can experience an increase in urinary output and this in turn can result in dehydration; good hydration levels can slow down the development of diabetic ketoacidosis, helping to maintain healthy blood sugar levels (Burge *et al.*, 2001).

Dehydration is a risk factor that is associated with falls in older people (DH, 2001). Dehydration can cause disorientation, dizziness, headache and tiredness (Kleiner, 1999), increasing the risk of dizziness, fainting and falling. Adequate hydration in the older population could be part of an effective falls prevention strategy, reducing the risk of falls.

Failure to ensure that the patient is adequately hydrated can lead to a number of pathophysiological changes that can put the health and well-being of the individual at risk. It is therefore vital that this aspect of care is given the priority it deserves. There may be instances where the patient requires an intravenous infusion to replace fluid loss or to hydrate the patient. An alternative to intravenous fluid replacement (and in particular in the frail elderly person) is **hypodermoclysis** (Dasgupta *et al.*, 2000). Hypodermoclysis involves the insertion of a small cannula (a butterfly cannula) into the subcutaneous tissues (often this is in the abdomen). The cannula is secured using an occlusive type of dressing and the prescribed infusion begins. The rate and duration of fluid to be transfused is determined by prescription and the care and management of the patient is in accordance with local policy. It is vital that all fluids (input and output) are recorded on the fluid balance chart.

Nausea and vomiting

There are many reasons why a person may feel nauseous and/or vomit. Johnson *et al.* (2006) point out that most patients will experience **nausea** and/or **vomiting** during the disease process, this may be as a result of the disease pathology or the consequence of treatment. Nausea and vomiting may indicate pathophysiological changes that are occurring within the body. Both nausea and vomiting can be particularly upsetting for the patient as well as for their families; they can also impact on the person's ability to perform the activities of living.

Nausea

Crumbie (2007) described nausea as an unpleasant sensation that produces a feeling of discomfort in the region of the stomach with a feeling of a need to vomit. Nausea can be short-lived or long-lasting. A person may experience nausea alone, with no vomiting, and they may vomit without nausea coming before the act of vomiting. Some people experience nausea and then go on to vomit. Nausea, therefore, does not always lead to vomiting.

Nausea is a symptom of many conditions; it can be due to physical or psychological issues. It is not an illness and not all of the causes are necessarily related to the stomach; for example, those patients who are receiving chemotherapy may experience nausea. Nausea can be caused by adverse drug reactions; nausea is also a common symptom of pregnancy. Usually, the presence of nausea means that there may be an underlying pathological condition occurring in the body. The following could also cause nausea:

- diabetes mellitus
- influenza
- gastroenteritis
- renal failure
- adrenal insufficiency
- peptic ulcer
- vertigo

Treatment of nausea will depend on the cause of it. Avoidance of foods in the short-term may help to reduce the feelings associated with nausea. Removing strong smells or avoiding strong smells such as perfume or aftershave can also help to alleviate nausea. Some people experience nausea when they are, for example, travelling in a car, and stopping the car and sitting still can help alleviate the feelings of nausea that are caused by perceived movement and actual movement.

The nurse may advise the patient to eat small meals throughout the day as opposed to three large meals, and encourage the patient to eat slowly avoiding foods that are hard to digest. If it is the smell of food that is provoking the nausea then foods should be eaten cold or at room temperature, avoiding the smell of food as it is cooking or has been cooked.

An **antiemetic** (for example metochlopromide), medicines that are given to prevent or stop nausea and vomiting, may also be administrated. There are also a number of mechanical aids that are used to help prevent nausea (and vomiting). These devices work by applying continuous pressure on specific acupressure points located on the wrist and can be used by children and adults.

Vomiting

Vomiting is a complex physiological activity (Woodruff, 2004). Excessive vomiting can have a profound effect on a person's fluid balance and their electrolytes (Brooker, 2007). The vomiting centre (sometimes this is also known as the emetic centre) situated in the medulla oblongata of the brain is responsible for the initiation of vomiting. Both physical and psychological impulses can excite the vomiting centre causing the patient to vomit. Some causes of excitement of the vomiting centre include:

- fear/anxiety
- odours
- pain
- unpleasant sights
- side effects of some drugs
- radiotherapy
- hypercalcaemia

The sensitivity of the vomiting centre varies in different people and as such the nurse should treat each person on an individual basis. Vomiting can be defined as the forceful expulsion of gastric contents through the mouth and/or nose.

It is important to determine, if possible, the cause of vomiting; this should be the first line of treatment and possibly remove the causative factor. Caring for the patient who is vomiting will include the following:

- ask the patient if they have tried and tested methods of dealing with vomiting and if appropriate implement these
- ensure the patient is nursed upright (unless contraindicated)
- nurse the patient in the lateral position if the patient is unconscious and unable to protect his or her own airway
- administer prescribed antiemetic medication
- ensure privacy (ensure curtains are drawn and doors closed)
- provide easy access to vomit bowl and tissues (ensure receptacle is available to dispose safely of used tissues)
- remove the dirty vomit bowl and replace with a clean one as soon as possible
- offer the patient physical comfort by being with them holding the vomit bowl or mopping the brow
- observe, measure, record and report vomitus
- provide the patient with the opportunity to use a mouthwash
- provide the patient with the opportunity to 'freshen up' after they have finished vomiting
- change any soiled clothing/bedding
- try to avoid strong odours such as food, perfumes and aftershaves that may induce nausea and vomiting

If the extent of vomiting or retching has been excessive, the patient may complain of exhaustion or headache, and muscle soreness can also occur. An explanation of why the person may feel like this, as well as the administration of a prescribed analgesic can help to provide comfort.

Excessive vomiting and anorexia as a result of this will impinge on a person's hydration status leading to dehydration and loss of weight. Attention must be paid to the effects of excessive vomiting as extreme gastric secretion can lead to electrolyte imbalance and an ensuing acid–base (i.e. acidosis) discrepancy. The management of this will depend on the extent of vomiting and the patient's overall condition.

Caring for the patient with oedema

The abnormal collection of fluid in the interstitial spaces is known as oedema (Kumar and Clark, 2005). This aspect of the chapter provides an overview of the nursing care required for the patient with oedema in order to maintain a safe environment and provide comfort. The causes of pulmonary and peripheral oedema have been discussed earlier in this chapter.

Pulmonary oedema

Many patients who are diagnosed with pulmonary oedema will be acutely ill and they (and their families) may be highly anxious and afraid. The nurse must provide care that takes both the physical and psychological aspects of the condition into account for both the patient and family.

The first line of treatment should be to determine the cause of pulmonary oedema and to take steps to eliminate or reduce this; attempts should be made to reverse the specific cause(s). For example, if the cause is left-sided heart failure then measures should be taken to improve the pumping action of the left side of the heart.

Signs and symptoms of pulmonary oedema

The signs and symptoms can include some or all of the following:

- dyspnoea/orthopnoea
- wheeze
- tachycardia and tachypnoea
- hypotension
- cardiogenic shock
- sweating
- pallor/cyanosis
- nausea
- anxiety
- dry or productive cough (if productive pink frothy sputum)

Investigations to confirm diagnosis

It is important to remember that pulmonary oedema can result in mild to severe dyspnoea; therefore, when obtaining a history from the patient in order to make a diagnosis the nurse must bear this in mind and questioning of the patient should be kept to an absolute minimum. The nurse should ask questions that are only absolutely necessary and framed in such a way that the patient need only nod or shake the head in order to make a response. After a detailed history has been undertaken with data being obtained from the primary source (the patient) or secondary sources (i.e. other health care professionals, the patient's spouse, family or friends) then the following investigations may be required:

- chest X-ray
- blood gas analysis
- estimation of cardiac enzymes
- liver function tests
- estimation of urea and electrolytes
- electrocardiograph

Nursing management

Ongoing treatment of the specific cause of pulmonary oedema should continue and the patient's airway must also be managed if dyspnoea becomes so severe that this is in danger; in the acute phase the patient may need to be resuscitated. The key aim should be to improve oxygenation, and this can be done by the administration of prescribed oxygen therapy via facemask. As pulmonary oedema indicates that there is an abnormal collection of fluid in the interstitial spaces, it is imperative that there is strict control of fluid balance and in some cases a urinary catheter may need to be inserted to provide close monitoring of urinary output. Below is an overview of the management of the patient with pulmonary oedema; this, it should be noted, is not a comprehensive list and care will be dictated by the patient's condition and response to therapeutic interventions, and as such the patient requires close monitoring and the provision of skilled nursing care.

■ reassurance, psychological and physical support and explanations (for the patient and family) with regards to care interventions
■ provide the patient with a nurse call bell, leave this in close proximity
■ provide easy access to sputum pot and tissues (ensure receptacle is available to dispose safely of used tissues)
■ nurse the patient upright (unless this is contraindicated) supported by pillows
■ administration of prescribed humidified oxygen via face mask
■ administration of prescribed medication, for example diuretics (i.e. furosemide) and with caution diamorphine, to alleviate anxiety, pain and distress
■ strict monitoring of fluid balance (may include hourly urine measurements if a urinary catheter is in situ)
■ fluid restriction if indicated
■ monitoring, measuring and reporting of oxygen saturation, blood pressure, respiratory rate, depth and rhythm, monitoring of pulse frequency dictated by the patient's condition
■ assistance with all activities of living as appropriate

Peripheral oedema

Whilst pulmonary oedema, as its name suggests, causes problems associated with breathing as a result of excessive fluid in the lungs, peripheral oedema presents as a collection of excessive fluid within the tissues that pools in the dependent regions, for example the legs, ankles, feet and sacral region (Riley, 2007); sacral oedema tends to occur more in those patients who are bed bound. The pooling of fluid can be associated with lack of mobility, the consequence of gravitational pull, as well as the physiological factors that are related with oedema formation as described earlier in this chapter.

Pitting oedema is the more serious type of oedema. The area of skin, for example the ankles, when lightly pressed remains indented (a pit forms); this is a more serious type of oedema than the type that does not pit. Riley (2007) suggests that peripheral oedema does not appear or become visible until the body has retained 4 L of fluid. If, for example, a patient retains 5.5 L of fluid this is equivalent to 5.5 kg of weight; hence a way of determining if the patient, along with meticulous fluid balance monitoring, is retaining fluid is to record daily weight.

Skin that has become oedematous predisposes the patient to the development of pressure sores (decubitus ulcers) and infection, particularly when the skin over the oedematous area has broken down. This risk can become more evident when nurses who handle patients with oedema have long or sharp fingernails, watches, pens, badges and scissors that can potentially catch the patient's skin and cause more trauma, hence the importance of short nails and the covering of items of equipment in the nurse's pockets. It is important that the patient's fingernails are also kept short to prevent them from inadvertently causing damage to their skin. The principles of care for the patient who has peripheral oedema include:

- a clear explanation of the condition to the patient and if appropriate family
- assessment of skin condition in association with local policy for skin assessment
- careful washing and patting dry (not rubbing) of the oedematous skin
- fluid balance monitoring
- daily weight
- administration of prescribed diuretics (for example furosemide)
- elevation of oedematous ankles when sitting out of bed to aid drainage of the pooled fluid
- assistance with those activities of living that the patient is unable to carry out independently

Conclusion

Understanding the complex concepts and processes of fluid and electrolyte balance is vital if safe and effective care is to be provided to patients who may sometimes, as a result of fluid and electrolyte imbalance, be critically ill. The nurse has a pivotal role to play when helping people who are experiencing pathophysiological changes associated with fluid and electrolyte imbalance.

This chapter has explained how the dynamics of fluid balance can have a profound effect on an individual's health and well-being. The subtle changes associated with fluid balance have to be recognised by the nurse quickly in order to avert harm; this can be done in many ways using all the senses as well as implementing the fundamentals of science.

It is not possible in a chapter of this size to address in depth all concerns associated with fluid and electrolyte balance and the associated disorders. The reader is advised to access more detailed texts and other forms of information related to fluid and electrolytes with the key aim of providing care that is safe, effective and founded on a sound evidence base.

Multiple choice questions

1. Fluid moves between compartments by a process called:
(a) diffusion
(b) osmosis
(c) active transport
(d) ATP

2. Most of the body fluid is found in the:
(a) extracellular compartment
(b) interstitial space
(c) vascular space
(d) intracellular compartment

3. A cell in a hypertonic solution will:
(a) crenate and die
(b) swell and burst
(c) remain the same
(d) grow faster

4. The major cation outside the cell is:
(a) potassium
(b) sodium
(c) calcium
(d) phosphate

5. Pulmonary oedema is:
(a) accumulation of fluid in the lungs
(b) accumulation of fluid in the heart
(c) accumulation of sodium in the lungs
(d) accumulation of potassium in the heart

6. The term _hypodermoclysis_ means:
(a) the insertion of intravenous cannula in order to administer medication
(b) the injection of an intramuscular medication
(c) excess body fat
(d) the insertion of a small cannula into the subcutaneous tissues

7. Oedema is defined as:
(a) a collection of fluid around the brain
(b) the abnormal collection of fluid in the interstitial spaces

(c) distension of the abdomen
(d) swelling around the eye

8. The term *dyspnoea* means:
(a) difficulty with swallowing
(b) difficulty with breathing
(c) difficulty passing urine
(d) an anxiety attack

9. The consumption of water at regular intervals can help:
(a) dilute bile and stimulate gall bladder emptying
(b) prevent gallstone formation.
(c) both of the above
(d) none of the above

10. Fluid balance is:
(a) the measuring of all fluids and solids
(b) a state where the amount of fluid taken into the body equals the amount of fluid that leaves the body
(c) the amount of all fluid excreted by the body
(d) the amount of all fluid entering the body

Answers: 1.b, 2.d, 3.a, 4.b, 5.a, 6.d, 7.b, 8.b, 9.c, 10.b

Test your knowledge

❖ List the functions of water.

❖ Explain how fluid and electrolytes move between compartments.

❖ List the major electrolytes and their functions.

❖ How would you encourage an older person to increase their fluid intake in order to prevent them from becoming dehydrated?

❖ Outline the nursing care of a person who is feeling nauseous and vomiting

❖ Describe how you would monitor a bed-bound person's fluid intake.

Glossary of terms

Amines: Organic compounds that contain nitrogen.

Anions: Negatively charged ions.

Antiemetic: Medication given to prevent vomiting or to ease nausea.

Cations: Positively charged ions.

Compartments: Spaces.

Dehydration: Excessive fluid loss from the body.

Detoxification: Removal of toxic substance from the body.

Electrolytes: Substance that dissociate in water to form ions.

Extracellular: Space found outside the cell.

Hypertonic: Solution that has large amounts of solutes dissolved in it.

Hypodermoclysis: Insertion of a small cannula into the subcutaneous tissues.

Hypotonic: Solution that has a low concentration of solutes.

Interstitial: Space between cells.

Intracellular: Space inside the cell.

Isotonic: Solution that has the same osmolality as the body fluids.

Metabolism: Chemical process of the cell.

Nausea: An unpleasant sensation that produces a feeling of discomfort in the region of the stomach with a feeling of a need to vomit.

Oedema: Abnormal accumulation of fluid in the interstitial space.

Osmolality: Osmotic concentration of a solution.

Osmosis: Movement of water through a selective permeable membrane from an area of high volume to an area of low volume.

Osmotic pressure: Pressure created by water as it moves across a selective permeable membrane.

Plasma: Fluid component of the blood.

Stoma: Any opening, a mouth.

Tonicity: Term used instead of osmolality.

Vomiting: A disagreeable experience that occurs when the stomach contents are reflexly expelled through the mouth or nose.

References

Brooker, C. (2007). Promoting hydration and nutrition. In: Brooker, C. and Waugh, A. (eds) *Foundations of Nursing Practice: Fundamentals of Holistic Care*. London: Mosby, pp. 531–568.

Burge, M.R., Garcia, N., Quails, C.R. and Schade, D.S. (2001). Differential effects of fasting and dehydration in the pathogenesis of diabetic ketoacidosis. *Metabolism*, 50(2), 171–177.

Carter, P.J. (2007). *Essentials for Nursing Assistants: A Humanistic Approach to Caregiving*. Philadelphia: Lippincott.

Casimiro, C., Garcia-de-Lorenzo, A. and Usan, L. (2002). Prevalence of decubitus ulcer and risk factors in an institutionalized Spanish elderly population. *Nutrition*, 18(5), 408–414.

Chan, J., Knutsen, S.F., Blix, G.G., Lee, J.W. and Fraser, G.E. (2002). Water, other fluids and fatal coronary heart disease. *American Journal of Epidemiology*, 155(9), 827–833.

Crumbie, A. (2007). Caring for the patient with a disorder of the gastrointestinal system. In: Watson, M. and Crumbie, A. (eds) *Watson's Clinical Nursing and Related Sciences*, 7th edn. Edinburgh: Bailliere Tindall, pp. 427–495.

Dasgupta, M., Binns, M.A. and Rochon, P.A. (2000). Subcutaneous fluid infusions in a long-term setting. *Journal of the American Geriatric Society*, 48(7), 795–799.

Department of Health (2001). *National Service Framework for Older People*. London: DH.

Department of Heath (2007). *Improving Nutritional Care: A Joint Action Plan from the Department of Health and Nutrition Summit Stakeholders*. London: DH.

Gray, M. and Krissovich, M. (2003). Does fluid intake influence the risk for urinary incontinence, urinary tract infection and bladder cancer? *Journal of Wound, Ostomy and Continence Nursing*, 30(3), 126–131.

Green, S.M. and Simpson, P.M. (2007). Eating and drinking. In: Hogston, R. and Marjoram, B.A. (eds) *Foundations of Nursing Practice: Leading the Way*, 3rd edn. Basingstoke: Palgrave, pp. 121–153.

Hodgkinson, B., Evans, D. and Wood, J. (2003). Maintaining oral hydration in older adults: A systematic review. *International Journal of Nursing Practice*, 9, S19–S28.

Johnson, A., Harrison, K., Currow, D., Luhr-Taylor, M. and Johnson, R. (2006). Palliative care and health breakdown. In: Chang, E., Daly, J. and Elliott, D. (eds) *Pathophysiology Applied to Nursing Practice*. Sydney: Mosby, pp. 449–471.

Kleiner, S.M. (1999). Water: An essential but overlooked nutrient. *American Dietetic Association*, 99(2), 201–207.

Kumar, P. and Clark, M. (2005). *Clinical Medicine*, 5th edn. Edinbrugh: W.B. Saunders.

Lemon, P. and Burke, K. (2004). *Medical – Surgical Nursing; Critical Thinking in Client Care*, 3rd edn. New Jersey: Pearson Education.

McCance, K.L. and Huether, S.E. (2006). *Pathophysiology: The Biological Basis for Disease in Adults and Children*, 5th edn. St. Louis: Elsevier Mosby.

Metheny, N.M. (1996). *Fluid and Electrolyte Balance*, 3rd edn. Philadelphia: Lippincott.

Reid, J., Robb, E. and Stone, D. (2004). Improving the monitoring and assessment of fluid balance. *Nursing Times*, 100(20), 36–39.

Registered Nurse Association of Ontario (2005). *Prevention of Constipation in the Older Adult Population*. Ontario: RNAO.

Riley, J. (2007). Breathing and circulation. In: Brooker, C. and Waugh, A. (eds) *Foundations of Nursing Practice: Fundamentals of Holistic Care*. London: Mosby, pp. 463–500.

Stotts, N.A. and Hopf, H.W. (2003). The link between tissue oxygen and hydration in nursing home residents with pressure ulcers: Preliminary data. *Journal of Wound, Ostomy and Continence Nursing*, 30(4), 184–190.

Thibodeau, G.A. and Patton, K.T. (2007). *Anatomy and Physiology*, 6th edn. St. Louis: Elsevier Mosby.

Water UK (2005). *Wise up on Water: Hydration and Healthy Ageing*. London: Water UK.

Woodruff, R. (2004) *Palliative Medicine Evidence Based Symptomatic Supportive Care for Patients with Advanced Cancer*, 4th edn. Oxford: Oxford University Press.

Chapter 18

The skin and associated disorders

Ian Peate

Test your prior knowledge

- Name the layers of the skin.
- Describe the role of the skin in health.
- How might the nurse help to prevent skin cancer?

Learning outcomes

On completion of this section, the reader will be able to:

■ Discuss the anatomy and physiology of the skin.

■ Describe the various functions of the skin.

■ Discuss the appendages.

Introduction

This chapter introduces the reader to the structure and function of the skin. The skin (including its appendages), the only visible largest organ of the body, is also known as the **integumentary** system. An overview of the anatomy and physiology of the skin is provided; the function of the skin is also discussed, and a number of skin conditions are considered along with the nursing management of a patient with a skin disorder. There are a number of appendages of the skin, hair follicles, eccrine and apocrine glands and the nails; a brief discussion of these will also be provided. This chapter considers preventative strategies that the nurse may wish to introduce to prevent conditions such as skin cancer.

Skin disease affects 20–30% of the population at any one time (All Parliamentary Group on Skin, 1997); it can affect a person's ability to carry out their activities of living and it can also have an impact on their sense of well-being. The nurse on a daily basis observes the patient's skin whilst they carry out nursing care; it is vital therefore that they have an understanding of the function of the skin in order to recognise problems that may occur. There are many areas of nursing practice where the nurse will come into contact with people who suffer with problems of the skin and the nurse is ideally placed to offer these people support with respect to some of these conditions.

Some skin conditions have the potential to cause stigma, such as eczema and psoriasis; the nurse as advocates can dispel any misunderstanding regarding contagion and enhance the individual's social well-being. Appearance and image are often associated with success and achievement, and the blemish-free individual that is usually portrayed in the media (in most Western societies) is the image to which many strive; this is not always possible for those with skin conditions. Society places much emphasis on physical appearance and for those who have skin problems this can become increasingly challenging. People with skin problems may experience difficulties in other aspects of their lives, for example, from a sexual relation perspective and also concerning issues surrounding self-esteem and self-concept, altered body image can have profound effect on the individual, their partner and their family (Marks, 2003). Patients may report feeling ostracised, stigmatised and isolated; some people with skin disorders according to Lewis-Jones (1999) feel 'unclean, like a leper'. Mitchell and Kennedy (2006) note that skin disease is not just a cosmetic nuisance, emphasising that it can have a profound impact on a person's life; they suggest that it can help to think of the five 'Ds' in association with dermatology:

■ **Disfigurement**
■ **Discomfort**
■ **Disability**
■ **Depression**
■ **Death**

Emotional problems	■ Low self-esteem ■ Feeling unclean ■ Problems with relationships ■ Feeling stared at ■ Being regarded as infectious or contagious
Clothing restrictions	■ Avoiding short sleeves ■ Avoiding the wearing of dark clothing due to skin shedding ■ Avoiding the wearing of summer clothing when the skin is exposed ■ Clothing can become stained or ruined when using greasy oily skin preparations
Social restrictions	■ Skin becomes itchy in hot places where people congregate ■ Avoiding swimming or sports facilities ■ Avoiding communal changing rooms
Financial implications	■ Routine prescriptions are expensive but essential ■ No allowances are made to replace clothing or bedding ■ No allowances are made for fuel bills due to extra laundering and bathing

Source: Adapted from Page (2006).

Table 18.1 Some of the problems that patients with skin conditions may experience

Page (2006) summarises some of the problems that patients with skin conditions may experience (see Table 18.1).

Dermatology is the study of the skin and its diseases; dermatologists are specialist practitioners who diagnose and treat diseases of the skin, nails and hair. The nurse can help enhance the quality of life for the person who has a skin problem.

The anatomy and physiology of the skin

The skin in humans (as with most other mammals) consists of two layers: the outer layer – the epidermis; and an underlying layer made of fibrous tissue – the dermis. Below the dermis is subcutaneous fat. At a cellular level the skin is composed of a number of types of cells; these cells and their functioning are essential to for maintaining health and the promotion of well-being (see Figure 18.1).

The skin is estimated to weigh between 2.5 and 4 kg in an adult and is thickest at the palms and soles (approximately 1 mm thick) and at the eyelids it is at its thinnest – approximately 0.1 mm; there are over one million nerve endings in the skin, and it covers a surface area of 2 m^2 (Hughes and Van Onselen, 2001).

The skin has a number of vital functions and these have been summarised in Box 18.1.

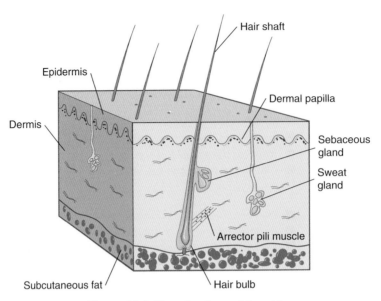

Figure 18.1 The structure of the skin.

Epidermis

The epidermis is the outer layer of the skin and is composed primarily of keratinocytes (approximately 95% of cells), including other specialised cells, for example melanocytes, Langerhans cells and Merkel cells. Table 18.2 outlines the functions of these cells.

The epidermis is composed of stratified epithelium and it has no blood vessels. The cellular nourishment (including oxygenation) and the removal of waste products occur through diffusion from the vascular network in the superficial dermis.

The prime functions of the epidermis are to provide a physical and biological barrier to the environment; the penetration of irritants is prevented by the epidermis, as is the loss of water and the

---

Box 18.1 The key functions of the skin

■ Protection from harmful external factors (such as microbes, ultraviolet light and chemicals)
■ Internal homeostasis (a balanced internal environment)
■ Shock absorber
■ Thermoregulation
■ Insulation
■ Sensation
■ Lubrication
■ Protection and grip
■ Calorie reserve
■ Synthesis of vitamin D
■ Body odour
■ Psychosocial

Cells	Functions
Melanocytes	These cells are located in the basal layer of the epidermis. The melanocytes produce the pigment melanin; melanin is found in the eyes, hair and skin. Melanin is responsible for providing protection and the absorption of ultraviolet rays. Melanin is the primary determinant of human skin colour
Langerhans cells	Langerhans cells are one part of the body's immune system, they activate the immune response and in particular the T-helper cells. They play an important role in contact allergies
Merkel cells	These cells are found in small numbers in the basal layer. They have roles to play in sensation, they are associated with sensory nerve endings and are found in specific areas such as the palms, soles and genitalia. Their exact function is unclear

Source: Adapted from Gawkrodger (2003) and Lawton (2006a).

Table 18.2 The functions of melanocytes, Langerhans and Merkel cells

management of internal homeostasis (Lawton, 2006a). Waugh and Grant (2006) suggest that there are three key factors associated with the various layers of the epidermis:

- division and migration of epidermal cells to the skin surface on a regular basis
- keratinisation of the epidermal cells
- rubbing away of the epidermal cells (desquamation)

The layers of the epidermis are shown in Figure 18.2.

The basal layer (also called the stratum basale) is located close to the cells that are nearest to the dermis at the dermo-epidermal junction; it is at this point that cell division takes place. Cells migrate upwards from the dermo-epidermal junction and over a period of approximately 21–18 days they **keratinise** prior to being shed.

Cells in the next layer are the *prickle cell layer* (stratum spinosum), and they provide protection against shearing forces or trauma to the skin; these cells are moving upwards above the basal layer.

Fine granules are formed from within the *granular layer* (stratum granulosum). These granules are the precursor of keratin, which eventually replaces the cytoplasm of the cells.

Clear cell layer (stratum lucidium) is only present in areas where the skin is thick, for example the soles and palms. These cells have large amounts of keratin; they are flattened and closely packed. When injury or trauma occurs, the skin production of these cells is increased and calluses or corns are formed.

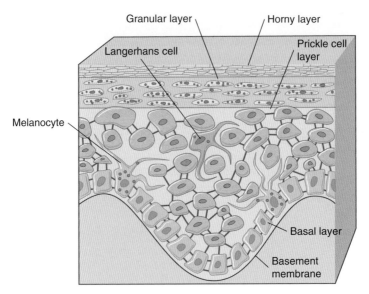

Figure 18.2 The layers of the epidermis.

Horny layer (stratum corneum) is the uppermost part of the epidermis and is made up of thin, flat and non-nucleated cells. These are dead cells. These cells are shed from the skin.

Dermis

The dermis is chiefly composed of a network of connective tissue (mainly collagen) underlying the epidermis of the skin, and it acts as the anchor that joins the dermis and epidermis. The connective tissue gives strength and elasticity as well as providing a supportive meshwork for the specialised structures throughout the dermis. This layer of the skin is much thicker than the epidermis; the key function is to support and sustain the epidermis. The dermis provides a protective pad for the deeper structures, protecting them from trauma, and it also nourishes the epidermis and has a vital role to play in wound healing; without the cells contained within the dermis wound healing will not take place (Moulin *et al.*, 2000).

Lawton (2006b) describes the dermis as comprising numerous specialised cells, for example mast cells and fibroblasts as well as:

- blood vessels
- lymphatics
- nerves
- sweat glands
  (see Figure 18.3).

Just as the epidermis has layers so too does the dermis; the dermis has two layers (Lawton, 2006b).

The first layer, *superficial papillary dermis*, is made up primarily of loose connective tissue that contains blood vessels in the form of capillaries; elastic fibres and collagen are also components. The depth of the superficial papillary dermis depends on age and anatomical location.

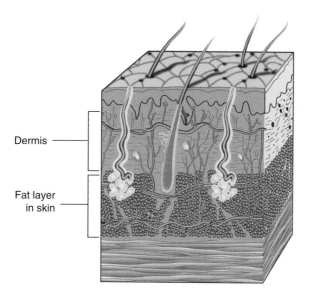

Figure 18.3 The structure of the dermis.

The second layer is called the *reticular dermis*. This layer is thicker than the superficial papillary dermis, dense connective tissue and larger blood vessels are interlaced with elastic fibres (providing pliability) and thick bundles of collagen are present in this layer, the collagen provides strength and intracellular matrix makes up most of the dermis. There are also mast cells and fibrobalsts as well as nerve endings and lymphatics vessels. These structures are surrounded by a viscous gel that bathes the structures allowing nutrients, hormones and waste products to pass through the dermis. The viscous gel helps to provide bulk, allowing the dermis to act as a buffer.

Blood supply

Thermoregulation is primarily controlled by a complex network of blood vessels within the dermis. Lying close to the epidermal border is the superficial plexus which is made up of a number of inter-connecting arterioles; these vessels wrap themselves around the structures in the dermis, and through this interconnecting network oxygen and nutrients are supplied to the cells. At the border with the subcutaneous layer, is the deep plexus. These vessels in comparison to those in the superficial plexus are more substantial; they connect vertically to the superficial plexus (Lawton, 2006b).

Lymph vessels

The lymph vessels play an important role in draining excess tissue fluid and plasma proteins from the dermis; this results in internal homeostasis – ensuring that there is the correct volume and composition of tissue fluids (Page, 2006). Lymph also searches for foreign matter such as bacteria and antigenic substances.

Nerves

Nerves (found also in the basal layer of the epidermis) detect mechanical and thermal changes; free sensory nerve endings (the Merkel cells) are found in both layers detecting pain, irritation and temperature. The skin is supplied with approximately one million nerve fibres; sensory perception is an important protective mechanism of these cells. Specialist receptors responding to pressure and vibration (Pacinian corpuscles) and touch/sensitivity (Meissner's corpuscles) are also found in the dermis. Autonomic nerves supply the blood vessels and sweat glands and the Arrector pili muscles (Gawkrodger, 1992; Lawton, 2006b).

The subcutis

The subcutis is a subcutaneous layer that lies below the dermis. The layer, composed mainly of fat (adipose tissue), provides the skin with support and acts as a shock absorber. The subcutis is also responsible for providing the body with insulation and storage of nutrients; the subcutis is interlaced with blood vessels and nerves.

The appendages

Lawton (2006c) suggests that there are three important components of the skin known as the appendages of the epidermis:

- the sweat glands
- hair follicles and sebaceous glands
- nails

Sweat glands

Sweat glands are coiled tubes of epithelial tissue; they open out to pores on the skin surface (see Figure 18.4). Each gland has individual nerve and blood supplies; they secrete a slightly acidic fluid

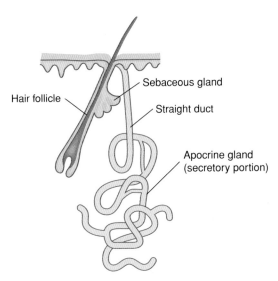

Figure 18.4 Sweat gland.

containing water and salts (excess excretory products). Keratin maintains its suppleness because of the action of sweat. There are two types of sweat glands – eccrine and apocrine. Reaction to heat and fear and the production of secretions by the eccrine glands is in response to the sympathetic nervous system. These glands are found all over the body; however, there are more sites where they are more numerous, for example the forehead, axillae, soles and palms.

The apocrine glands are also coiled; they are not as numerous as the eccrine glands and are found in more localised sites – the pubic and axillary regions, the nipples and perineum – and are not functional until puberty; it is understood that they secrete **pheromones** released into the external environment. A **viscous** material is excreted that causes body odour when acted upon by the surface bacteria.

Hair follicles and sebaceous glands

Hair is found on all surfaces of the body except the palms, soles and lips; its amount, distribution, colour and texture vary depending on its location and males and females, young and old and ethnic groups. It contributes to an individual's unique appearance. Hair colour is determined by the melanocytes that are within the hair bulb and hair growth is influenced by genetic and hormonal factors.

Hair is a keratin structure of the epidermis; each hair is a thread of keratin and is formed from cells at the base of a single follicle (Timby, 2005). It has several functions:

- sexual
- social
- thermoregulation
- protection

The key role of hair is to prevent heat loss. The whole skin surface is provided with hair follicles; each pore is an opening to a follicle and they are situated deep in the dermis above the subcutaneous layer. When heat leaves the body through the skin, it becomes trapped in the air between the hairs. Attached to each gland is a small collection of smooth muscle called the Arrector pili; these muscles contract and become erect in response to cold, fear and emotion. The contraction of the muscle can be seen on the skin in the form of 'goose bumps'.

The hair follicles are accompanied by sebaceous glands, and **sebum** (a liquid substance) is secreted by these glands providing lubrication to the skin as well as ensuring that the skin and hair are waterproof. Sebum is a slightly acidic substance that has antibacterial and antifungal properties (Page, 2006). The distribution of the sebaceous glands varies; they are most prominent on the scalp, face, upper torso and anogenital region, and during puberty these glands are at their most active (Lawton, 2006c). Page (2006) suggests that sebum production is influenced by sex hormone levels. Figure 18.5 demonstrates what is known as a pilosebaceous unit; the pilosebaceous unit is composed of the follicle, the hair shaft, the sebaceous and the Arrector pili.

Nails

The final appendage is the nails; these too are made of keratin and their tough texture is because the keratin is formed in concentrated amounts; they can be described as horn-like, and there are no nerve endings in nail. They act as protectors; fingernails and toenails afford some protection to the digits. Nails also make it easier to grab or grasp things. Lawton (2006c) suggests that the nails act as a counterforce to the fingertips which have many nerve endings allowing an individual to receive a lot of information about the objects we touch.

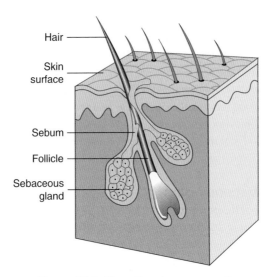

Figure 18.5 The pilosebaceous unit.

The rate of nail growth varies; on average, nails grow at a rate of 0.1 cm per day (1 cm per 100 days). Fingernails require 4–6 months to regrow completely; toenails take longer to grow, between 12 and 18 months to regrow completely. The rate of growth depends upon factors such as the age of the person, the time of year, amount of exercise undertaken and hereditary factors (Haneke, 2006). Nail growth can be impeded by trauma and inflammation; changes in the integrity of the nails can be the result of injury or infection and in some instances evidence of systemic diseases, for example chronic cardiopulmonary disease or fungal infection (Timby, 2005). Figure 18.6 demonstrates the structure of the nail.

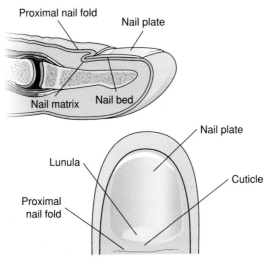

Figure 18.6 The structure of the nail.

Learning outcomes

On completion of this section, the reader will be able to:

- Describe some of the pathophysiological changes that may occur to the skin.
- Highlight the role and function of the nurse when caring for those who may suffer with a skin condition.

Disorders of the skin

There is an old saying – a picture is worth a thousand words – this saying is particularly true when caring for people with skin, hair and nail disorders. It is important that you understand what some of the most common skin lesions look like. When discussing skin conditions, the term *lesion* describes a small area of disease, whereas a rash or eruption describes an area of skin that is widespread. The reader may benefit from consulting a colour skin atlas to enhance their skills of observation (White, 2003; Wolff *et al.*, 2005).

Many skin lesions can be diagnosed at sight; however, there is still the need to adopt a systematic approach to diagnosis and this will entail a detailed nursing and medical history as well as a physical examination. To confirm diagnosis other investigations may also be needed. Page (2006) provides details of what a full history should entail (see Box 18.2). The nurse needs to use effective and sensitive

---

Box 18.2 Some components of the history

- Any known allergies
- Onset, initial site and duration of the condition
- Associated symptoms, for example itch, redness, oozing
- Actions that might make the condition worse, for example exposure to heat or cold, any stress including activities
- Family history, for example genetic predisposition
- Associated systemic symptoms, for example asthma
- Current prescribed medications, including any medications that are being applied to the skin as well as any oral preparations
- Current over-the-counter medications, including any medications that are being applied to the skin as well as any oral preparations
- Social history, this should include details about occupation, hobbies, amount of exercise, housing, smoking, alcohol intake and use of illicit drugs
- Impact of the disorder on them as an individual, their self-esteem, self-image, their ability to manage on a daily basis and any coping mechanisms used
- Impact of the disorder on others they live with or work with

Source: Adapted from Page (2006).

Extrinsic	Intrinsic
Extremes of heat	Genetic/hereditary factors
Allergens	Internal disease
Chemicals	Medications
Irritants	Infections
Trauma	Psychological factors
Friction	
Infections	
Sunshine	
Sun lamps	
Source: Adapted from Hunter *et al.* (2002).	

Table 18.3 Some intrinsic and extrinsic factors that can predispose a person to skin disease

communication skills to help reveal the diagnosis and also the person's description and understanding of the disorder as well as their perception and the perceptions of others of living with it.

Gawkrodger (2003) reports that the type, incidence and prevalence of skin disorders is closely associated with and depends on a person's social, economic, geographical and cultural circumstances. There are a number of factors that can predispose a person to skin disorders, both extrinsic and intrinsic (see Table 18.3).

Skin disorders can be minor or life-threatening with a number of people seeking their own remedies to some of the problems they encounter. There are, however, a number of conditions that require more intensive interventions; these interventions can take place in the patient's own home, in the primary care setting or there may be a need for the person to be admitted to hospital. The next section of the chapter spends some time on some types of skin disorders.

Skin cancer

Sunlight is the main cause of skin cancer and the incidence of this cancer has increased steadily over the years (DH, 2000). In the UK, skin cancer is the second most common form of cancer (Foss and Farine, 2007). There are three forms of skin cancer:

- malignant melanoma
- basal cell carcinoma (BCC)
- squamous cell carcinoma (SCC)

Malignant melanoma

This is the most dangerous form of skin cancer and in all cases of skin cancer this accounts for 10% of them (Wolff *et al.*, 2005). The cells of the body that become cancerous in malignant melanoma are the melanocytes. Melanoma usually develops in a **naevus** (also known as mole); it can metastasise rapidly via the circulatory and lymphatic systems.

This type of skin cancer spreads rapidly and because of the speed in which it spreads this makes it the most dangerous type. These cancers are more common in young people and are closely related to sunburn and overexposure (Foss and Farine, 2007).

Risk factors

There is one key risk factor for melanoma, i.e. sun or sunbeds (ultraviolet light). There are, however, some people who are more at risk than others. More women than men get melanoma; it is the seventh most common cancer in women. The disease is rare in those who are aged under 14 years; in those aged 15 years, the incidence steadily rises with age, and the highest incidence is in those aged 80 years and over. Risk increases the more moles a person has.

Those who are fair skinned are more at risk than those who are dark skinned; however, dark skinned people can and do get malignant melanoma. Those who are fair and have a tendency to freckle in the sun are most at risk as are those who do not tan at all; these people are usually those who peel before getting a tan. People with melanoma are twice as likely to have been badly sunburned at least once in their lives; sunburn as a child is even more damaging than sunburn as an adult because during childhood the skin is at its most vulnerable. Risk is also associated with geography and where the person was born. Those who are fair skinned and were born in hot country, for example Australia, have an increased risk of melanoma for life, in contrast to those who went to live there as a teenager or compared to those with similar skin colour who live in cooler climates. The skin would have been exposed to the effects of the sun whilst the person was young, when the skin was at its most delicate. A family history, i.e. a family member who has had melanoma places a person at risk. Box 18.3 provides a summary of risk factors associated with melanoma.

Signs and symptoms

There are a number of warning signs that may indicate malignant melanoma (Page, 2006):

Box 18.3 A summary of key factors that put a person at risk of developing malignant melanoma

- Exposure to sun
- Use of sunbeds
- Being female (evidence to suggest that hormones play a part if risk is inconclusive)
- Age
- Presence of moles
- Being fair skinned
- History of sunburn, having been sunburned at least once and risk rises if this occurred as a child
- Geographical factors (where the person was born)
- Family history

Characteristic	Points
Change in size[a]	2
Change in colour (for example, getting darker, becoming patchy or multi-shaded)[a]	2
Change in shape[a]	2
7 mm or more across in any direction	1
Inflammation	1
Oozing or bleeding	1
Change in sensation (for example, itching or pain)	1

[a]Denotes the major features.

Source: Adapted from NICE (2006).

Table 18.4 Assessing changes in moles (lesions)

- new or existing moles getting bigger
- the shape of the mole is changing; if there is a change in the edge of the mole, it becomes irregular in shape around the edges
- the colour of the mole changes – it gets darker or becomes patchy or multi-shaded
- the mole becomes itchy or painful
- if it starts to bleed or becomes crusty
- if there is any surrounding or underlying inflammation

Diagnosis

A patient's history as well as full physical examination is required. The nurse should examine and observe the whole of the body. Hutchinson's freckle (also known as lentigo maligna) is a premalignant melanoma condition (Mitchell and Kennedy, 2006). Hutchinson's freckle can be seen on the face or other areas of the body that are exposed to the sun; in some patients, the condition has been slowly enlarging for a number of years.

The only method used to confirm diagnosis of a malignant melanoma is to take a biopsy of the lesion and subject it to histological testing (**histology**). Usually, the specimen is obtained under a local anaesthetic but this will depend on the body where the lesion is. Urgent referral must be made if the lesion is suspected to be cancerous; the lesion is measured and usually photographed in order to make comparisons at a later stage. A seven-point scale is advocated by National Institute for Health and Clinical Excellence (NICE, 2006) in order to help make the decision to refer to a specialist (see Table 18.4). Within the scale, there are three major features and four minor ones.

Two points are given for any of the major features and one for the minor features; if the mole (the lesion) scores three points or above then urgent referral is required. However, NICE (2006) suggests that if there is any cause for concern, regardless of the score, then the person should be referred to a specialist.

Dermatoscopy may be performed in order to examine the lesion. This is a painless test that has the ability to magnify the area up to ten times.

Nursing care and management

Precancerous moles can be treated by excision under local anaesthetic; early malignant melanomas can also be treated in this way. The longer a suspicious mole is left, the more difficult it can be to treat with a poorer **prognosis**. If the mole is removed the patient will have **sutures** in place and they will need to stay in situ for up to a week; the patient returns to the centre where the lesion was removed and usually receives the results of the histology. If the histology reveals that lesion was non-cancerous then no further treatment is needed; however, if there is evidence of cancerous cells more tests will be required.

One of the proposed tests will be one that determines how deep the melanoma is – this is called staging. The deeper the cancerous cells, the more likely it is that the cancer has spread within the body (Thompson *et al.*, 2005). The following tests may also be required:

- blood tests
- chest X-ray
- ultrasound scan
- bone scan
- CT scan

Wide local excisions may be required depending on the individual's unique circumstances, for example, how much of the mole (lesion) was left behind and how deep the melanoma has grown into the tissues. In some circumstances, if a large area of skin has been excised this may require skin grafting.

Lymph node removal, if there is lymph involvement, may be needed and there is some evidence to suggest that treatment can also include **chemotherapy**, another type of treatment that may be offered is interferon treatment. Chemotherapy and interferon (biological therapy) is also known as **adjuvant** treatment. **Radiotherapy**, the use of high-energy radiation, to kill cancer cells can also be used; again this will depend on the individual needs and circumstances. Sharpe (2006) suggests that there is no improvement regarding survival when adjuvant therapy is used; however, disease-free intervals may be prolonged.

Often patients are anxious and concerned about the results of test and the decisions they will have to make. The nurse has a duty to provide the patient with physical and psychological support before, during and after all interventions; this may include providing information in a manner that the patient understands, and is able to assimilate and then able to make an informed decision.

Regular follow-up is needed and the frequency at which this is required will depend on the individual circumstances. The aim of follow-up is to see how the patient is coping and determine if they need any further physical or psychological support, if there is recurrence around the scar, if there is any spread to the lymph nodes or other parts of the body or if there are any new melanomas.

Basal cell carcinoma and squamous cell carcinoma

BCC is a type of skin cancer of the epidermis. BCC is slow to develop and commonly occurs on the face. SCC occurs to the outermost layers of the skin. Often it appears as a scaly or crusty patch of skin bigger than 1 cm (but may be smaller); it does not heal. Both these types of cancer are called non-melanoma skin cancers and are the most common type of cancer in the UK (NICE, 2006). Usually, they appear on body parts that are exposed, for example:

- face
- neck
- ears
- forearms
- fingers
- hands

These types of skin cancer are more common in the older population (DH, 2002). Prognosis for those with this type of cancer is very good.

The main treatment for BCC and SCC is surgery (Motley *et al.*, 2003). The type of surgery is classed as a minor surgery and involves the use of a local anaesthetic to remove the cancer. Radiotherapy may be used to treat large areas of skin cancer or if the cancer is in a difficult place to operate on or if the patient is unable, due to ill health or incapacity, to have surgery performed safely (Sharpe, 2006). Chemotherapy is another option, but for BCC and SCC this is rarely used. Creams that contain chemotherapeutic medications may, however, be used and in particular where those cancers are only on the top layer of the skin.

In all cases of skin cancer, malignant or non-malignant, and for all patients, the nurse should be prepared to provide health promotion advice. Nurses in any situation can encourage regular checking of the skin; they are ideally placed to provide information concerning skin self-examination (Oliviera *et al.*, 2004). Effective treatment depends on early detection of skin cancer and a prompt diagnosis (NICE, 2006).

Health promotion advice – skin cancer

Nurses, when they have the opportunity should be proactive in providing health promotion advice concerning the damaging effects of the sun and the avoidance of skin cancer to those who may need it, for example those working outdoors and younger members of the population.

Not everyone's skin offers the same protection in the sun and because of this it is important to know about skin types. Those with skin types I–IV need to take most care in the sun, particularly those who have skin types I and II. Those who have skin types V and VI generally only need to protect their skin when the sun is particularly strong or they go out in the sun for a long period of time. Table 18.5 details the classification of skin types. Box 18.4 provides some advice the nurse can give to patients concerning sun protection.

Skin cancer is a significant increasing health problem for the nation; prevention according to Sharpe (2006) is a long-term issue and will require major attitude and behavioural changes of the population.

Eczema

According to Mitchell and Kennedy (2006), the word *eczema* comes from the Greek meaning to boil over. The terms eczema and **dermatitis** are used synonymously; they can be described as acute or chronic (Waugh and Grant, 2006) and the severity can vary. The condition can affect all age groups. There is no specific diagnostic test for eczema (Hoare *et al.*, 2000) and the diagnosis is based on clinical

Type	Characteristics
Type I	Pale skin, burns very easily and tans rarely. Generally these people have light coloured or red hair and freckles
Type II	These people usually burn but may gradually tan. Often they have light hair, blue or brown eyes. Some may have dark hair but still have fair skin
Type III	Generally tan quite easily, but with long exposure to the sun burn. Usually, they have dark hair with brown or green eyes
Type IV	Tan very easily, but with long exposure to the sun will burn. Often they have olive skin, brown eyes and dark hair
Type V	Naturally brown skin with dark hair and brown eyes. These people burn only with prolonged exposure to the sun and their skin further darkens easily
Type VI	Have black skin with dark brown eyes and black hair. These people burn only with extreme exposure to the sun and their skin further darkens easily

Source: Adapted from British Association of Dermatologists (2007).

Table 18.5 Skin types

assessment. With the correct treatment the inflammation can be reduced; however, there is currently no cure for eczema.

As with most skin conditions, that are visible, eczema can have a profound effect on an individual's self-esteem. The patient may also experience disturbed sleep as a result of the clinical manifestations. For younger patients, there may be a significant impact on their behaviour and development as a result of disturbed sleep, lowered self-esteem and social isolation (ostracism). Frequent visits to the doctor, the need to apply messy **topical** applications and the use of special clothing can add to the burden of the disease. Eczema can have a profound effect not only on the patient but also on their family.

Gawkrodger (2003) explains that the inflammatory response seen in eczematous skin conditions are provoked by changes as a result of internal (endogenous) or external (exogenous) factors or both. Hoare *et al.* (2000) state that there are at least ten forms of eczema. Wolff *et al.* (2005) describe the characteristics of both acute and chronic eczema. Acute eczema is characterised by:

- **pruritus**
- **erythema**
- **vesiculation**

and chronic eczema by:

- pruritus
- **xerosis**
- **lichenfication**

Box 18.4 Some points related to sun protection

■ Select a waterproof sunscreen, one with an adequate sun protection factor (SPF). An SPF of 15 multiplies the period of time it takes to burn by 15. An SPF of at least 15 should be used by everyone. Those who have paler skin should use a higher SPF rating. The sunscreen should screen out both ultraviolet A (UVA) and ultraviolet B (UVB) rays. A lip balm with a high SPF should also be applied to the lips

■ The sunscreen should be rubbed in well and applied approximately 15–30 minutes before going out in to the sun. Every 2 hours throughout the day the sunscreen should be reapplied and also after swimming

■ Avoid excessive exposure to the sun. Light-coloured loose fitting clothing should be worn as this will help the person feel cooler. Garments should be closely woven as lightweight clothing provides little protection to UV light which will pass through lightweight clothing. A wide brimmed hat protects the head and neck

■ The sun should be avoided between 1100 hours and 1500 hours and this is particularly important in those countries that are close to the equator

■ Sunglasses should be worn as prolonged exposure can cause damage to the lens of the eyes resulting in an opaqueness (cataract). Sunglasses that conform to British standards are advocated

■ The skin's sensitivity is increased when cosmetics are worn in the sun, therefore they should be avoided

■ UV light can be reflected by water, snow and buildings; therefore, it is important to apply sunscreen when sitting in the shade. Cloud is no barrier to UV light, and it is still possible to burn on a cloudy day, as UV light can penetrate cloud

Source: Adapted from Foss and Farine (2007).

■ **hyperkeratosis**
■ **fissure formation (rare)**

Endogenous eczema

Atopic eczema

This condition is described as a chronic **relapsing** inflammatory skin condition; the patient tends to scratch and itch at a red rash that is often found in skin creases such as the elbows and behind the knees. Archer (2000) suggests that other features include:

■ crusting
■ scaling
■ cracking
■ swelling of the skin

The cause of atopic eczema is unknown. The condition is also associated with other diseases such as hay fever and asthma. Adults make up nearly one-third of community cases of atopic eczema (Hoare *et al.*, 2000).

Pathophysiological changes are the result of complex interactions between:

■ the skin barrier
■ genetic responses
■ environmental issues
■ pharmacological factors
■ immunological causes

Microscopically, atopic eczema appears as an excessive fluid between the cells in the epidermis (this is known as spongiosis); when the condition worsens the fluid erupts into the epidermis and forms vesicles – small collections of fluid, and vesiculation occurs (Mitchell and Kennedy, 2006). In atopic eczema, a hypersensitivity response occurs in reaction to an antigen and antibody effect; however, Wolff *et al.* (2005) suggest that the antigen–antibody response is still not fully understood. A genetic predisposition and a combination of allergic and non-allergenic factors appear to be influencing features.

Discoid eczema

Also called nummular eczema, the aetiology of this type of eczema is unknown. It appears to peak twice per year in autumn and winter (Wolff *et al.*, 2005) and is more common in middle aged and older people; it usually lasts for only a few weeks (Page, 2006). Characteristically, the disease appears as coin-shaped plaques with small papules and vesicles on an erythematous base, more common on the lower legs.

Seborrhoeic eczema

The main areas affected are the hairy areas of the body, and the patient may complain of itching and have a red scaly rash (Mitchell and Kennedy, 2006). The disease is more common in men and may be associated with patients who are immunosuppressed, for example those with human immunodeficiency virus (HIV). This type of eczema can become complicated as a result of fungal infection.

Varicose eczema

This type of eczema commonly affects the lower limbs and can occur with or in the presence of varicose ulcer (Page, 2006). The aetiology is associated with chronic venous stasis; often the area involved becomes red and itchy and the patient may also have varicose veins and oedema (Gawkrodger, 2003).

Diagnosis

It has already been stated that diagnosis is made on clinical examination; referral to a dermatologist may be required. Other diagnostic tests include:

■ blood tests
■ patch test
■ allergy tests

Exogenous eczema

In industrial settings, exogenous eczema is common (Mitchell and Kennedy, 2006; Page, 2006). It is usual for this type of eczema to erupt at the point of contact and the way in which the patient presents will depend on the cause of irritant. The immune system overreacts to a substance that would otherwise be harmless.

There are many irritants that can cause allergic contact dermatitis, for example, the wearing of earrings or jewellery that contains nickel may cause allergic contact dermatitis and hypersensitivity will occur; perfumes and cosmetics can also cause contact dermatitis. Dermatitis may be triggered by the wearing of disposable gloves, for example, an allergenic reaction to disposable gloves can occur, if this is the case the user should be advised to use hypoallergenic, commercially supplied, disposable gloves. Hunter *et al.* (2002) suggest that in such cases the person may have to consider a change in occupation; occupations that are considered high risk include:

- hairdressing
- catering
- health care
- printing
- engineering
- agriculture
- horticulture
- construction
- cleaning

Nursing care and management

The care and management of the various types of eczema are similar. In atopic eczema, one of the main complications is infection (bacterial and fungal) as a result of a break in the skin as occur in atopic eczema where the skin is rough or broken. When the skin is infected, it contains pustules that are green or yellow in colour, with large blisters; the patient may feel unwell and have a raised temperature. The role of the nurse is to prevent infection in this instance and this can be done by educating the patient, explaining how the infection may be caused and spread by scratching.

The nurse should explore with the patient what it is that causes or makes the eczema worse; the answers to these questions can lead the nurse to test the patient for certain things, for example, to recommend a patch test. If an allergen or irritant has been identified then this should, if possible, be avoided. The following outlines the general approach to the management of atopic eczema; however, it should be noted that approaches to care should be tailored to meet individual needs:

- Remove, if possible, the irritant or allergen that causes the antibody–antigen reaction.
- Offer support to the patient and their family to empower educate and motivate. The overall aim should be to raise self-esteem and self-awareness and as such to prevent stigma.
- If the eczema, for example, is varicose eczema then the patient may be advised to wear support hosiery or if appropriate and possible, surgical intervention may be required.
- Creams, ointments and oils can be used to act as emollients to reduce the drying and itching effects of the disease.
- Aqueous cream may be used as a substitute for soap. Soaps can have the effect of further drying the skin. Perfumed products should be avoided.
- If infection occurs then **antibiotics** or **antifungal** medication may need to be prescribed. These medications are often given systematically but may be applied topically.

- In some instances, topical steroid preparations can be used to reduce inflammation, but these preparations should be used with caution and should not be used for longer than is necessary.
- Topical preparations containing both antibiotics and steroids are available but these should only be used for the short-term.
- Antihistamines may be prescribed.

The other issues that the nurse will need to consider, for example, are:

- Encourage rest as sleeping may be difficult for some patients.
- Dietary advice may be needed if the allergen is a food product; a multidisciplinary approach is advocated with referral to a dietician.
- Complementary therapies may help some patients. Complementary therapies are just complementary, and not a substitute to conventional medicine; however, the nurse must respect the patient's wishes.
- When applying medications the nurse must, at all times, wear gloves not only to combat the risk of cross infection but also to avoid absorbing the patient's medicines.

Psoriasis

There are several forms of psoriasis; this skin disorder is a non-infectious, inflammatory disorder that can appear as a red raised demarcation of skin patches with silvery whitish scales (Mitchell and Kennedy, 2006); the condition can vary from mild to severe. The aetiology is unknown.

The patient may also experience an itch. If itching occurs the scales are easily shed. It occurs most frequently on the back, the elbows, knees and scalp. This skin condition has the potential to also cause the patient feel ashamed and dirty.

Pathophysiologically, the cells of the basal layers of the epidermis reproduce and the more rapid upward progression of these cells through the epidermis results in an incomplete maturation of the upper layer (Waugh and Grant, 2006); there is an overproduction of skin cells. Sometimes psoriasis is associated with arthritis and this is called psoriatic arthropathy. The rash associated with psoriasis can occur when the patient is experiencing an episode of arthritis.

Thirty-five per cent of the patients with this condition have a family history (Mitchell and Kennedy, 2006); Page (2006) points out that there are other precipitating/aggravating factors:

- infection (streptococcal throat infection)
- some medications, i.e. antimalarials, antidepressants, beta-blockers
- sunlight (can help or hinder)
- hormones – psoriasis can become better or get worse during pregnancy or menstruation
- psychological stress, i.e. a bereavement, a life event such as divorce or sitting examinations
- trauma, i.e. burns, the site of an injury or a surgical scar

Hunter *et al.* (2002) suggest that the classification of psoriasis is made on clinical presentation. Skin biopsy, skin swab, throat swab and blood tests as well as clinical examination will be required to confirm diagnosis (Page, 2006). Treatment will include psychological support for the patient and the family.

There are a range of topical therapies that are available to manage psoriasis. The nurse has a role to play in motivating and encouraging the patient to apply the therapies and to apply them meticulously, adhering to the treatment regimen. The following is a list of some of the topical therapies. It must be noted that whatever treatment is chosen this is not a cure for the disease and there is no single treatment that will suit everyone and individual assessment is required (Mitchell and Kennedy, 2006):

■ Emollients with the aim to lubricate the skin and ease scaling as well as providing patient comfort.
■ Coal tar ointment – these preparations have an antipruritic and anti-inflammatory effect (these preparations may stain clothing).
■ Dithranol – this preparation is used to suppress cell proliferation.
■ Vitamin D analogues such as calcipotriol, tacalcitol and calcitriol; these are used amongst other things to inhibit cell proliferation.
■ Phototherapy can be used to inhibit cell division for some forms of psoriasis.
■ Methotrexate – this medicine is often used in the treatment of cancer; it causes inhibition of cell division.
■ Retinoids – these preparations influence the activity of the epidermis.
■ Topical steroids – used only for a short period.

Conclusion

The skin, also called the integumentary system, is the largest organ in the body and has several important functions. This chapter has provided an overview of the skin and has discussed a number of pathological changes that can occur resulting in disease or illness. Some of the more common skin conditions have been discussed with an emphasis on skin cancer. The reader is advised to consult other texts to fully appreciate the scope and potential the nurse has in helping people with skin conditions; this chapter has merely touched on the topic. The nurse has a vital role to play in assisting the individual with problems associated with the skin; however, this can only be achieved with insight and understanding.

As well as the physiological disturbances resulting in problems of skin there are also important psychological ramifications that must be given much consideration. The nurse has a role to play in empowering and motivating the patient in order to adhere to prescribed treatment regimens that can often be messy and potentially damage clothing and bedding. Many patients and their families with skin conditions voice concerns about social isolation and ostracism; education and explanation may help to reduce these feelings; the nurse is ideally placed to do this, acting as a key resource.

Multiple choice questions

1. The average adult has how many square metres of skin?
(a) 3 m^2
(b) 4 m^2
(c) 5 m^2
(d) 2 m^2

2. Skin is thickest on:
(a) the lips
(b) the earlobes
(c) the hands
(d) the nose

3. Dermatoglyphics is another word for:
(a) the dermis
(b) the epidermis
(c) subcutaneous fat
(d) finger prints

4. Each hair follicle is made of:
(a) sebum
(b) sweat
(c) keratin
(d) muscle

5. The most dangerous form of skin cancer is:
(a) basal cell carcinoma
(b) malignant melanoma
(c) squamous cell carcinoma
(d) sarcoma

6. The integumentary system is also known as:
(a) the skin
(b) the muscles
(c) the gastrointestinal tract
(d) the nervous system

7. An emollient is:
(a) an antibiotic
(b) a steroid
(c) an alcohol-based medication
(d) a substance that moisturises, soothes and softens the skin

8. The term *topical* means:
(a) to inject
(b) to ingest
(c) to apply to the skin
(d) to insert

9. What are the stages involved in primary wound healing?
(a) scab formation and scarring
(b) scarring
(c) cell proliferation
(d) inflammation, proliferation and maturation

10. Which of the following is not an antibiotic?
(a) hydrocortisone
(b) cefuroxime
(c) erythromycin
(d) trimethoprim

Answers: 1.d, 2.c, 3.d, 4.c, 5.b, 6.a, 7.d, 8.c, 9.d, 10.a.

Test your knowledge

- Describe the nursing care of patient with atopic eczema.
- Outline the role and function of the nurse when providing advice to a patient or group of patients concerning skin cancer avoidance.
- Describe the pathophysiological changes that occur during wound healing.

Glossary of terms

Adjuvant: Agents that modify the effects of other agents.

Antibiotics: Chemical compounds that stop the growth of microorganisms.

Antifungal: Medications used to treat fungal infections.

Chemotherapy: The use of chemical substances to treat diseases, primarily to treat cancer.

Dermatitis: Inflammation of the skin.

Dermatoscopy: A magnifier with a light allowing illumination of the lesion.

Erythema: Redness.

Extrinsic: Originates externally.

Fissure: A groove or tear.

Histology: The study of tissue, microscopic anatomy.

Hyperkeratosis: Excess keratins are produced resulting in thickening of the skin.

Integumentary: The external covering of the body.

Intrinsic: Originates internally.

Keratin: A tough insoluble protein.

Keratinise: To convert into keratin.

Lichenfication: Thickening of the skin as a result of chronic scratching.

Naevus: A pigmented lesion of the skin.

Pheromones: A chemical that triggers an innate behavioural response in another.

Prognosis: A prediction about how a patient's disease will progress.

Pruritus: Itching.

Radiotherapy: The medical use of radiation to treat cancer.

Relapsing (relapse): Occurs when the patient is again affected by a condition that has occurred in the past.

Sebum: An oily substance made of fat and the debris of fat producing cells.

Sutures: Stitches.

Topical: A medication applied to the body surface.

Vesiculation: Collection of fluid in the skin.

Viscous: Relating to the thickness of a fluid.

Xerosis: A term used to describe dry skin.

References

All Parliamentary Group on Skin (1997). *An Investigation into the Adequacy of Service Provision and Treatments for Patents with Skin Diseases in the UK*. London: All Parliamentary Group on Skin.

Archer, C.B. (2000). The pathophysiology and clinical features of atopic dermatitis. In: Williams, H.C. (ed) *Atopic Dermatitis*. Cambridge: Cambridge University Press.

British Association of Dermatologists (2007). *Know Your Skin Type*. Available at http://www.bad.org.uk/public/cancer/Skin_Types_Poster.pdf. Last accessed May 2007.

Department of Health (2000). *The NHS Cancer Plan: A Plan for Investment A Plan for Reform*. London: DH.

Department of Health (2002). *Compendium of Clinical and Health*. London: National Centre for Health Outcomes Development.

Foss, M. and Farine, T. (2007). *Science in Nursing and Health Care*, 2nd edn. Harlow: Pearson.

Gawkrodger, D.J. (1992). *Dermatology: An Illustrated Colour Text*. Edinburgh: Churchill Livingstone.

Gawkrodger, D.J. (2003). *Dermatology: An Illustrated Colour Text*, 3rd edn. Edinburgh: Churchill Livingstone.

Haneke, E. (2006). Surgical anatomy of the nail apparatus. *Dermatology Clinic*, 24(3), 291–296.

Hoare, C., Li Wan Lo, A. and Williams, H. (2000). Systematic review of treatments for atopic eczema. *Health Technology Assessment*, 4(37), 1–191.

Hughes, E. and Van Onselen, J. (2001). *Dermatology Nursing: A Practical Guise*. Edinburgh: Churchill Livingstone.

Hunter, J., Savin, J. and Dahl, M. (2002). *Clinical Dermatology*, 3rd edn. Oxford: Blackwell Scientific.

Lawton, S. (2006a). Anatomy and function of the skin. Part 2 – The epidermis. *Nursing Times*, 102(32), 28–29.

Lawton, S. (2006b). Anatomy and function of the skin. Part 2 – Dermis and adjacent structures. *Nursing Times*, 102(33), 26–27.

Lawton, S. (2006c). Anatomy and function of the skin. Part 4 – Appendages. *Nursing Times*, 102(34), 26–27.

Lewis-Jones, S. (1999). Quality of life – skin disease and disability. *Dermatology in Practice*, 7(3), 8–10.

Marks, R. (2003). *Roxburgh's Common Skin Diseases*. London: Arnold.

Mitchell, T. and Kennedy, C. (2006). *Common Skin Disorders*. Edinburgh: Churchill Livingstone.

Motley, R., Kersey, P. and Lawrence, C. (2003). Multiprofessional guidelines for the management of cutaneous melanoma. *British Journal of Dermatology*, 146, 7–17.

Moulin, V., Auger, F.A., Garrel, D. and Germain, L. (2000). Role of wound healing myofibroblasts on re-epithelialization of human skin. *Burns*, 36(1), 3–12.

National Institute for Health and Clinical Excellence (2006). *Improving Outcomes for People with Skin Tumours Including Melanoma: The Manual*. London: NICE.

Oliviera, S.A., Dusza, S.W., Phelan, D.L., Ostroff, J.S., Berwick, M. and Halpern, A.C. (2004). Patient adherence to self examination. Effect of nurse intervention with photographs. *American Journal of Preventative Medicine*, 26(2), 152–155.

Page, B.E. (2006). Skin disorders. In: Alexander, M.F., Fawcett, J.N. and Runciman, P.J. (eds) *Nursing Practice, Hospital and Home: The Adult*, 3rd edn. Edinburgh: Churchill Livingstone, pp. 525–552.

Sharpe, G. (2006). Skin cancer: Prevalence, prevention and treatment. *Clinical Medicine*, 6, 333–334.

Thompson, J.F., Scolyer, R.A. and Kefford, R.A. (2005). Cutaneous melanoma. *Lancet*, 365, 687–701.

Timby, B.K. (2005). *Fundamental Nursing Skills and Concepts*, 8th edn. Philadelphia: Lippincott.

Waugh, A. and Grant, A. (2006). *Ross and Wilson Anatomy and Physiology in Health and Illness*, 10th edn. Edinburgh: Churchill Livingstone.

White, G. (2003). *Color Atlas of Dermatology*, 3rd edn. London: Mosby.

Wolff, K., Allen-Johnson, R. and Suurmond, S. (2005). *Fitzpatrick's Color Atlas and Synopsis of Clinical Dermatology*, 5th edn. New York: McGraw-Hill.

Chapter 19

The ear, nose and throat, eyes and their associated disorders

Carl Clare

KEY WORDS

- Pinna
- Tympanic membrane
- Eustachian tube
- Cochlea

- Septum
- Turbinates
- Epiglottis
- Larynx

- Iris
- Retina
- Sclera
- Humour

Test your prior knowledge

- ❖ Which part of the ear contains the sensory organ for balance?
- ❖ Which structure is completely removed from the throat during a laryngectomy?
- ❖ Which part of the eye is affected by a cataract?

> ## Learning outcomes
>
> On completion of this section, the reader will be able to:
>
> ■ Describe the functions of each of the three sections of the ear.
> ■ Explain the functions of the nose in respiration.
> ■ Describe the functions of the true vocal cords and the false vocal cords.
> ■ Describe the roles of the two types of photoreceptors of the eye.

Introduction

Disorders of the structures of the head and neck range from the relatively minor to some of the most challenging a nurse may be asked to care for. The special senses of the ear, nose and eye are something that are often taken for granted, but conditions that affect these senses can have a massive impact on the daily activities of a person. The aim of this chapter is to introduce the reader to the physiology and associated disorders of the special senses and in line with the speciality of ear, nose and throat (ENT) care, the physiology and disorders of the throat, will also be reviewed.

Physiology of the ear, nose and throat

Ear

The ear is divided into three sections (see Figure 19.1):

■ external
■ middle
■ inner

Each of these three sections is integral in the process of hearing and the inner ear is also essential in the maintenance of the sense of balance.

External ear

The external ear consists of the pinna, the external ear canal and the tympanic membrane.

■ **Pinna** – a skin covered flap of elastic **cartilage** shaped somewhat like the end of a horn surrounding the end of the external auditory canal.
■ External ear canal – a slightly 'S' shaped tube lined with skin, fine hairs, sebaceous (oil) glands and ceruminous (wax) glands. The purpose of the oils and the wax is to lubricate the ear canal, kill bacteria and, in conjunction with the hairs, keep the canal free of debris (Lewis *et al.*, 2007).

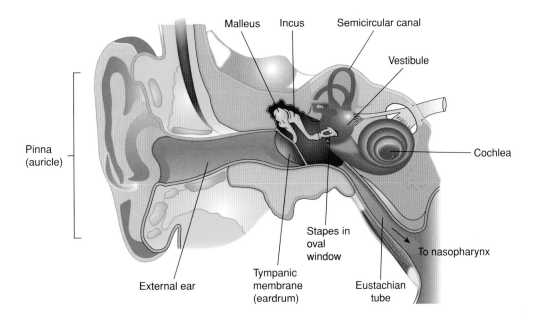

Figure 19.1 The ear.

- **Tympanic membrane** – composed of **epithelial cells**, **connective tissue** and **mucous membrane**. It acts as a partition between the external and middle ears and is responsible for the transmission of sound from external to middle ear.

Middle ear

The middle ear is an air space lined with mucous membrane; it is connected to the nasopharynx by the **eustachian tube**, thus allowing for the equalisation of air pressure between the middle ear and the throat (and therefore atmospheric air). This equalisation of pressure ensures free movement of the tympanic membrane in response to sound waves conducted along the external ear canal.

Within the middle ear are three bones (the ossicles or **ossicular chain**):

- hammer (malleus)
- anvil (incus)
- stirrup (stapes)

These interlink with each other and are connected with the tympanic membrane. Vibrations of the tympanic membrane are conducted along the bones to the oval window; these vibrations are then transmitted via the oval window into the fluid of the inner ear. Movement in this fluid leads to stimulation of the hearing receptors.

Inner ear

The inner ear is also known as the **labyrinth** due to the complicated series of canals it contains (Jenkins *et al.*, 2007). The inner ear is composed of two main, fluid-filled parts:

■ Bony labyrinth – a series of cavities within the temporal bone that contain the main organs of balance (the **semicircular canals** and the **vestibule**) and the main organ of hearing (the **cochlea**).
■ Membranous labyrinth – a series of sacs and tubes that are contained within the bony labyrinth. Movement of the fluid within the membranous labyrinth contained within the cochlea stimulates the hearing receptors leading to the generation of nerve impulses that are transmitted to the hearing centres of the brain (Guyton and Hall, 2006).

Nose

The nose is the first part of the respiratory tract and also contains the receptors for the sense of smell. The functions of the nose are threefold (Jenkins *et al.*, 2007):

■ warming, moistening and filtering inhaled air
■ detecting **olfactory** stimuli
■ resonance chamber that modifies the quality of speech

The nose can be divided into external and internal sections (Jenkins *et al.*, 2007):

■ External nose – a framework of bone and cartilage covered by muscle and skin and lined with a mucous membrane. This framework is attached to the frontal and maxillary bones of the skull. The external nose is divided into two airways (**nares** or nostrils) of roughly equal size by the **septum**, which forms part of the framework of bone and cartilage.
■ Internal nose – a large chamber lined with **ciliated** mucous membrane and containing coarse hairs that filter out large particles from inhaled air. Finer particles that enter the nose become trapped in the sticky **mucus** created by the membrane and are then transported to the nasopharynx by the ciliary system. The internal nose is divided into two by a continuation of the septum. Each side contains three shelves formed by projections of bone known as the **turbinates** (Figure 19.2); these increase the surface area that inhaled air must pass over (Guyton and Hall, 2006). The internal nose has an extremely rich vascular supply, which in conjunction with the turbinates maximises the humidification and warming of the air passing through. The internal nose also contains openings (**ostia**) from the **sinus cavities** (contained within the bones of the skull).

Throat

The throat consists of the oropharynx and the hypopharynx (Reynolds, 2004) (Figure 19.3).

Oropharynx

Tonsils

The tonsils are five collections of **lymphatic nodules** mostly located in a ring around the junction of the oral cavity and the oropharynx (Tortora and Grabowski, 2003).

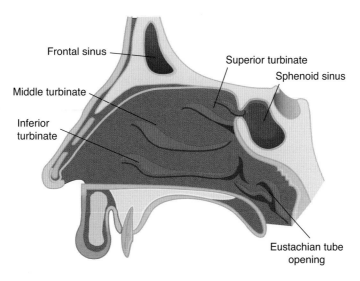

Figure 19.2 The nose.

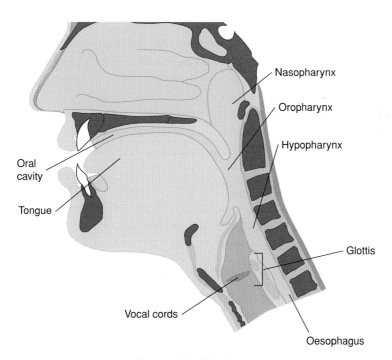

Figure 19.3 The throat.

- Two palatine tonsils located at the back of the oral cavity.
- Two lingual tonsils located at the base of the tongue.
- A single pharyngeal tonsil (adenoid) is located at the junction of the nasal cavity and the nasopharynx.

The role of the tonsils is to participate in the fight against inhaled or ingested foreign substances.

Hypopharynx

Larynx

The **larynx** is a short tube that connects the lower hypopharynx with the trachea. It is composed of a mucous membrane covering several pieces of cartilage including:

- thyroid cartilage (Adam's apple)
- **epiglottis** – a large piece of cartilage that covers the opening of the glottis during swallowing, thus protecting the airway
- cricoid cartilage – a ring of cartilage that forms the inferior wall of the larynx and connects to the first cartilage ring of the trachea

The mucous membrane of the larynx is formed to create two pairs of folds:

- Ventricular folds – (false vocal cords) when they are brought together they enable the holding of the breath against the pressure in the thoracic cavity, such as when lifting a heavy object (Tortora and Grabowski, 2003).
- **Vocal cords** (folds) – (true vocal cords) situated below the ventricular folds, the vocal cords are fundamental to the generation of speech. Sound is generated by the vibration of these cords but the mouth, nasal cavity and nasal sinuses are also required to create recognisable speech (Guyton and Hall, 2006).

Physiology of the eye

The eyeball (**globe**) is made up of three layers (Lewis *et al.*, 2007) (Figure 19.4):

- a tough outer layer – fibrous tunic
- a middle layer – vascular tunic
- the retina – sensory tunic

Fibrous tunic

This layer is composed of the **cornea** and the **sclera**, and contains no blood vessels. The cornea is a curved, transparent coat which helps focus light onto the retina. The sclera (the 'white' of the eye) covers the entire eyeball, except where the cornea is present; it gives shape and protection to the eyeball. The anterior sclera (but not the cornea) is covered by the **conjunctiva** which produces a lubricating mucus that prevents the eye from drying out (Marieb and Hoehn, 2007).

Vascular tunic

The vascular tunic (**uvea**) is composed of the iris, the ciliary body and the choroid.

- **Choroid** – a highly vascular membrane; its blood vessels supply nutrition to all the tunics of the eye (Marieb and Hoehn, 2007).

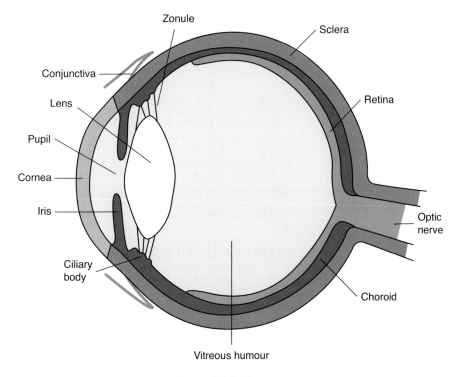

Figure 19.4 **The eye.**

- **Ciliary body** – at the front of the eye the choroid becomes the **ciliary body** – a thickened ring of smooth muscles that circle the lens, and have an important role in controlling the shape of the lens. The choroid is connected to the lens by a suspensory ligament (**zonule**).
- **Iris** – coloured part of the eye lying between the cornea and the lens; it contains a hole (the **pupil**) through which light can enter the eye. The size of the pupil is controlled by the contraction and relaxation of two separate layers of muscle fibres contained within the iris.

Sensory tunic

The **retina** has two layers; however, only the neural layer is directly involved with vision (Marieb and Hoehn, 2007). Within this neural layer are the **photoreceptors**:

- **rods** for peripheral and dim light vision
- **cones** for bright light and colour vision

Impulses generated as a result of stimulation of these photoreceptors are transmitted to the visual cortex via the **optic nerve**.

Internal structure

Internally, the eye is divided into two chambers by a barrier formed from the lens and the zonule:

- **Anterior segment** – in front of the lens and zonule. This chamber is filled with **aqueous humour** which is constantly formed and drained (Guyton and Hall, 2006). Aqueous humour provides the lens and the cornea with nutrients and oxygen.

■ **Posterior segment** – filled with a gel-like substance called **vitreous humour**. The thick vitreous humour supports the back of the lens, holds the retina against the choroid and contributes to **intraocular pressure**, thus helping to maintain the shape of the eye (Jenkins *et al.*, 2007).

Lens

The lens is the main apparatus for focusing light onto the retina (Guyton and Hall, 2006). The thickness of the lens is varied by the contraction and relaxation of the ciliary muscles depending on whether the eye is focusing on near or far objects.

Movement of the eye

Movement of the eye is controlled by the extrinsic eye muscles; neuromuscular coordination ensures the simultaneous movement of both eyes (Lewis *et al.*, 2007).

Disorders of the ear, nose and throat, and eye

Learning outcomes

On completion of this section, the reader will be able to:

■ Describe the nursing care of a patient following ear surgery.

■ Describe the nursing care of a patient following nasal surgery.

■ Explain the difference between a tracheostomy and a laryngectomy.

■ Discuss the two types of glaucoma.

Disorders of the ear, nose and throat
Ear

Ear wax

Impaction of ear wax in the external ear canal is a common complaint often related to patient attempts to remove ear wax with fingers or cotton buds. Impaction of ear wax reduces the ability of sound to travel the length of the external ear canal and the responsiveness of the tympanic membrane to sound waves leading to a temporary reduction in the ability to hear. This is especially common in older patients who have a tendency to produce more, and drier wax (Lewis *et al.*, 2007).

One method for the removal of ear wax is the **syringing** of the external ear canal often preceded by the use of a cerumenolytic (substance that actively helps to break down wax) or a wax softener (Somerville, 2002).

Otitis externa

This is diffuse inflammation of the external ear canal, often associated with regular swimming ('swimmers ear') (Agius *et al.*, 1992). The condition is characterised by pain, itching and a discharge from the ear canal. The discharge is usually watery at the beginning but becomes **purulent** as the condition progresses.

The spread of infection can lead to **pyrexia** and systemic symptoms such as **malaise**. The infection is usually caused by a mixture of microorganisms and swabs should be sent for microbiological culture and sensitivity.

Nursing care of this condition includes:

- Careful removal of any debris from the external ear canal.
- Packing of the external ear canal with ribbon gauze soaked with **topical antibiotics** and a steroid preparation (Kilner *et al.*, 2000).
- If the infection has become systemic (entered the blood stream) or extensive the patient may require oral antibiotics, analgesia and bed rest.
- The patient should be discouraged from scratching the affected ear and advised to prevent water from entering the ear canal (McKenzie *et al.*, 1986).

Tympanic membrane rupture

Rupture of the tympanic membrane due to improper ear syringing technique, blows to the side of the head or blast injuries are often self-healing as long as infection is not present.

Patients should be advised to avoid:

- the entry of water into the ear
- introducing of foreign objects such as cotton buds

Persistent deafness may indicate damage or displacement of the ossicular chain and may require surgical intervention.

Otitis media

Acute otitis media is a condition that is often associated with upper respiratory tract infections and **sinusitis** (Finkelstein *et al.*, 1994). The infection tracks up into the middle ear via the eustachian tube leading to infection and the collection of **pus**. The infection and the pressure resulting from the collection of pus may lead to a range of potential symptoms including:

- pain
- pyrexia
- malaise
- headache
- nausea and vomiting
- **tinnitus**
- reduction in hearing
  (Beers *et al.*, 2006).

Treatment for acute otitis media includes:

- antibiotics
- pain relief
- **antipyretics**
  (Stafford and Youngs, 1999).

- Nasal decongestants may reduce inflammation of the eustachian tube and allow drainage of the middle ear into the nasopharynx (McKenzie *et al.*, 1986).

■ Application of warmth to the affected ear in order to reduce pain.
■ Avoid water entering the ear canal.

Untreated, or repeated episodes of acute otitis media may lead to chronic infection of the middle ear which may eventually spread to the mastoid process of the temporal bone of the skull (mastoiditis) (Tortora and Grabowski, 2003). Tympanic membrane rupture is common and destruction of the bones of the ossicular chain is also possible (McKenzie *et al.*, 1986). Symptoms include:

■ purulent discharge
■ pain – may be associated with redness and swelling of the bone behind the pinna (mastoid process) (Reynolds, 2004)
■ pyrexia
■ hearing loss
■ nausea and vomiting
■ **vertigo**

Treatment for the chronic complications of otitis media is usually surgical and depends on the structures that are affected:

■ myringoplasty – repair of the tympanic membrane, often using grafted tissue
■ ossiculoplasty – reconstruction of the ossicular chain
■ tympanoplasty – myringoplasty and ossiculoplasty performed at the same time
■ mastoidectomy – removal of infected tissue from the middle ear and mastoid bone – often performed with a tympanoplasty

The nursing care of patients following surgery of the ear is detailed in Box 19.1.

Box 19.1 Nursing care of the patient following ear surgery

■ Recovery period – nurse flat on the opposite side to the operation side with no pillows
■ Advise the patient to avoid sudden movements of the head
■ Administer analgesia as prescribed
■ Pillows are introduced for comfort when the patient feels able to tolerate them, most patients are able to tolerate sitting up after 24 hours (McKenzie *et al.*, 1986)
■ Following operations on the inner ear observe for signs of **neurological** damage (neurological observations at least 4 hourly for the first 24 hours)
■ Facial nerve damage may occur at the time of the operation or subsequently due to inflammation or oedema. The patient should be asked to show their teeth or smile to assess for **facial palsy**
■ Patient should avoid coughing, sneezing, and or blowing their nose, or straining during bowel movements for 7–10 days as this will lead to an increased pressure in the ear via the eustachian tube. If coughing or sneezing is unavoidable then the patient is advised to keep the mouth open to reduce the pressure on the middle ear (Lewis *et al.*, 2007). **Laxatives** may be provided to avoid straining during bowel movements
■ Most patients can be discharged after 2–3 days but should be advised to avoid water entry into the ear, crowded places (where respiratory infections may be contracted), and changes in air pressure (such as flying or high altitudes) until advised by the surgeon (Lewis *et al.*, 2007)

Otosclerosis

Formation of new bone around the footplate of the stapes; often **hereditary** and is associated with a gradual deterioration in hearing. The treatment is stapedectomy – the removal of part of the stapes and insertion of a prosthesis (Cherry, 1997).

Ménière's disease

Ménière's disease is a disorder of the inner ear characterised by episodes of:

- vertigo
- nausea and vomiting
- tinnitus
- varying hearing loss
- **aural** fullness (a feeling of 'stuffiness' in the ear)
- 'drop attacks' – a feeling of being pulled to the ground; alternatively some patients feel as though they are whirling through space

The duration of an episode may be hours or days. The nursing care of a patient experiencing an acute episode of Ménière's disease includes:

- reassurance and counselling
- quiet, darkened, environment
- comfortable position (often **semi-recumbent**)
- avoid sudden head movements
- fluorescent and flickering lights, and watching television should be avoided as they can exacerbate symptoms
- vomit bowls should be provided
- all drugs should be administered **parenterally**
- nurse call bell should be put in patient's reach and the patient advised not to mobilise without assistance

Treatment of the disease requires long-term medication (**antihistamines**, antivertigo drugs and **anticholinergics**). Patients who experience a reduced quality of life (frequent incapacitating attacks and/or loss of employment) may require surgery (Lewis *et al.*, 2007).

Nose

Epistaxis (nose bleed)

Often associated with trauma to the nose, or upper respiratory tract infections. Control is achieved by applying pressure to the upper part of the nose by pinching it between the finger and the thumb whilst the patient sits with their head tilted forward to avoid blood draining into the throat and being swallowed. Nasal packing may be required and in some cases this may be modified by the use of a **foley catheter** or **postnasal pack** to provide a firm base against which to pack the nose (McKenzie *et al.*, 1986). Further care for difficult-to-control bleeds may include:

- frequent observations (blood pressure and pulse half hourly)
- assessment of blood loss and blood transfusion if **hypovolaemia** is suspected

> **Box 19.2 Nursing care of the patient following nasal surgery**
>
> - In the immediate postoperative period patients will normally have a nasal pack in place. This is removed 24–48 hours after the operation
> - Monitoring of the patients' airway is essential in the immediate postoperative period due to the risk of blood or nasal packing entering the respiratory tract
> - When the patient is fully conscious their head should be raised above the level of the heart and they should be encouraged to sleep with at least three pillows (Robinson, 2006). This reduces bleeding and swelling. Ice packs may also be used to reduce swelling if allowed by the surgeon
> - Administer analgesia and antibiotics as prescribed
> - Patient should avoid sneezing, blowing their nose, or straining during bowel movements for 10–14 days as this may lead to bleeding (Sigler and Schuring, 1993). If sneezing is unavoidable then the patient is advised to keep the mouth open to reduce the pressure on the nose. **Laxatives** may be provided to avoid straining during bowel movements
> - After the removal of nasal packs steam inhalations or a saline spray will help to keep the nasal mucosa moist and loosen any crusts

- cold compresses applied to nose and back of the neck to reduce blood flow to the nose
- antihypertensive drugs for **hypertensive** patients
- **cauterisation** or surgical **ligation** of blood vessels (Cherry, 1997)

Deviated nasal septum

A condition that may be **congenital** or acquired (due to trauma); the patient may present with nasal obstruction. Treatment is normally surgical:

- Submucous resection (SMR) – removal and resection of the parts of the septum causing the deviation.
- Septoplasty – septum is completely freed and the removal of areas around its margin may allow it to be repositioned in the midline.

The nursing care of patients following surgery of the nose is detailed in Box 19.2.

Nasal polyps

These are soft fleshy swellings inside the nose: the end product of prolonged oedema of the nasal **mucosa** caused by prolonged infection or allergy. The patient may present with nasal obstruction, nasal discharge and headaches. The treatment is the surgical removal of the **polypi** (ethmoidectomy) and treatment of the underlying cause.

Sinusitis

Following a viral infection of the nose the natural resistance of the mucosa is reduced and a **secondary bacterial infection** occurs which rapidly spreads into the sinuses. The swelling of the mucosa may close off the ostia of the sinuses; thus the infected mucus is unable to escape. The symptoms include:

- pain
- nasal obstruction

- malaise
- pyrexia
- localised tenderness

If untreated there is the possibility of complications such as:

- spread of infection to the eyes
- **intracranial** infection or abscess formation
- osteomyelitis (infection of the bone)

The treatment of sinusitis includes:

- nasal decongestants to reduce the mucosal swelling and allow drainage
- antibiotics
- pain relief
- antral lavage – introduction of a **trocar** and **cannula** into the maxillary (antral) sinus to allow the cavity to be flushed with normal saline (Sigler and Schuring, 1993)
- abscesses require surgical intervention

The nursing care includes:

- warm, well-ventilated environment
- fluid intake of at least 3 L a day (McKenzie *et al.*, 1986)
- good oral hygiene
- steam inhalations
- bed rest may be required for 24–48 hours
- whilst recovering the patient should avoid extremes of temperature, crowded environments and smoking (Sigler and Schuring, 1993)

Throat

Tonsillitis and quinsy

Tonsillitis is a condition characterised by inflammation of the tonsils leading to the patient presenting with:

- bilateral sore throat
- **dysphagia**
- pyrexia
- malaise

Treatment is usually:

- antibiotics
- encourage a fluid intake of 1–3 L per day (McKenzie *et al.*, 1986)
- pain relief
- good oral hygiene
- recurrent bouts of tonsillitis may require surgical removal of the tonsils (tonsillectomy)

The development of a **peritonsillar abscess** (quinsy) associated with tonsillitis may follow and patients may present with:

- inflamed tonsil with swelling due to the collection of pus
- worsening dysphagia often with an associated inability to swallow saliva
- worsening pain on one side of the throat
- **trismus** – an inability to open the mouth due to spasm of the jaw muscles

This is considered a much more serious condition and surgical drainage (with antibiotic cover) is recommended (Cherry, 1997).

Tracheostomy

Tracheotomy is the surgical procedure of making an incision into the anterior tracheal wall for the purpose of creating an airway; a **tracheostomy** is the opening (**stoma**) that is created by the tracheotomy (Lewis *et al.*, 2007). Tracheostomies are created for several reasons:

- relief of upper airways obstruction
- protection of the lungs from the **aspiration** of food or **regurgitation** of the stomach contents
- **respiratory insufficiency**
- long-term ventilation
- following a laryngectomy

Most tracheostomies are temporary and a plastic or metal tube is inserted into the stoma to maintain the patency of the airway (Figure 19.5). Following a laryngectomy the trachea is brought to the surface of the neck and a permanent stoma is formed (Feber, 2006).

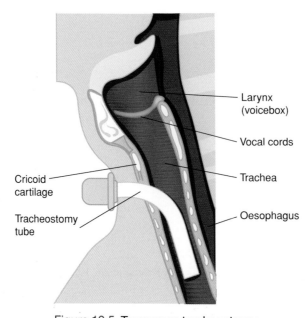

Figure 19.5 Temporary tracheostomy.

Potential complications following tracheostomy formation include:

- tube dislodgement – avoided by correctly securing the tube with tapes and **sutures**
- tube obstruction – due to the build-up of secretions or the formation of a mucus plug which is then coughed into the tube
- surgical emphysema – the escape of air into the soft tissue of the neck, characterised by a 'crackling' sensation when **palpated**
- **pneumonia**
- tracheo-oesophageal fistula – created by excessive or prolonged inflation of a cuffed tracheostomy tube leading to **necrosis** of the tracheal wall and the development of a hole (**fistula**) between the trachea and the oesophagus; the fistula allows the entry of food and fluids into the lungs

The nursing care of a patient following the creation of a tracheostomy:

- Nurse upright to reduce oedema formation.
- Frequent observations – blood pressure, pulse, respirations and oxygen saturations should be noted every 15 minutes for the first 2 hours then reducing to half hourly for 2 hours and then hourly for 24 hours.
- A low pressure cuffed tracheostomy tube (Box 19.3) should be placed in the operating theatre and should be left inflated for the first 24 hours to reduce the chance of bleeding. To reduce the chance of **pressure necrosis** the cuff pressure should be checked every 8 hours (Lewis *et al.*, 2007). The correct cuff pressure is maintained by the use of a pressure gauge.
- Suctioning – this is dependent on patient requirements (patients will produce secretions at different rates) but usually is done every 15–30 minutes for the first 24 hours (Stokes, 1985). The type and quantity of the suctioned mucus should be monitored and recorded (Lewis *et al.*, 2007).
- **Humidification** – as the air entering the patients' lungs is no longer warmed and humidified by the upper airway the provision of humidification is essential to prevent the formation of crusts which may block the tracheostomy tube.
- Dressings should be kept clean and dry as wet dressings encourage the growth of bacteria and may lead to wound infections or, if inhaled, respiratory infections (Feber, 2006).
- The tracheostomy tube is first changed after 48 hours – this is a procedure that should only be carried out by two nurses at least one of whom should be experienced in this procedure.

Box 19.3 Cuffed and uncuffed tracheostomy tubes

- **Cuffed** tracheostomy tubes have an inflatable cuff towards their **distal** end; this is used to create an airtight seal in the trachea. They are generally used in patients who require a tracheostomy for ventilation (for instance, in intensive care) or for patients who are at risk of aspirating food or body fluids (for instance, immediately posttracheostomy formation there is a risk of bleeding from the operative site). Cuffed tracheostomy tubes have a low pressure cuff and therefore there is no requirement to deflate the cuff regularly so long as the pressure is checked with a pressure gauge.
- **Uncuffed** tracheostomy tubes (as in Figure 19.5) are much more common. However, in the acute setting it is recommended that a cuffed tracheostomy tube of the correct size is kept by the bedside for use in an emergency situation (such as resuscitation)

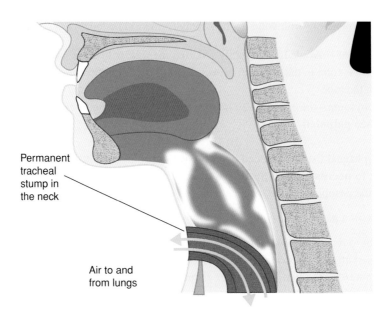

Figure 19.6 Laryngectomy.

Longer term care of the patient with a tracheostomy is geared towards enabling the patient to perform their own care (including tube care, tube changes, suctioning and dressing changes).

Laryngectomy

Laryngectomy is the removal of the entire structure of the larynx (Figure 19.6) and is the standard treatment for advanced laryngeal cancer (Scottish Intercollegiate Guidelines Network (SIGN), 2006).

During a laryngectomy the trachea is brought to the surface of the neck and a permanent tracheostomy is formed through which the patient breathes; therefore, there is no connection between the mouth and nose and the lungs. Immediately postoperatively the stoma will be protected by a tracheostomy tube and the care of the patient is similar to that of a patient with a temporary tracheostomy. The greater trauma to the trachea raises the risk of bleeding and oedema formation, and it is therefore common practice for oxygen saturations to be monitored with **pulse oximetry** continuously for 24 hours and then overnight for 2–3 days. Once the risk of bleeding and oedema formation has reduced, about 5–10 days postoperatively, the tracheostomy tube is removed and replaced with a silicone stoma button or stud to prevent the closure of the stoma as scar tissue forms (Feber, 2006). Patients are normally discharged 14 days postoperatively.

The loss of the normal humidification and warming mechanisms of the mouth and nose will lead to the drying of the mucus lining of the lower respiratory tract and a significant increase in water loss via exhaled air. This leads to changes in respiratory mechanisms and a significantly increased risk of respiratory infections (Feber, 2006). The loss of moisture will lead to the creation of thick secretions and crust formation which may completely block the stoma and thus threaten life. Humidification is essential for laryngectomy patients and once the patient is discharged they must use a passive heat and moisture exchanger (**HME**) worn over the stoma; these are usually made of foam that traps the heat and moisture in expired air; this is then transferred into the inspired air.

The loss of the patients' voice following laryngectomy can have significant psychological effects and several communication methods are available (Lewis *et al.*, 2007):

- Voice prostheses (speaking valve) – a valve placed between the trachea and the oesophagus which diverts expired air into the oesophagus when the tracheostomy is manually blocked; thus air passes into the mouth.
- Electrolarynx – a battery-powered device held against the mouth that creates speech with the use of sound waves.
- Artificial larynx – similar to an electrolarynx except that the device is held to the neck rather than the mouth.
- Oesophageal speech – this involves the patient swallowing air, trapping it in the oesophagus and releasing it to create sound.

It is important that laryngectomy patients wear a medical alert bracelet identifying them as a '**neck breather**' in the event of an emergency situation.

Disorders of the eye
Cataracts

A cataract is **opacity** within the lens and has several causes (Stollery *et al.*, 2005):

- congenital
- age related – occurring in patients over the age of 60 years
- traumatic – penetrating or blunt trauma
- toxic – radiation therapy or drugs such as topical steroids
- secondary – to diseases of the eye or systemic disease such as diabetes mellitus

Patients may report:

- decrease in vision
- 'misty vision'
- abnormal colour perception
- glare – dazzling by bright lights due to abnormal light refraction

The treatment of cataracts is surgical and requires the removal of the diseased lens and replacement with a **prosthetic** lens (Riaz *et al.*, 2006). The procedure is normally carried out under local anaesthetic and the patient is given **sedation**. Postoperatively, the patient can be discharged when the effects of sedation have worn off (Lewis *et al.*, 2007). Postoperative self-care advice may include:

- administration of antibiotic and steroid eye drops as prescribed
- cover the eye with an eye patch and protective shield for 24 hours, then only at night
- avoid situations that increase intraocular pressure (stooping, coughing or lifting)
- a reduction in **visual acuity** in the immediate postoperative period is not unusual – it may take up to 2 weeks for vision to improve
- once full healing has occurred (approximately 6–8 weeks) a prescription for glasses will be required as the prosthetic lens is not able to correct for near vision (e.g. reading)

Macular degeneration

Macular degeneration is characterised by a gradual loss of central vision but peripheral vision is maintained. There are two types of macular degeneration (Stollery *et al.*, 2005):

- Dry macular degeneration – associated with small, round, white yellow areas (**drusens**) in the macula. There is currently no treatment available.
- Wet macular degeneration – caused by the development of abnormal blood vessels below the retina. Current treatments are controversial and include dietary changes to include high levels of vitamins C and E, beta-carotene and zinc (Chopdar *et al.*, 2003). A small number of patients may be suitable for photodynamic therapy (**PDT**) (National Institute for Health and Clinical Excellence, 2003) which involves the injection of a dye into the blood vessels; subsequent excitation of the dye by a 'cold' laser (which does not damage the retina) **coagulates** the targeted blood vessels.

Glaucoma

Glaucoma is a term relating to a series of disorders characterised by:

- increased intraocular pressure (IOP)
- optic nerve **atrophy**
- loss of peripheral vision – 'tunnel vision'   (Lewis *et al.*, 2007).

Loss of vision is related to a loss of balance in the generation and reabsorption of aqueous humour; the subsequent rise in IOP leads to damage to the head of the optic nerve. The treatment of glaucoma is dependent on the particular type:

- Open angle glaucoma – the mechanisms for the drainage of aqueous humour become blocked. The onset is subtle and without symptoms until the patient finally notices the loss of peripheral vision, by which time the visual loss is usually large (Stollery *et al.*, 2005). Primary treatment is the reduction of IOP with eye drops. Laser treatment is effective in the short-term but surgery remains the main option for treatment.
- Acute closed angle glaucoma – the lens bulges forward and restricts aqueous humour drainage. The onset is rapid and the patient may report:
  - ☐ headaches
  - ☐ nausea and vomiting
  - ☐ eye pain
  - ☐ blurred vision.

This is an ocular emergency and requires immediate medical attention. The patient will require laser iridotomy (creation of a hole in the iris) as a matter of urgency (Stollery *et al.*, 2005). Nursing care includes:

- nursing the patient in a quiet, darkened, environment
- providing vomit bowls, tissues and mouth washes as required
- administer analgesia as prescribed
- cold compresses to the forehead to reduce pain
- administration of prescribed drugs including an intravenous infusion of mannitol (Nethralaya, 2004), **antiemetics** and eye drops
- reassurance and explanation

Retinal detachment

Retinal detachment is the detachment of the neural layer from the rest of the retina. Patients may experience:

- flashing lights
- **floaters** – small dark particles in the vision caused by small haemorrhages
- loss of vision – related to the area of detachment

Treatment is by surgery (Stollery *et al.*, 2005):

- Laser therapy or **photocoagulation** is used to seal tears or holes in the retina and prevent the further accumulation of subretinal fluid, which would otherwise make the detachment worse.
- **Plombage** (scleral buckling) – a small square of material is sutured onto the sclera over the site of the hole, thus pushing the retinal layers back together.
- **Encirclement** – silicone band around the eyeball. Used where there is a large area of detachment or multiple holes.

Subretinal fluid is drained during all the procedures listed above to allow the separated layers to come into contact again.
   Nursing care includes:

- Bed rest to prevent further detachment occurring before and after surgery.
- Patient may be required to be nursed in a position that causes the detachment to lie against the underlying layers and also encourage the subretinal fluid to be reabsorbed.
- Analgesia – patients will experience eye pain after surgery.
- Eye care – the eyelids and conjunctiva are usually swollen after surgery.

Retinopathy

The leading cause of retinopathy in the UK is diabetes mellitus (Pachaiappan *et al.*, 2006) and can be divided into two types:

- **Non-proliferative** retinopathy – **aneurysms** of the capillaries of the eyes, retinal **haemorrhages** and hardened **exudates** of **lipids** (Stollery *et al.*, 2005).
- **Proliferative** retinopathy – the retina has become **ischaemic**, in response there is a development of new blood vessels in the eye; however, new blood vessels are fragile and have a tendency to bleed. These blood vessels also grow into the vitreous humour. Eventually, fibrous bands develop which pull on the retina and cause retinal detachment.

Treatment of retinopathy includes (Stollery *et al.*, 2005):

- control of cholesterol levels
- advice on diet and **glycaemic control**
- laser therapy to the retina – dead retinal tissue does not encourage new blood vessel formation. Therefore, a laser beam is used to create multiple small areas of dead retinal tissue (**scotomas**) which will not have an effect on vision but will reduce the growth of new blood vessels

■ vitrectomy – removal of the vitreous humour – this removes blood vessels and haemorrhages; vitreous humour is not naturally replaced by the body, however, replacement with aqueous humour will occur

Conclusion

Disorders of the head and neck can lead to the loss of an ability to maintain the activities of daily living and may even threaten life. When faced with these possibilities the patient will often be anxious and frightened. In this situation being cared for by a nurse with knowledge of both the condition and the care required will help the patient to reduce these feelings. This chapter has introduced the reader to the physiology of the eye, ear, nose and throat. With this knowledge the reader has then been introduced to some of the conditions associated with these structures. Knowledge of the physiology and the associated conditions of these structures enables the nurse to deliver care as a valued member of the multidisciplinary team. Whilst this chapter cannot hope to cover all the conditions associated with the special senses and the throat it gives the reader a firm base from which to deliver competent and knowledgeable care and to develop their knowledge in these fascinating areas.

Multiple choice questions

1. What connects the middle ear and the nasopharynx?
(a) oropharynx
(b) eustachian tube
(c) larynx
(d) ear canal

2. What is the inner ear also known as?
(a) network
(b) warren
(c) maze
(d) labyrinth

3. What is the purpose of the turbinates in the inner nose?
(a) cooling and moistening air
(b) filtering and cooling air
(c) warming and moistening air
(d) filtering and warming air

4. How many tonsils does the body have?
(a) 5
(b) 4
(c) 6
(d) 3

5. What is the retina otherwise known as?
(a) fibrous tunic
(b) vascular tunic
(c) sensory tunic
(d) choroid tunic

6. Following ear surgery what should a patient be advised to do?
(a) avoid coughing
(b) wash the ear regularly
(c) blow their nose
(d) avoid lying down

7. Epistaxis is another name for what?
(a) hay fever
(b) nose bleed
(c) nasal polyps
(d) infection of the nose

8. Oxygen administered to a laryngectomy patient must be what?

(a) high flow

(b) low flow

(c) humidified

(d) dried

9. Following a cataract operation patients should be advised to:

(a) avoid stooping

(b) avoid coughing

(c) avoid lifting

(d) all of the above

10. Following an operation to treat retinal detachment patients should be:

(a) encouraged to mobilise

(b) kept on bed rest

(c) not allowed any pillows

(d) nursed upright

Answers: 1.b, 2.d, 3.c, 4.a, 5.c, 6.a, 7.b, 8.c, 9.d, 10.b.

Test your knowledge

❓ Name the three bones (ossicles) in the middle ear.

❓ Name the two types of humour in the eyes.

❓ What is a quinsy?

❓ Give three reasons for a patient to have a tracheostomy.

❓ What are the two types of retinopathy?

Glossary of terms

Aneurysm: Dilatation of the wall of a blood vessel.

Anticholinergics: A class of drugs that block the action of acetylcholine and thus inhibit the transmission or effect of parasympathetic nerve action.

Antiemetics: A class of drugs that reduces nausea and vomiting.

Antihistamines: A class of drugs that inhibit the effect of histamines.

Antipyretics: A class of drugs that reduce fever.

Aspiration: Inhalation of a foreign body (such as food).

Atrophy: A reduction in size or activity.

Aural: Related to the ear.

Cannula: A flexible tube containing a stiff, pointed trocar. Once inserted into the body the trocar is removed allowing fluid to pass along the cannula.

Cartilage: A supporting connective tissue made up of various cells and fibres.

Cauterisation: Coagulation of tissues by heat or caustic substances.

Cilia: Small, hair-like processes on the outer surface of some cells.

Coagulation: The process of transforming a liquid into a solid (especially blood) or the hardening of tissue by physical means.

Congenital: Present at birth.

Connective tissue: Tissue that supports and binds other body tissue.

Distal: Away from the beginning.

Dysphagia: Difficulty in swallowing.

Epithelial cells: Cells that cover the internal and external organs of the body.

Exudate: A discharge of fluid or cells.

Facial palsy: Paralysis of some or all of the muscles of the face.

Fistula: An abnormal passage from an internal organ to the surface of the skin or between two organs.

Foley catheter: A rubber catheter with an inflatable balloon tip.

Glycaemic control: Control of blood sugar levels.

Haemorrhage: Bleeding.

Hereditary: Transmitted from parent to child.

Humidification: Increasing the water content of inhaled air.

Hypertension: High blood pressure.

Hypovolaemia: Low levels of fluid in the circulation.

Intracranial: Within the skull.

Intraocular pressure: Pressure within the eye.

Ischaemic: Decreased blood supply to a body organ or part.

Laxatives: A class of drugs that promote evacuation of the bowel.

Ligation: Tying off a blood vessel to stop or prevent bleeding.

Lipids: Free fatty acids in the blood (e.g. cholesterol).

Lymphatic nodules: Collection of lymphoid tissue.

Malaise: A feeling of body weakness.

Mucosa: Mucous membrane.

Mucous membrane: Thin sheet of tissue lining a part of the body that secretes mucus.

Mucus: The secretions of mucous membranes.

Necrosis: Tissue death.

Neurological: Pertaining to the nervous system.

Olfactory: Pertaining to the sense of smell.

Opacity: Referring to the opaque quality of a substance.

Opaque: Does not allow the passage of light.

Palpation: Using the fingers or hands to examine by touch.

Parenterally: Not by the digestive system.

Pneumonia: A condition characterised by acute inflammation of the lungs.

Polypi: Plural of polyp.

Postnasal pack: Packing the upper nasopharynx with gauze or sponge to prevent the flow of blood into the nasopharynx. Also, provides a firm base against which to pack the nasal cavity if required.

Pressure necrosis: Tissue death caused by prolonged or excessive pressure.

Prosthesis: An artificial replacement for a missing part of the body.

Pulse oximetry: Non-invasive measurement of the oxygen content of the blood.

Purulent: Producing or containing pus.

Pus: A creamy exudate that is usually due to bacterial infection, often yellow in colour.

Pyrexia: Fever.

Regurgitation: Return of swallowed food to the mouth.

Respiratory insufficiency: Inability to breathe due to weakness of the muscles of respiration.

Sac: A pouch.

Secondary bacterial infection: Bacterial infection following viral infection.

Sedation: State of calm or sleepiness brought about by drugs.

Semi-recumbent: Reclining position.

Stoma: An opening. Usually used to refer to a surgically created opening.

Sutures: Stitches.

Syringing: A procedure of introducing a fluid into a cavity to flush out debris or foreign bodies.

Tinnitus: Ringing noise in the ear.

Topical antibiotics: Antibiotics applied to the skin or a mucous membrane.

Trocar: Sharp, pointed rod that fits inside a tube (cannula).

Vertigo: Dizziness.

Visual acuity: Detailed central vision.

References

Agius, A.M., Pickles, J.M. and Burch, K.L. (1992). A prospective study of otitis externa. *Clinical Otolaryngology and Allied Sciences, 17*(2), 150–154.

Beers, M., Porter, R.S., Jones, T.V., Kaplan, J.L. and Berkwits, M. (eds) (2006). *The Merck Manual of Diagnosis and Therapy*, 18th edn. New Jersey: Merck.

Cherry, J.R. (1997). *Ear, Nose and Throat Surgery*. London: Cavendish Publishing Ltd.

Chopdar, A., Chakravarthy, U. and Verma, D. (2003). Age related macular degeneration. *BMJ, 326*(7387), 485–488.

Feber, T. (2006). Tracheostomy care for community nurses: Basic principles. *British Journal of Community Nursing, 11*(5), 186–193.

Finkelstein, Y., Ophir, D., Talmi, Y.P., Shabtai, A., Strauss, M. and Zohar, Y. (1994). Adult-onset otitis media with effusion. *Archives of Otolaryngology – Head and Neck Surgery*, *120*(5), 517–527.

Guyton, A.C. and Hall, J. (2006). *Textbook of Medical Physiology*, 11th edn. Philadelphia: Elsevier Saunders.

Jenkins, G.W., Kemnitz, C.P. and Tortora, G.J. (2007). *Anatomy and Physiology. From Science to Life*. Hoboken, NJ: John Wiley & Sons.

Kilner, T., Docking, P. and Hayward, E. (2000). Ear, nose and throat emergencies. In: Dolan, B. and Holt, L. (eds) *Accident and Emergency: Theory into Practice*. Edinburgh: Baillière Tindall, pp. 447–458.

Lewis, S.L., Heitkemper, M.M., Dirksen, S.R., O'Brien, P.O. and Bucher, L. (2007). *Medical – Surgical Nursing: Assessment and Management of Clinical Problems*, 7th edn. St. Louis: Mosby Elsevier.

Marieb, E.N. and Hoehn, K. (2007). *Human Anatomy and Physiology*, 7th edn. San Francisco: Pearson Benjamin Cummings.

McKenzie, G.J., Chawla, H.B. and Gordon, D. (1986). *The Special Senses*, 2nd edn. London: Churchill Livingstone.

National Institute for Health and Clinical Excellence (NICE) (2003). *TA68 Macular Degeneration (Age Related) – Photodynamic Therapy: Summary*. London: NICE.

Nethralaya, S. (2004). *Clinical Practice Patterns in Ophthalmology*. London: Taylor & Francis.

Pachaiappan, K.J., Patel, V., Morrissey, J. and Gadsby, R. (2006). Lipid management in type 1 diabetes. *Diabetic Medicine*, *23*(Suppl 1), 11–14.

Reynolds, T. (2004). Ear, nose and throat problems in accident and emergency. *Nursing Standard*, *18*(26), 47–53.

Riaz, Y., Mehta, J.S., Wormald, R. et al. (2006). Surgical interventions for age-related cataract. *Cochrane Database of Systematic Reviews*, Issue 4. Art. No.: CD001323. DOI: 10.100214651858.CD001323.pub2.

Robinson, R. (2006). Ear, nose, and throat disorders. In: Nettina, S. (ed) *Lippincott Manual of Nursing Practice*, 8th edn. London: Lippincott Williams & Wilkins, pp. 586–620.

Scottish Intercollegiate Guidelines Network (SIGN) (2006). *Diagnosis and Management of Head and Neck Cancer. A National Clinical Guideline*. Edinburgh: SIGN.

Sigler, B.A. and Schuring, L.T. (1993). *Ear, Nose, and Throat Disorders*. St. Louis: Mosby – Year Book Inc.

Somerville, G. (2002). Mini-review: The most effective products available to facilitate ear syringing. *British Journal of Community Nursing*, *7*(2), 94–101.

Stafford, N. and Youngs, R. (1999). *ENT: Colour Guide*. Edinburgh: Churchill Livingstone.

Stokes, D. (1985). *Learning to Care on the ENT Ward*. Sevenoaks, Kent: Hodder and Stoughton Ltd.

Stollery, R., Shaw, M. and Lee, A. (2005). *Opthalmic Nursing*, 3rd edn. Oxford: Blackwell Publishing.

Tortora, G.J. and Grabowski, S.R. (2003). *Principles of Anatomy and Physiology*, 10th edn. Hoboken, NJ: John Wiley & Sons.

Appendix

Reference values in venous serum (adults)

Analysis	Reference range	
	SI units	Non-SI units
Albumin	36–47 g/L	3.6–4.7 g/100 mL
Alkaline phosphatase	40–125 U/L	—
Amylase	<100 U/L	—
Bilirubin (total)	2–17 μmol/L	0.12–1.0 mg/100 mL
Calcium	2.12–2.62 mmol/L	4.24–5.24 mEq/L or 8.50–10.50 mg/100 mL
Chloride	95–107 mmol/L	95–107 mEq/L
Cholesterol (total)	<5.5 mmol/L	—

HDL-cholesterol
  Male
  Female
	
	0.5–1.6 mmol/L
	0.6–1.9 mmol/L
		
		19–62 mg/100 mL
		23–74 mg/100 mL

Copper	13–24 μmol/L	83–153 μg/100 mL

Analysis	Reference range	
	SI units	Non-SI units
Creatine kinase (total)		
Male	30–200 U/L	—
Female	30–150 U/L	—
Creatinine	55–120 μmol/L	0.62–1.36 mg/100 mL
Ferritin		
Male	17–300 μg/L	17–300 ng/mL
Female	14–150 μg/L	14–150 ng/mL
Glucose (fasting)	3.6–5.8 mmol/L	65–104 mg/100 mL
Glycated haemoglobin (HbA$_1$)	5.0–6.5%	—
Immunoglobulin A	0.5–4.0 g/L	50–400 mg/100 mL
Immunoglobulin G	5.0–13.0 g/L	500–1300 mg/100 mL
Immunoglobulin M		
Male	0.3–2.2 g/L	30–220 mg/100 mL
Female	0.4–2.5 g/L	40–250 mg/100 mL
Iron		
Male	14–32 μmol/L	78–178 μg/100 mL
Female	10–28 μmol/L	56–156 μg/100 mL
Magnesium	0.75–1.0 mmol/L	1.5–2.0 mEq/L or 1.82–2.43 mg/100 mL
Osmolality	280–290 mmol/kg	280–290 mosm/L
Phosphate (fasting)	0.8–1.4 mmol/L	2.48–4.34 mg/100 mL
Potassium (plasma)	3.3–4.7 mmol/L	3.3–4.7 mEq/L
Potassium (serum)	3.6–5.1 mmol/L	3.6–5.1 mEq/L
Protein (total)	60–80 g/L	6–8 g/100 mL
Sodium	132–144 mmol/L	132–144 mEq/L
Total CO_2	24–30 mmol/L	24–30 mEq/L

(Continued)

Analysis	Reference range	
	SI units	Non-SI units
Transferrin	2.0–4.0 g/L	0.2–0.4 g/100 mL
Triglycerides (fasting)	0.6–1.7 mmol/L	53–150 mg/100 mL
Urate		
Male	0.12–0.42 mmol/L	2.0–7.0 mg/100 mL
Female	0.12–0.36 mmol/L	2.0–6.0 mg/100 mL
Urea	2.5–6.6 mmol/L	15–40 mg/100 mL
Zinc	11–22 μmol/L	72–144 μg/100 mL
Haematological values		
Bleeding time (Ivy)	Less than 8 minutes	—
Body fluid (total)	50% (obese) to 70% (lean) of body weight	—
Intracellular	30–40% of body weight	—
Extracellular	20–30% of body weight	—
Blood volume		
Male	75 ± 10 mL/kg	—
Female	70 ± 10 mL/kg	—
Coagulation screen		
Prothrombin time	8.0–10.5 seconds	—
Activated partial thromboplastin time	26–37 seconds	—
Erythrocyte sedimentation rate[a]		
Adult male	0–10 mm/h	—
Adult female	3–15 mm/h	—
Fibrinogen	1.5–4.0 g/L	0.15–0.4 g/100 mL
Folate		
Serum	1.5–20.6 μg/L	1.5–20.6 ng/mL
Red cell	95–570 μg/L	95–570 ng/mL
Haemoglobin		
Male	130–180 g/L	13–18 g/100 mL
Female	115–165 g/L	11.5–16.5 g/100 mL

Analysis	Reference range	
	SI units	Non-SI units
Leucocytes (adults)	$4.0–11.0 \times 10^9$/L	$4.0–11.0 \times 10^3$/mm^3
Differential white cell count		
Neutrophil granulocytes	$2.0–7.5 \times 10^9$/L	$2.0–7.5 \times 10^3$/mm^3
Lymphocytes	$1.5–4.0 \times 10^9$/L	$1.5–4.0 \times 10^3$/mm^3
Monocytes	$0.2–0.8 \times 10^9$/L	$0.2–0.8 \times 10^3$/mm^3
Eosinophil granulocytes	$0.04–0.4 \times 10^9$/L	$0.04–0.4 \times 10^3$/mm^3
Basophil granulocytes	$0.01–0.1 \times 10^9$/L	$0.01–0.1 \times 10^3$/mm^3
Packed cell volume (PCV) or haematocrit		
Male	0.40–0.54	—
Female	0.37–0.47	—
Platelets	$150–350 \times 10^9$/L	$150–350 \times 10^3$/mm^3
Red cell count		
Male	$4.5–6.5 \times 10^{12}$/L	$4.5–6.5 \times 10^6$/mm^3
Female	$3.8–5.8 \times 10^{12}$/L	$3.8–5.8 \times 10^6$/mm^3
Red cell lifespan (mean)	120 days	—
Red cell lifespan $T\frac{1}{2}$ (^{51}Cr)	25–35 days	—
Reticulocytes (adults)	$25–85 \times 10^9$/L	$25–85 \times 10^3$/mm^3
Vitamin B$_{12}$	130–770 pg/mL	—

[a]Higher values in older patients are not necessarily abnormal.

Index

Small Animal Anesthesia & Analgesia

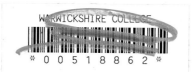